History of the Treatment
of Spinal Injuries

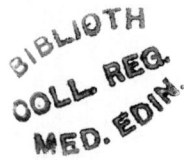

History of the Treatment
of Spinal Injuries

John Russell Silver

Emeritus Consultant
National Spinal Injuries Centre
Stoke Mandeville Hospital, United Kingdom

Foreword by Sir Roger Bannister

Kluwer Academic / Plenum Publishers
New York, Boston, Dordrecht, London, Moscow

ISBN 0-306-48032-8

©2003 Kluwer Academic / Plenum Publishers, New York
233 Spring Street, New York, New York 10013

http://www.wkap.nl/

10 9 8 7 6 5 4 3 2 1

A C.I.P. record for this book is available from the Library of Congress

Permissions for books published in Europe: *permissions@wkap.nl*
Permissions for books published in the United States of America: *permissions@wkap.com*

Printed in the United States of America

Dedication

This book is dedicated to all those people with spinal injuries whose courage and cheerfulness served as a constant inspiration for this work.

Foreword

In this book Dr Silver who has devoted his life to the treatment of spinal injuries achieves a unique balance of historical perspective and neurological expertise.

Early in the last century several great neurologists directed their piercing intellects towards this neglected problem. The British pioneers were Head, Riddoch and Holmes in the First World War but interest lapsed after 1918. Early attempts at treatment in Germany by Wagner and Foerster were stifled in the 1930s by the rise of Hitler: he removed all Jewish doctors from official posts, many in neurology and psychiatry. They were "decertified" and demoted to "attendants of the sick" and only able to treat Jewish patients. Meanwhile many Aryan doctors joined the S.S., broke their Hippocratic oath, and placed service to the state ahead of their service to their patients: eventually this led to human experimentation and death camps, which were organised by doctors who decided who should live and who should die.

Ludwig Guttmann lost his post working as assistant to the distinguished German neurologist Otto Foerster whom Dr Silver interestingly describes as "a thoroughly unpleasant man". Guttmann had to work as director of the Jewish Hospital and in 1939 fled to Oxford where until 1944 he was employed in the Neurosurgical Unit under Sir Hugh Cairns, who refused to promote him. Then when no one else would employ him he was made the first Director of the new Stoke Mandeville Spinal Injuries Unit. After 11 years, since 1933, without proper clinical responsibility, he seized the chance of clinical power and independence, even though the field of spinal injuries was unpopular because results of treatment were so poor. His control of Stoke Mandeville was utterly complete. He appointed staff and was able to accept suitable patients and reject others, at will.

Dr Silver worked with Dr Guttmann for 4 years and so developed the expertise to become the Consultant in charge of the Liverpool Regional Paraplegic Centre. His experiences entitle him to make a judgement of Dr Guttmann that we should accept. It is measured and, I think, fair.

Dr Guttmann owed much to Dr Munro in America and did not have original ideas. The major problems that then led to death of paraplegics were bedsores and bladder and kidney infections. These Guttmann meticulously tackled, at first catheterising patients himself to prove that infection could be avoided. He felt passionately about clinical research and used X-ray techniques to measure the depth of bedsores. All aspects of care were analysed and woe betide any member of the whole hospital staff from doctors to porters who were found deficient or were dilatory in obeying his instructions. Patients who did not cooperate and submit were in danger of expulsion. But his methods worked. Whereas patients in three wartime spinal units, if they survived, were no better on discharge after two years, Guttmann's patients were usually rehabilitated to lead useful lives, even if wheelchair bound. The most successful competed in the para-Olympics which he devised and which eventually became a recognised and worthwhile part of the Olympic Movement. Guttmann's dictates were widely repeated in the medical world – for example of pastes and cream for bedsores he commented, "you can put anything you like on a bedsore except the patient". Patients were turned two hands day and night. He himself at times got up at night to make sure it was happening.

Dr Silver was proud to have worked with him as were many others who survived the experience. Does it matter, if like Harvey Cushing the founder of modern neurosurgery, he sought to blame others when something went wrong but always took the credit when things went right. Silver muses philosophically that some very successful people are extremely difficult with socially unattractive traits, being egotistical, stubborn, disagreeable, and bullies. But Silver accepts Guttmann as a dynamic, even charismatic, leader who by his percepts and example changed world wide the treatment of spinal injuries. If his faults were obvious, so were his triumphs and how much the latter outweigh the former, which I suggest can be accepted mainly as a result of his frustration under Foerster and his rejection by Oxford. It is thanks to Guttmann's refusal to accept defeat that thousands of paraplegics, instead of turning their faces to the wall, fought on and recovered hope for their future in fulfilled and useful lives.

I can commend this book highly both to neurologists and to students of medical history.

Sir Roger Bannister

Preface

Injury of the spinal cord has been known since antiquity. The spinal cord cannot be repaired. Treatment consists of preventing complications until the spine has stabilised and the patient can be rehabilitated to an independent life. Surgeons have concentrated upon carrying out an operation on the spine. There was no improvement in treatment until the beginning of the 20th century. This book explores the development of treatment in the Ancient World and the Middle Ages until Paré. After Paré medical traditions separated and the developments and leading figures are discussed.

In the 19th century the controversies over surgery in the United Kingdom between Cooper and Bell are described. The First World War led to the setting up of the first spinal unit in the United Kingdom with outstanding work by Head, Riddoch and Holmes. This work ceased and patients were looked after on a custodial basis at the Royal Star and Garter Home. The Second World War led to the development of modern treatment in the United Kingdom and Guttmann's role is evaluated.

In the United States Munro developed the first spinal unit in 1936 and pioneered treatment. Initially Canada followed and then excelled the United States.

In Germany, the leading country in Europe medically at the end of the 19th century, work started with Wagner and Kocher and was developed by the anatomical and physiological work of Foerster. The failure of treatment to evolve in Germany was due to the advent of the Nazi party with its policies of euthanasia, anti-intellectualism and anti-semitism.

In France the descriptive work of Dupuytren, Duchenne and Charcot is presented. The therapeutic work of Dejerine and Marie, who set up the first French spinal units in the First World War, is evaluated.

Consistency in nomenclature proven to be difficult with respect to the following two points:

1. The nomenclature of the hospitals keeps changing. For example, Queen Square started off as the National Hospital for the Relief and Cure of the Paralysed and Epileptic, and then it changed to the National Hospital for Nervous Diseases. It is now the National Hospital for Neurology and Neurosurgery but is commonly referred to as Queen Square. Other hospitals have closed down such as the King George V Hospital, central London. There is another King George V Hospital at Ilford which is now known as the King George Hospital which is totally confusing for the researcher and I am sure for the reader.

2. The difficulty of how to refer to traumatic injuries of the spinal cord as so many different descriptions are used: paraplegia, tetraplegia, spinal injury, traumatic spinal cord injury.

I have tried to make the nomenclature uniform throughout but quotations cannot be altered and the task proved impossible.

John Silver

Acknowledgements

This book is based on an M.D. thesis for London University undertaken as a part-time self-funded student at the Wellcome Institute.

In the production of this book I have been helped by a number of people particularly Mr A Gresford and Miss Joanna Lawrence who have guided me in turning my thesis into a book.

I should like to thank Dr Hugh Baron for his meticulous monitoring of my ideas, his encyclopaedic knowledge of 20th century medicine, for restraining my wilder prejudices and pointing me in the direction of references. I would also like to thank Professor W.F. Bynum, Professor H. Cook, Dr A. Hardy, the late Professor R. Porter, Mr M. Samuelson, Professor P. Thane and Professor M. Tremblay.

The greater part of the book details historical facts that took place more than 60 years ago. Nevertheless the recollections and discussions with the following proved an original source of living history: Dr H. Baker, Professor R. Bowden, Mrs G. Buck, the late Dr J. Colover, Dr C. Dumurgier, Dr I. Eltori, Mr D.K. Evans, Dr H. Frankel, Mr N. Gibbon, Mrs E. Goddard, the late Dr A. Hardy, Dr P. Harris, Mr D. Le Vay, Mr M.R. McClelland, Professor B. McKibbin, Dr M. Maury, the late Dr V.C. Medvei, Dr P. Nathan, Professor R. Roaf, Professor A. Rossier, Miss J. Scruton, Dr N. Watson and Dr G. Weisz.

I also wish to thank the archivists and librarians who were particularly helpful: Mr J. Evans, Archivist at the Royal London Hospital, Mr S. Wilson, Archivist at Queen Square, the Public Record Office, the British Red Cross, the Coal Industry Social Welfare Organisation, the Royal Society of Medicine, the Rockefeller Library Queen Square, the Royal College of Physicians, the Royal College of Surgeons, Stoke Mandeville Hospital, and the Wellcome Institute.

I am grateful for the meticulous translation of the German and French texts by Dr Frank Beck, Karin Band and Marie-France Weiner and the outstanding patience of my secretaries, Lindsay Cornell and Marie-France Weiner. I owe a special debt to Helena Bradbury for her patience and forbearance in struggling through both the thesis and the book. Without her, the thesis would not have been completed and the book would not have been started.

Lastly but no means least I owe a great debt of gratitude to my wife, Marilyn, for putting up for the last 5 years with my moments of abstraction and preoccupation with this work.

Contents

List of Figures

List of Tables

Introduction

I qualified in 1954 at the Middlesex Hospital Medical School, London University. As a student, my interest in orthopaedics was generated by Mr Josiah Grant Bonnin (1909-1989), Orthopaedic Surgeon at the Central Middlesex Hospital. My first job was in accident surgery at the Luton & Dunstable Hospital, dealing almost entirely with major trauma from Watling Street. After a six month appointment I was anxious to see 'cold' orthopaedics and visited both the Royal National Orthopaedic Hospital, Stanmore, which specialised in the correction of scoliosis and the repair of peripheral nerve injuries, and the National Spinal Injuries Centre at Stoke Mandeville Hospital where Dr Ludwig Guttmann (1899-1980) had already established an international reputation for the treatment of spinal injuries. The ward rounds, teaching sessions and the whole atmosphere at Stoke Mandeville were remarkably stimulating and uplifting. I decided to pursue a career in spinal injuries and after obtaining full registration, I returned to work at the National Spinal Injuries Centre. I believed that Guttmann had pioneered the treatment of spinal injuries and that prior to his work, all spinal patients died rapidly after injury from renal sepsis and overwhelming pressure sores.

I spent my National Service as an orthopaedic junior specialist in the Royal Air Force. Following this, I expanded my neurological training by spending three and a half years on the neurology, neurosurgery and physiology units at the Middlesex Hospital, returning to Stoke Mandeville in a research post on the spinal unit until appointed consultant in charge of the Liverpool centre in 1965.

At that time, although aware that there were spinal units at the Veterans' Hospitals in the United States, I had always uncritically accepted that priority for the development of treatment rested at Stoke Mandeville, particularly because when Dr Ernest Bors (1900-1990), the leading spinal injury specialist in the Veterans' Hospitals, visited the unit in 1963 he paid tribute, describing Stoke Mandeville as being the Mecca of spinal injury work. This belief persisted until, in 1969, at a meeting at the Ministry of Health held to discuss the setting up of additional spinal units in the United Kingdom, Harold Jackson Burrows (1902-1981) told me that the original work had all been done in the United States by Donald Munro (1889-1973) from 1936 onwards.

During the Second World War, although there were spinal units in the United Kingdom, treatment was not successful. Realising how advanced the Americans were, Guttmann, who was not working in spinal injuries at the time, had been sent with Frank Holdsworth (1904-1969), an orthopaedic surgeon from Sheffield, to visit Dr Munro in order to observe his methods and set up spinal units in the United Kingdom incorporating Munro's ideas. Holdsworth opened a unit at Sheffield and Guttmann at Stoke Mandeville.

Jackson Burrows' opinion should be taken seriously as, at the time, he was National Advisor on orthopaedics and had been Dean of the Institute of Orthopaedics for 21 years, President of the British Orthopaedic Association and on the Council of the Royal College of Surgeons. He had edited a book on modern trends in spinal injuries, in which Guttmann wrote a chapter.

Guttmann told me and this has been confirmed by his secretary, Miss Joan Scruton (Scruton, 1999), and his colleague, Dr Hans Frankel (Frankel, 1999), that he visited the United States in the early days.

I have read many of Munro's papers and books, the first of which were written in 1936. He started his first spinal unit at the City Hospital, Boston in 1936' and subsequently was responsible for the Veterans' Service at Cushing Hospital during the Second World War. There was an established pattern of treatment in the United States in the Veterans' Hospitals prior to the opening of the Unit at Stoke Mandeville in 1944 and Munro's work was recognised.

It is a philosophical question, and of great interest, as to who has the primacy for discovery. If an idea is published in an obscure journal and it is ignored at the time but a hundred years later someone else develops the idea and everyone follows it, who deserves the credit for discovery?

The evidence to be evaluated is:

What have people achieved and published?

What recognition did they receive at the time and was it accepted as mainstream treatment?

Do subsequent investigators acknowledge where the work comes from?

Many years later, to evaluate what the respective roles were.

I am dealing with this matter historically. Initially there was one medical tradition in Europe but latterly separate schools grew up in France, Germany, the United Kingdom and then in the United States. I have considered each country separately because during the wars there was little communication and ideas evolved independently. There was also a great deal of chauvinism. Writers only quoted their own work and, if they did quote other doctors, it was only those from their own country.

There is no way of healing the spinal cord. The basis of treatment is:

One doctor in charge who takes a comprehensive approach to the management of the patient

Early transfer to a specialised centre where patients can be rehabilitated

Prevention of complications: pressure sores, urinary tract infections, by meticulous treatment until the fracture has stabilised

Maintenance of nutrition

Treatment will be analysed as to how these precepts are followed, whether it was applicable at the time and how it refers to the present day.

No comprehensive textbook has been written on the history of the treatment of paraplegia but articles have dealt with fragments. Frankel (1971) on intermittent catheterisation gives a historical review of bladder management, as does Guttmann, in his textbook on spinal cord injuries, (Guttmann, 1973).

Chapter 1

Historical Survey

1.   ANTIQUITY

1.1   Egypt

In Egypt, paraplegia following injury of the spine was first described in The Edwin Smith Surgical Papyrus in about 3000 B.C. (Bennett, 1964). The Egyptian surgeons carefully distinguished between patients with open wounds or sprains of the cervical vertebrae in whom the spinal cord was not involved, and patients with dislocations and fractures of the spine who had lost power and sensation in all four limbs. They noted that the patient would have priapism (erection), and incontinence of urine and semen.   They also described bloodshot eyes, no doubt due to involvement of the sympathetic nervous system.   Surgeons were unwilling to treat patients with paraplegia because of its poor prognosis.   Doctors then, as now, were unwilling to be associated with a hopeless case.

1.2   Classical Greece

After the decline of the Egyptian Empire, the next to leave a record of their medical practice were the Greeks, foremost amongst them, Hippocrates (c. 460-370 B.C.).   Medicine was dissociated from religion and a systematic record of practice was presented.   No distinction was made between fractures and dislocations of the spine. He was the first to describe traction in the treatment of these injuries and even attempted to reduce the dislocation by means of hyperextension, placing the patient on his back with a bladder beneath the spine, inflating it by means of a pipe. Greek thought spread throughout the Ancient World, particularly to Alexandria and was eventually incorporated into Roman philosophy. The Romans had little original to contribute in this sphere and Galen (c. 129-210 A.D.) merely repeated the teachings of Hippocrates (Bennett, 1964).

1.3   The Jewish Tradition

The Talmud was codified between the second and fifth centuries. It discussed spinal cord injury in humans and the effect of a spinal cord injury upon animals, which was a serious matter, as Jews are not allowed to eat diseased animals (Preuss, 1993).

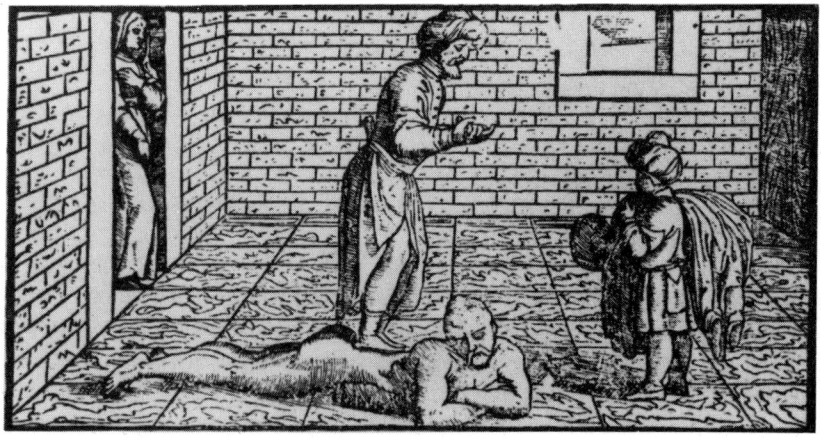

Figure 1. Reduction of a dislocation of the spine when the physician stands upon the gibbosity with his heels, Avicenna 980(?)-1037 (Bennett, 1964).

1.4   Greece

Paul of Aegina (AD 625-690) employed a windlass for traction of the spine. After he had achieved reduction he used a piece of wood to splint the fractured spine. This he recommended when there was a fractured spine with compression of the cord. He suggested that an incision should be made above the site of injury, and that the piece of bone compressing the cord should be removed if possible. He also advised removal of a fractured spinous process if this was causing pain. It would appear that he actually carried out this operation, or knew of surgeons who had. He was aware of the serious nature of the operation and admonished his readers to warn those concerned about the full dangers of the operation (Bennett, 1964).

1.5   Moslem Medicine

The fall of the Roman Empire led to an almost total abolition of the practice of medicine in Western Europe. Greek and Roman traditions were preserved in the Eastern Empire and in the Arabian Empire, by Christian, Jewish and Moslem physicians. Avicenna (AD 980–1037) followed the teachings of Paul of Aegina and maintained that a fracture of the body of the vertebra was fatal when accompanied by paralysis. At that stage a significant but retrograde development occurred. Galen taught that surgery is only a mode of treatment – the surgeon lost his position of equal status with the physician (Bennett, 1964).

1.6   Hindu Medicine

Surgery was well developed in India in the first centuries of the Christian era. A complete scientific textbook of surgery, the Sushruta Samhita (Kaviraj, 1911), was written in the third or fourth century. There is a description of treating dislocations of the neck and how to manage fractures of the spinal column. Sushruta believed fractures of the spine to be hopeless. The practice of surgery declined so that by the 17th century foreign visitors to India remarked how surgery was virtually non-existent. Medicine was largely based on a holistic system of Ayurveda with concentration on medical conditions such as winds and vapours. There was thus no medical tradition of treating spinal injuries.

1.7   Chinese Medicine

China is an old civilisation. There were two periods in Chinese medicine. Traditional medicine dated from 2697 BC–1800 AD when attempts were made at dissection and there was some description of hospitals for the paralytic but no record of spinal injuries. Modern medicine dating from 1800 AD saw the introduction of western medicine initially by the Jesuits and latterly by British, Russian and American doctors. Western hospitals were established in 1913 and an orthopaedic hospital in 1928 but there is no description of spinal injuries (Wong & Wu, 1932).

2.   PRE-RENAISSANCE

In Europe prior to the Renaissance, medical schools associated with the universities were gradually re-established, the first at Salerno, where Roland of Parma (circa 1230) studied. He used manual extension for the treatment of fractured spines and was the first to emphasise one of the keystones of modern practice: the necessity for early treatment. Following this important pre-Renaissance school, several Italian surgeons wrote textbooks on treatment, one of which, by Lanfranc of Milan (not known -1315), was translated into English (Bennett, 1964). He repeated the advice given by the Egyptian surgeons with regard to paralysis 'If thou seest evil signs in that case, go away therefrom' (Bearsted, 1930).

3.   THE RENAISSANCE

The Renaissance was the beginning of modern medicine. Accurate dissections of the human body by Leonardo da Vinci (1452-1519) (O'Malley & Saunders, 1952) and Vesalius (1514-1564) (Saunders & O'Malley, 1950), whose anatomical studies enabled William Harvey (1578-1657) and others to think rationally about their work, laid the scientific basis for the practice of surgery.

4.   THE 16TH CENTURY

4.1   Ambroise Paré (1564-1598)

Ambroise Paré was the first modern surgeon.   A barber surgeon by training, he rose to be head surgeon to the army and head physician to four French Kings.   He wrote a textbook of surgery and recommended laminectomy when the spinal cord was compressed. Contrary to Paul of Aegina, he recommended that the fractured spinous process should not be removed if it was still attached to the periosteum.   He described and illustrated methods of reducing the dislocated spine, advising initial manual reduction and then the use of pieces of wood to achieve a more satisfactory reduction.   He was aware of the fatal nature of this injury, but did not specify the cause of death.

There was little progress in treatment following Paré's work.   Such advances as were made were stimulated by the wars that necessitated having a large number of surgeons to treat the wounded throughout Europe.   In

Germany, Fabricius Ab Aquapendente (1533-1619) suggested open reduction of fracture dislocation of the spine, pointing out the practical difficulties of intractable haemorrhage that could be arrested by the use of twisted oakums. (Bennett, 1964).

After Paré, medical traditions separated. The literature will be pursued under separate chapters on the United Kingdom, United States, Canada, German-speaking world, and France.

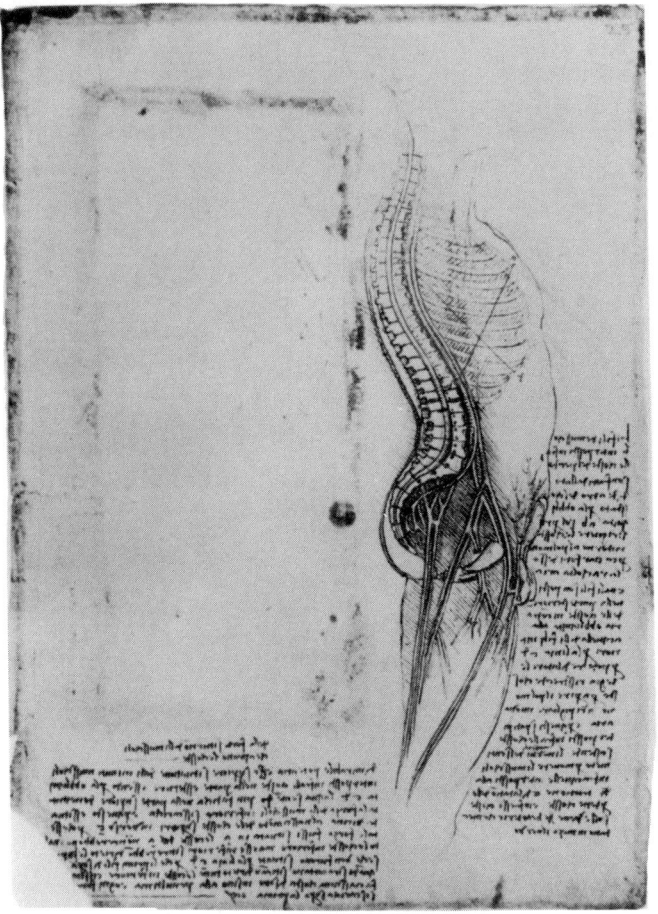

Figure 2. Sagittal section of the body demonstrating the spinal cord, pelvic vessels and nerves, and muscles between the ribs. The spinal cord is carried the entire length of the neural canal instead of terminating at its customary level at the lower border of the first lumbar vertebra. In addition, there is an excessive number of pre-sacral vertebrae (O'Malley & Saunders, 1952).

Chapter 2

The United Kingdom

PART 1: THE 19th CENTURY

1. INTRODUCTION

In the 19th century, London was the centre of a fascinating medical tradition started by John Hunter (1728-1793) and continued by his pupil, Charles Bell (1774-1842). This was the era of the London private medical schools, often called anatomy schools. Stimulated by the economic wealth of the country, new medical schools were founded at the Middlesex and University College Hospitals but they did not have the fine academic tradition of Scotland.

London was a very busy place with horse drawn traffic. People fell under the wheels of the carriages and fell from the masts of ships, resulting in many spinal injuries. There was a ferment of ideas but the management of these cases gave rise to a controversy between Astley Cooper and Charles Bell.

2. THE 19th CENTURY

2.1 Sir Astley Paston Cooper (1768-1841)

Cooper, the doyen of British surgeons, a popular teacher and author of many textbooks, was very interested in the management of spinal injuries.

11

In 1824, he described how a violent blow to the loins could produce paralysis of the lower extremities. This paralytic state could be dealt with by cupping, but if at the end of a week or 10 days the paralytic state still continued, blisters should be applied. He gave an account of an instructive case when he was living with Mr Henry Cline (1750-1827), presumably as a pupil:

"A girl received a severe blow in the neck, after this it was found that, whenever she attempted to look at any thing above her head, she was put under the necessity of putting her hands behind it, and gradually elevating it to the object. When she wanted to look at any thing beneath her head, she put her hands under her chin and lowered her head to the object." (Cooper, 1824)

This presumably was a case of instability of the atlas with some cord involvement produced whenever the head was moved.

"The child lived twelve months after the accident. On examination of the body after death, Mr Cline found the atlas broken through; there was a transverse fracture of the atlas but no displacement. When she endeavoured to raise her head, the dentiform process quitted its natural situation and carried back a portion of the atlas; when her head inclined forward, pressure was produced upon the spinal marrow, as it was likewise when the body was agitated. Mr Henry Cline was the first person who attempted to give relief in this accident. Being an excellent anatomist and a most reasonable surgeon, he saw no reason why cases of this kind should not be treated as cases of fracture with depression of the skull. Accordingly he cut down upon the arch of the spinal marrow, where the compression was greatest, and with a small trephine of his own invention he sawed through the arch of the spinous process, and took off the pressure on the spinal marrow, by raising the depressed portion of the arch. It is well known, that in cases of fracture where the displacement has been slight, union of the bone has been produced."

Cooper discussed the difficulties of the operation, pointing out that "in many of these cases the spinal marrow is itself torn through. In some cases of fracture, with displacement, it is completely torn".

Mr Frederick Tyrell had attempted the operation since Cline:

"Both cases have terminated unfavourably. Whether future experiments may be attended with better success it is impossible to say. The proposal was plausible; the operation was easily performed, and as to the result, if the spinal marrow were not torn, there seems no reason why a person should not recover after such an operation."

Cooper was not a blind advocate of laminectomy.

"We are obliged, however, to speak doubtingly on this subject, since the first experiments have been unsuccessful. If you could save one life in ten, aye, one in a hundred, by such an operation, it is your duty to attempt it, notwithstanding any objections, which some foolish persons may have urged against it."

He advocated Cline's operation saying:

"He was blamed for making this trial, I am not sure he would have been ultimately successful; but in a case otherwise without hope, I am certain such an attempt was laudable. Nothing is so easy as to condemn others; but let it be mentioned that the disposition to do so, is proof of a weak head and a bad heart and that it ought always to be discouraged in a profession in which character is all in all." (Cooper, 1823)

Cline was a surgeon and professor and eventually became President of the Royal College of Surgeons. Cooper had been apprenticed to him. By all accounts he was an interesting man who was regarded as the outstanding surgeon at St Thomas's. Although he had private means and no need for private practice, this did not stop him earning £10,000 a year from this, £200,000 in today's terms. Apart from surgery upon the spinal column, he made early experiments on blood transfusions.

Cooper (1823) described the symptoms and signs of paraplegia at different levels, stressing the incontinence of urine and faeces, making interesting observations on the preservation of circulation and inflammatory responses in the paralysed limbs. At that stage surgical and nursing care must have been of a high standard since not all patients with traumatic paraplegia died immediately. Patients with cervical injuries died within one week of injury and it was recognised that, in general, these cases were fatal. Patients with lumbar fractures died within one month, but Cooper recorded patients living as long as 2 years before dying of pressure sores. One patient was successfully rehabilitated so that he was able to dress and undress himself.

It is fascinating that Cooper, in his description of heroic surgery in ligating the aorta, recorded symptoms and signs of the first case of infarction of the spinal cord (Silver, 2003).

Unfortunately, Cooper's observations of the physical signs and prognosis in paraplegia were lost sight of because of his views on treatment by laminectomy. He denigrated anyone who opposed him and this led to his celebrated controversy with Sir Charles Bell.

2.2   Sir Charles Bell (1774-1842)

Bell was a highly cultured scientist, artist, philosopher, physiologist and anatomist. He wrote a textbook (Bell, 1824) discounting Cooper's views. In the introduction Bell asked pertinently:

"What shall we say of the recommendations daily given to students in our own times, who are taught to despise the study of books, and to neglect all authority but that of the person who is addressing them, and all practice or example, but that of the hospital to which chance has led them?" (Bell, 1824)

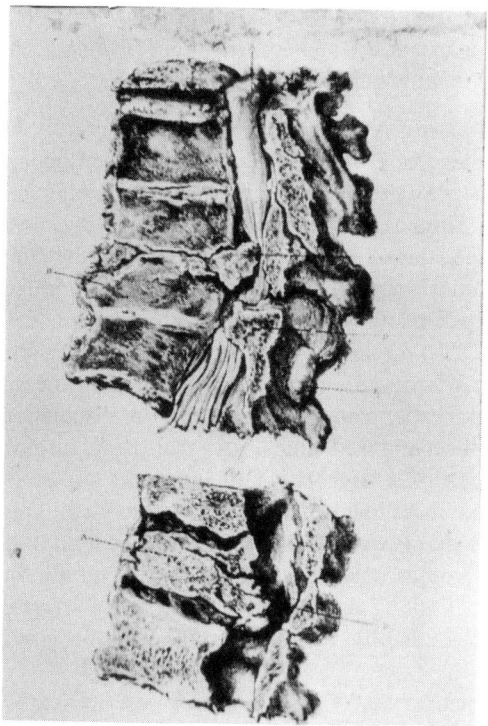

Figure 3. This beautifully drawn picture of the vertebral column by Sir Charles Bell shows the pathology of spinal cord injury. The damage is anterior and he stresses the futility of trephining posteriorly (Bell, 1824).

Bell's approach was modern. He pointed out that the damage to the spinal cord occurred at the moment of injury, and that it was not continuing pressure that damaged the cord. He emphasized that all the efforts of the surgeons should be devoted to making an accurate diagnosis in the first instance, and that the operation on the spinal column was both dangerous and useless. He said that, in cases of paraplegia, death was attributable to the retention of urine and subsequent inflammation. This was the first mention of renal failure as being a cause of death.

There was no method of anaesthetising the patient at that time. To carry out a laminectomy on a traumatised spinal column through bruised, bleeding, tissues would have been an extremely difficult technical task.

Bell's words, in the debate with Cooper, are profound, stimulating and still relevant today:

"For it must be acknowledged, that what are professionally called facts, are for the most part only those notions, which a man insensibly adopts in the course of his practice, and which takes colour from his education and previous studies. It is this, which makes the facts of one age differ from the facts of another age; and the opinions of men differently educated to vary on what they are inconsistent enough to call matters of fact."

Bell's view received wide acceptance in Britain. He made a lasting contribution to our knowledge of neurology, and there is a fascinating and beautiful description of an early case of missed injury of the spinal cord, which unfortunately has echoes today:

"March 29, 1816 – Marshall, a coal waggoner, was brought into the hospital from Edgeware; the account given by the people who had brought him was rather confused. They agreed that he had been riding on the fore-shaft of his cart, and, by a sudden jerk, was thrown off, and pitched on the back of his neck and shoulders. The man was somewhat intoxicated, and could not give a distinct description of what befell him. When carried into the hospital he was put up on his legs but he could not stand; and when supported by the shoulders, he dragged his legs after him. At this time he complained of pain in his loins but no injury was perceptible there. Between his shoulders, however, there was a degree of swelling and discolouration. Some of the people who were with him said that the wheel of the cart, which was empty, had gone over the small of his back; but after the first day he never complained of that part. Leeches were applied to the spine betwixt the shoulders and his bowels were opened." (Bell, 1838)

When he died, this man was found to have a complete separation of his last cervical from the first thoracic vertebra.

There was controversy between Bell, who recommended conservative treatment, and Cooper, who recommended surgery. Bell's views were accepted by John Bell (1763-1820) and Benjamin Brodie (1783-1862), but

Benjamin Bell (1749-1806) and John Flint South (1797-1882) favoured Cooper's views (Markham, 1951). Bell's views, possibly because of his distinguished contribution as a neurologist as well as a surgeon, held sway particularly in the United Kingdom.

2.3   Sir Benjamin Collins Brodie (1783-1862)

Brodie, like Bell, recommended conservative treatment in the management of spinal injuries with intermittent catheterisation but not blood letting. He was aware that paralysis of the bladder resulted in severe ascending infection of the kidneys. In a publication on tuberculosis of the spine, he stressed the risks of prolonged bed rest, leading to secondary contractures of the joints making it impossible for the patient to be mobilised (Brodie, 1850). He discussed Cline's operations and whether dislocations should be relocated. He thought that operations were not beneficial. He was aware of paralytic ileus as an immediate consequence of spinal injury (Brodie, 1865).

2.4   Thomas Blizard Curling (1811-1888)

The consequences of the pathological sequence resulting in paralysis of the bladder were delineated in the latter part of the 19th century.

Curling (1833, 1836) described the suppurative consequences of paralysis of the bladder on the kidneys, and pointed out that the survival time was proportional to the severity of the infection. Sir William Withey Gull (1816-1890), (1856, 1858), William Thorburn (1861-1923), (1889) and Charles Hilton Fagge (1838-1883), (1891) drew attention to renal pathology in this condition.

3.   THE LONDON HOSPITAL

At the London Hospital there was an interest in diseases affecting the nervous system with a series of doctors who, although general physicians and surgeons, devoted a considerable part of their energies to neurological problems. This tradition has continued to the present day.

James Parkinson (1755-1828), who gave the first description of Parkinson's disease, was a student there and subsequently worked as a general practitioner in the area. Sir Jonathan Hutchinson (1828-1913), Sir Victor Alexander Haden Horsley (1857-1916), Henry Head (1861-1940) and George Riddoch (1888-1947) all practised neurology at the London Hospital.

3.1   Sir Jonathan Hutchinson (1828-1913)

Hutchinson was a remarkable clinician and surgeon who made outstanding contributions to skin disease and to the manifestations of syphilis but particularly to neurology.

In a little known paper, Hutchinson (1866) gave a series of accounts of the clinical manifestations, treatment and pathological findings of those patients with spinal injuries. Many patients survived and left the hospital ambulant, having sustained severe injury of the spinal cord. Their bladders were treated with intermittent catheterisation. Hutchinson stated categorically that injury to the spinal cord was due to direct trauma and not to haematoma. He reiterated the views of Bell on the dangers of carrying out a laminectomy, recorded the dangers of pressure sores and recommended the use of a waterbed to prevent them. His views were modern and he drew attention to how badly patients were examined and how one should be sceptical of clinical observations:

> "Another source of fallacy is the difficulty of accurate observations. A man tells you 'I cannot move my legs' and you are unable to prove the contrary, though it is still possible that a very vigorous exertion of will might be able to set certain muscles in action; in other words, that voluntary motion, although seemingly in abeyance, is not absolutely lost. The same patient tells you that he 'can feel well' yet very probably, if you try accurate tests, such as the compasses or drawing a feather over the surface, you will find that his sensory function is very far from perfect. On account of our frequent neglect of such tests, we are compelled to receive with much qualification, recorded statements as to 'perfect sensation' being retained after these accidents." (Hutchinson, 1866)

He was such a meticulous observer of symptoms and signs that he recorded the first account of a prolapsed disc causing paraplegia following flexion of the spine from removal of a pile (Silver, 2001).

Patients with spinal injuries were treated on an individual basis. They were not congregated together and did not receive a standard regime of treatment.

3.2   James Sherren (1872-1945)

Sherren was appointed late in his life as surgeon to the London Hospital and was said to be an unusual, difficult man. He had an interest in neurological surgery and wrote a textbook entitled *Injuries of Nerves and their Treatment* (Sherren, 1908) in which he gave accounts of lesions of the cauda equina describing how, in penetrating wounds of the lumbar region, the cauda equina could be injured, possibly from a fall on to the buttocks. He discussed how the sphincter ani was paralysed and incontinence of faeces resulted, retention of urine was present at first followed by true incontinence in many cases and absence of sexual power. He was aware that the testes retained their sensation, despite the anaesthetic skin of the scrotum, as they were supplied from a higher level. The double nerve supply of the bladder was discussed. He gave an account of the incomplete recovery of a patient with a cauda equina lesion. He carried out nerve operations peripherally to improve function and delineated the dermatomes very accurately. The various diagnostic features were given and he thought there should be no difficulty diagnosing a pure cauda equina lesion. He reported that death seldom occurred as a direct result of an injury to the cauda equina but resulted most often from urinary infection. Early surgery was recommended.

4.   MARSHALL HALL (1790-1857)

Hall believed that he was one of the first to study the effects of spinal injuries (Manuel, 1996).

Although he was an outstanding clinician and neurologist, whose work on the reflex function of the nervous system and his delineation of spinal shock made important contributions to the study of spinal injuries, Hall was a controversial personality who, like Duchenne, did not hold a hospital appointment. When he wished to see patients with traumatic spinal injuries he had to travel (as did Duchenne) to different hospitals. The patients were not under his care.

5.   JOHN WHITAKER HULKE (1830-1895)

In 1891 Hulke presented 33 cases of fractures and dislocations of the vertebral column at the Middlesex Hospital over a period of 24 years, of which he personally treated 22. He carried out experimental work on the mechanics of production of the fracture.

"I do not remember, in the course of the Crimean Campaign, one single instance of survival of a gun shot injury of the vertebral column. In civil practice, however, a small number of such wounded escaped with life This is one of my series, the man was in fair health, but paraplegic, two and a half years after the date of the injury. In this case the course taken by the bullet was remarkable. Entering under the left collarbone, it traversed the apex of the lung (demonstrated by haemoptysis), and then, taking a circuitous route, fractured the 11th dorsal vertebra, severely damaging the spinal cord at that level." (Hulke, 1892)

He reviewed the symptomatology and discussed priapism and paralytic ileus, hyperpyrexia and treatment. He pointed out that:

"No class of cases demands the surgeon closer direct supervision, and in none is there greater necessity for his close personal attention to details of nursing, too frequently esteemed trivial and relegated to subordinate attendants" (Hulke, 1892)

He stressed the importance of immobilising the spine in the correct position by the use of partially filled sandbags. He discussed the difficulty of preventing bed sores, cystitis leading to suppurative nephritis, operative measures and manipulation to reduce dislocation and concluded that it was not a good idea to operate. He gave 16 case histories. One patient with a cervical injury recovered, 5 died between 3 days and 8 months after injury, one patient with a thoracic injury recovered, one survived and one was lost track of, 4 died between 2 and 237 days after injury. All 3 patients with lumbar injuries recovered.

Although Hulke only saw 22 patients in 24 years he recognised the vital necessity of close supervision by the responsible surgeon. This is the keystone of the management of spinal injuries. Without unremitting care throughout 24 hours by a responsible doctor, the patient will rapidly succumb.

6.   THE BOER WAR

The Boer War resulted in a large number of casualties, many of whom had spinal injuries. Unfortunately, the medical arrangements were a scandal.

6.1   Sir George Henry Makins (1853-1933)

Makins was a consulting surgeon to the South African Field Force. He wrote a book on the effects of injuries produced by bullets on the Expeditionary Force observed during four battles of the Boer War (Makins, 1913). He gave a rich description of the patients with spinal injuries who came under his care.

"Every degree of local injury to the constituent vertebrae and the contents of the spinal canal were met with considerable frequency. Pure, uncomplicated fractures of the bones were of minor importance. ...Injuries implicating the spinal medulla, on the other hand, were proportionately the most fatal of any in the whole body to the wounded who left the field of battle or Field hospital alive, and these cases formed one of the most painful and distressing features of the surgery of the campaign." (Makins, 1913)

Features and anatomy were discussed and he gave case descriptions. Hyperpyrexia in cervical injuries, with profuse sweating in the upper part of the body with dryness lower down, and the effect upon the heart (which presumably, was autonomic dysreflexia) were described.   Paralytic ileus in the low lesions, priapism, and pressure sores (which were present in all cases) were documented.   He described polyuria, anuria, post mortems, hysteria, compression of the cord, (which he dismissed) and the impingement of bone fragments and pressure from the bullets.   The ill effects of transport were recognised and he was against surgery except for the relief of pain.   He thought the condition was hopeless and concluded:

"Cervical and high dorsal injuries, as in civil practice, offered the worst prognosis.   In cases in which symptoms of total transverse lesion were present, as far as my experience went, it was, however, only a matter of importance as to the prolongation of a miserable existence.   All the patients eventually died; those with higher lesions, at the end of a few days; the lower ones, at the completion of an average of six weeks of suffering."

Makins gave a casualty rate of 9.6% but this is disputed by Colonel Sir Charters James Symonds (1852-1932) who dealt with the subject in the First World War:

"According to the Surgeon-General W. F. Stevenson, 58.3% of the cases in the Boer War died, and when there was actual lesion of the cord with fracture of the arch the death rate was 75%." (Symonds, 1917)

PART 2: THE FIRST WORLD WAR

7.   INTRODUCTION

It was the advent of the First World War with 2 000 000 casualties in Britain alone that forced the medical profession to systematically study and treat soldiers who had sustained spinal injuries.

Before this war, patients were admitted to the nearest hospital. Owing to the rarity of spinal injuries it took Hulke (1892) 24 years to put his series together. Lessons took a long time to be learned.

There were so many casualties in the First World War that they could not be treated in a haphazard manner. One of the problems in the Boer War had been the appalling transport facilities. Adequate arrangements had to be made to receive patients at the front, transport them and treat them. It was recognised that the best treatment for all casualties, whether abdominal or jaw wounds, was to send them to specialised centres. Phillip Vellacott (1872-1939) and Alfred Edward Webb-Johnson (1880-1958) writing about spinal injuries, concluded that:

> "Specialisation, as a rule, is advantageous to the patients, but in cases of this character doubt has been expressed whether the strain, especially in the early stages, is not too great for the patients and nurses. The heavy mortality in the early days has a depressing effect on both patients and nursing staff, but the advantages of concentration and specialisation were so great as far to outweigh the disadvantages and the lot of these men was much better than it could have been had they been distributed to all hospitals in the base." (Vellacott & Webb-Johnson, 1919)

8. CASUALTY RATES

The Great War was a conflict of unprecedented violence resulting in a large number of casualties, many of whom, inevitably, had spinal injuries. Initially peacetime methods of recording statistics were thought to be sufficient and were carried out by men trained in record-keeping routine, but with full mobilisation, record keeping fell to untrained men. Patients were rapidly transferred from one unit to another and central organisation was insufficient. The War Office introduced a record card, which was less than accurate.

Harvey Cushing gave an eyewitness account of the impossibility of keeping accurate records at the Front.

> "...and the wounded, bear in mind, are seriously and acutely hit, rushed on from one and all of the casualty clearing stations a few miles behind the lines as soon as transportation is possible. Records, if kept at all must necessarily be utterly inadequate...Indeed in rushes, no notes whatever can be made, and the wretched tags, insecurely attached to a button of the wounded soldier's uniform, are often lost or become rumpled and completely illegible.... There were two poor aphasic chaps from some Scotch regiment who were necessarily listed as 'unknown' since all identification marks had been lost in transit." (Cushing, 1936)

Around 20 million records were moved three times and used to provide information for future pension schemes and military and civilian medical services (Mitchell, 1931). The Ministry of Pensions took over the statistical organisation in 1920 and by December 1921 produced a figure that:

> "40% of those who served in the Great War were affected by war service in the sense of death or some form of war disablement, for which State compensation was given." (Mitchell, 1931)

In contrast, in the Second World War there were only 755 000 British casualties.

There is very imprecise information on how many men sustained spinal injuries in the First World War and survived long enough to be removed from the battlefield:

> "It is difficult, if not impossible, to form any opinion as to the number of cases of injury to the vertebrae and their contents which were met with during the war, as very many of these would fall into the category of killed or missing, but it is certain that the number was very large." (Thorburn, 1922)

Figures are sparse. In the last four months of 1914, 58 men from a force of 190 000 sustained paraplegia as a result of gunshot wounds. The Ministry of Pensions records that a total of 3531 paraplegics were discharged from treatment during the period 1st April 1919 to 31st March 1929 (Mitchell, 1931). This is clearly an underestimate.

9.   MEDICAL PERSONNEL

Before the First World War there had been an unhappy military tradition of maltreatment, unpreparedness and scandals in hospitals dating from the Napoleonic Wars, through the Crimean War and the Boer War. Each conflict resulted in scandal and public enquiry. As a result of this, hospitals were better organised in the First World War.

The total strength of the British Army in 1913 was 212 355, which rose to 4 796 088 in 1918 (Mitchell, 1931). In peacetime there were 1279 officers in the RAMC, which rose to 10 178 in 1918

> "The structure of the medical profession in Britain before the National Health Service (NHS) then, and the fact that consultancy work in general medicine and surgery constituted a form of specialization itself, did little to encourage the development of individual specialty careers of the American sort." (Cooter, 1993)

Postgraduate training was minimal in the United Kingdom. There were only a few trained neurologists and neurosurgeons, Gordon Holmes (1876-1965), Harvey Cushing (1869-1930) from the United States, Robert Foster-Kennedy (1884-1952), Sir Percy William George Sargent (1873-1933), a neurosurgeon, and Horsley, who went out to the Middle East and died of hyperpyrexia. Most army doctors had been busy general practitioners, totally unskilled and unprepared to deal with major trauma. They became bored by the long periods of light medical workload or inactivity, while awaiting casualties at the base hospitals. They were largely volunteers who returned to civilian duties in 1918 and rotated their duties so there was little continuity of care. This shortage of specialists made it difficult to deal with the huge number of casualties in an army, which had risen in numbers from 212 000 to 4.8 million.

Throughout the account the contribution of the following doctors will be discussed and evaluated and it would be useful to discuss their role and their personalities at this stage.

9.1 Personalities: Physicians

The First World War, through serendipity, enabled three outstanding neurologists, two of whom were already internationally recognised, to be responsible for spinal patients: Gordon Holmes, Henry Head and George Riddoch.

9.1.1 Gordon Holmes (1876-1965)

Holmes already had an established international reputation prior to the war as a neuropathologist and a neuroanatomist dating from his stay in Ludwig Edinger's laboratory (1855-1918) in Frankfurt-am-Main (Holmes, 1903).

He was well ahead of his time. He worked alongside Sargent, the neurosurgeon to the National Hospital for Nervous Disease (otherwise known as Queen Square) in a collaborative army hospital No 13 Unit at Boulogne. It was unknown at that time for surgeons and physicians to work in this way. No doubt Holmes learnt this from Horsley with whom he had worked before the war.

"Sargent had worked side-by-side with Holmes behind the front line in France during the First World War, and mutual respect had grown up. Percy Sargent was the only one who could pull Holmes's leg and tease him and Holmes would take it." (Critchley, 1979).

Macdonald Critchley (1900-1997), who was houseman to Holmes in 1923, described him as a Colossus who "…shone brightest among the galaxy of stars surrounding him". Holmes was "…tempestuous…volcanic …brusque (and) demanding". He "…exacted the utmost accuracy and dedication and he got it willingly". He "…expected (his students) to be on duty for twenty-four hours a day" and was "…a meticulous, obsessional observer".

"His clinical technique was thorough, and many would have said rough, even terrifying and yet he was so warm hearted that he could never understand why he was regarded as a bully, as indeed he was…"

He was known to:

"…Tear up the case-notes and scatter them across the ward; and throw on the desk his percussion hammer and his king size tuning fork."

"…As a colleague, Holmes was exciting. He rarely put in an appearance at medical committees. His few angry attendances were like war-drums announcing an impending battle over some issue, which evoked his tornado-like feelings…"

By all accounts, Holmes was a man not only of outstanding ability, but with great qualities of leadership, who burned on a short fuse and would not accept opposition to what he thought was proper treatment. As a neurologist, Holmes had overall responsibility for all patients with neurological disorders in France. Despite this he carried out meticulous research work late at night, on his own, investigating by simple cystometry, the bladder function of recently injured servicemen with spinal injuries.

9.1.2   Henry Head (1861-1940)

Head had worked with Holmes before the First World War on delineating sensory pathways and their work is still authoritative. Head remained at the London Hospital during the war. He was an outstanding clinician, neurologist and neurophysiologist.

After the war, when Head was offered the directorship of the London Hospital Medical Unit he insisted on academic and professional standards comparable to the German tradition and the United States. He wanted to set up a professorial unit with 8 full time physicians devoting their attention to the care of the patients. This was not welcomed in the private patient culture at the time as clinicians were not prepared to give up beds and the unit was not established.

It is striking that Holmes and Head were meticulous, obsessional and demanding men, who expected a great deal from their staff. They were both Fellows of the Royal Society. Not only had they carried out outstanding work before they came to treat patients with spinal injuries but when they were presented with unique material, patients with different cervical lesions which Cushing said he had never seen before (Cushing, 1936), they produced a series of detailed and meticulous papers, full of clinical observations and neurophysiological studies of the cord and bladder which govern our thinking to this day. Their descriptions have not been surpassed.

9.1.3   George Riddoch (1888-1947)

Riddoch was a younger man who was posted to the Empire Hospital, which was a private hospital for officers dealing with neurotrauma, under Head's direction.   He was an outstanding research worker who wrote an article on the reflex functions of the spinal cord (Riddoch, 1917), phantom limbs and central pain. After the war he was appointed to the staff of Maida Vale Hospital, the London Hospital and Queen Square.

Riddoch was a much under-rated figure.   There was virtually no neurosurgery being carried out in London until Sir Hugh Cairns (1896-1952), who was trained by Cushing in 1926-7, was stimulated by Riddoch to start neurosurgery initially at the London Hospital and later at Maida Vale.

At the beginning of the Second World War he was appointed neurologist to the Army, just as Holmes had been in the First World War.   He was Chairman of the committee on peripheral nerve injuries, which included spinal injuries and was on a head injuries committee.   Norman Dott (1897-1973) was trained by Cushing and Jefferson acknowledged his debt to Cushing. Both served on these committees and as a result the spinal injury units were set up throughout the country.   In turn, Jefferson trained George Frederick Rowbotham (1899-1975) who was in' charge of the unit at Newcastle.

Despite the time that has passed, Jack Colover, who was Riddoch's houseman and registrar between 1937 and 1939 at Queen Square, has told me that he was the outstanding neurologist with a great gift for research and teaching and was influential in getting Cairns appointed to the London Hospital (personal communication, 1999).   Peter Nathan, who also worked with Riddoch in 1939, has also confirmed the outstanding abilities of Riddoch (personal communication, 1999).

9.2   Personalities: Surgeons

9.2.1   Charters Symonds (1852-1932)

Charters Symonds was a remarkable man.   He was surgeon to Guy's Hospital and the first to perform an appendicectomy but unfortunately this was an isolated case and Treves received the credit for carrying out this operation on a large series. Symonds was very energetic and in 1886 was put in charge of the Ear, Nose and Throat Department. Symonds was a very great teacher of surgery. He retired early in 1913 at the age of 62 but carried on teaching at Lambeth Infirmary. In 1914 he went overseas to Malta as Consulting Surgeon in the army. His general expertise bore fruit in his paper on laminectomy (Symonds, 1917).

9.2.2   Sir William Thorburn (1861-1923)

William Thorburn was a member of the consultant staff of the Manchester Royal Infirmary who had an early interest in neurosurgery and studied the problem of spinal localisation and the correlation of paralysis to the segmental levels. He also described the significant posture of the arms in lesions of the cord at the seventh cervical level, having assembled a considerable number of cases with verified pathology on many of whom he carried out the autopsy himself.   These were published in 1889 in a monograph entitled *A Contribution to the Surgery of the Spinal Cord.* During the First World War, he studied surgery of the spinal cord and wrote the section in the official history of the medical services on spinal injury (Thorburn, 1922).

9.2.3   Sir John William Thomson Walker (1871-1937)

The general surgeons, by contrast, seemed to have a very ephemeral contact with spinal patients. In several cases there would be just one paper produced which was not based on any figures but was just speculation on the best form of treatment of the bladder.   The only one who seems to have maintained any contact at all with spinal cases is Thomson Walker who wrote a paper in 1917 on his experience at the King George V Hospital and the Royal Star & Garter. He wrote another paper in 1937 but this was just a recapitulation of his 1917 paper and, although he was the urological surgeon to the Royal Star & Garter, he said that his last experience was in 1929.

9.2.4   Phillip Northcott Vellacott (1872-1939)

Phillip Vellacott worked in the casualty clearing station for 2 years and kept records of more than 500 patients with spinal injuries but he contracted diphtheria and was invalided home.   His interest in spinal injuries ceased.

9.3   Personalities: Urologists

The urologists were of a lesser calibre.   Their accounts are diminished on two scores. They were not in overall charge of the patients and did not look further than the bladder or renal tract to describe other aspects of the management of the patients, which is vital if the patient is to be kept alive and rehabilitated.

9.4 Funding and general hospitals

At the beginning of the war, wounded soldiers were admitted to civilian hospitals such as the London Hospital. The hospital was paid four shillings daily for each military patient (MacPherson, 1921). This payment was raised to four shillings and ninepence in February 1918 and for military casualties in isolation hospitals to six or seven shillings per day. Voluntary hospitals and convalescent homes received a capitation grant of two shillings per day from the start of the war, which increased to three shillings in November 1914. In December 1916 a grant of sixpence was sanctioned for each unoccupied bed and in December, 1917 the maximum rate for occupied beds was increased to three shillings and threepence for Class A auxiliary hospitals and to two shillings and sixpence for Class B (convalescent homes) (MacPherson, 1921).

Doctors who tended wounded soldiers in auxiliary hospitals were paid fourpence daily for each equipped bed for patients from overseas, and threepence daily to others; with a limit of payment of seventeen shillings and sixpence daily to any one civil practitioner in the case of the former, and twelve shillings and sixpence daily for officer patients (MacPherson, 1921).

9.5 Specialised hospitals

In all fields early transfer to specialist centres led to much better results. As a result a plastic surgery unit was founded at Sidcup (Bamji, 1993), patients requiring abdominal surgery were segregated in specialised hospitals at the Front, amputees were seen at Queen Mary's Hospital, and the blind, neurosurgical, orthopaedic and psychiatric cases were segregated into specialised hospitals and received pioneering treatment with improved results.

The treatment of patients with traumatic injuries of the spinal cord followed this pattern and specialist hospitals were established at the King George V and Empire Hospitals followed by the Royal Star & Garter Home. Large numbers of spinal injury patients were now congregated together. Problems became immediately apparent. Improved treatment was partly the result of resentment on the part of the soldiers and relatives at the unprecedented casualties. Proper services for the wounded and the disabled had to be instituted, not necessarily for humanitarian but for political reasons. Something had to be done to care for these unfortunate victims on a long term basis:

> "There was widespread belief that each of these wounded men 'represented a centre of unrest, and that unless something could be done to improve their condition, or at least to have them feel that the government had done its best for them...(they) would have become centres of revolution'." (Cooter, 1993)

This was the catalyst for the beginning of centralised state medicine, which resulted in the setting up of the Ministry of Pensions and the British Association for Limbless Ex-Servicemen to look after the disabled, and the Association for the Blind.

10.   TREATMENT OF CASUALTIES

Today, a person who sustains a spinal injury is transferred within 60 minutes from the scene of the accident, possibly by helicopter. When they arrive at hospital, paramedics are in attendance, the fracture will have been immobilised with a collar on a scoop stretcher and intravenous fluids may well be running. This situation pertains even in modern warfare and was one of the developments of the Korean, Vietnam and Gulf wars. Early transfer by helicopter and optimum treatment of the severely injured patient has changed the outlook.

A supremely fit athlete, such as a mountaineer, immobilised on a mountainside, may die from hypothermia, even with proper modern equipment. A serviceman who sustains a spinal injury, who has lost blood and has major associated injuries, will succumb very rapidly without proper equipment and resuscitation. All writers acknowledge that many casualties were left to die on the battlefield and this would certainly apply to spinal injury cases (Keegan, 1998).

A spinal injury does not occur in isolation, patients with cervical injuries may have head injuries, those with thoracic lesions may have back or chest injuries, and those with lumbar lesions may have pelvic injuries. In gunshot wounds there may also be visceral damage.

11.   ANALYSIS OF CONTEMPORANEOUS PAPERS

Until this point individual papers have been discussed but in the First World War there were eleven contemporary British publications dealing with various aspects of treatment. The papers have been analysed and synthesised together to give an overall picture (Table 1).

Table 1. Review of the English First World War literature

PRINCIPLES OF TREAT-MENT	Medical Society 1916	Head & Riddoch 1920	Holmes 1915	Riddoch 1917	Symonds 1917	Thomson-Walker 1917/1937	Thorburn *et al.* 1918/ 1920-22	Vellacott *et al.* 1919	No. of Recom-mendations
Prevention of pressure sores							+		1/11
Careful catheterisation			+	+		+/+	+		5/11
Specialised staff	+		+						2/11
Early transfer to a spinal unit			+			+	+	+	4/11
Specialist rehabilitation facilities							+		1/11
Vocational training and reintegration							+		1/11
Physiotherapy							+		1/11
Opposition to early laminectomy							+		1/11
Management of fracture	+		+		+		+		4/11
Research, applied and basic		+	+	+				+	4/11
Statistics, living/dying	+		+		+	+	+	+	6/11

One of the papers, Medical Society (1916), is a discussion on gunshot wounds of the spine by doctors who were treating patients with spinal injuries. This is referenced under the individual authors: Adams, Armour (1869-1933), Buzzard (1871-1945), Collier (1870-1935), and Sargent. Another paper by Thomson-Walker (1937) summarises his wartime experience.

All the publications deal with servicemen, mainly from the Western Front but also from the Dardanelles, who sustained injuries to the spinal cord, mainly as a result of gunshot and shrapnel wounds. Two patients were injured in falls and two in aeroplane crashes.

11.1   Where patients were treated

In France patients were treated at the following hospitals: numbers 7, 13, 14, 20 and 24.   Holmes worked at No 13 and 14.

Cushing visited Holmes and Percy Sargent at No 13 General Hospital in Boulogne.   He recorded the vast number of casualties they had to deal with and was aware that the field of spinal injuries was new and had enormous potential for future research and treatment:

"After tea, Holmes and Sargent took me back to No 13, where I saw an amazing number of head and spinal wounded, for they often receive daily convoys of 300 recently wounded.   With the proper backing these two men have an unparalleled opportunity, not only to be of service to the individual wounded, but, when this is all over, to make a contribution to physiology, neurology, and surgery which will be epochal.

...Another group of injuries that were new to me were the transections of the spinal cord in the lower neck, which show, in addition to the total paralysis, an extraordinary lowering of body temperature – sometimes as low as 93 degrees F – with suppression of urine and death in two or three days, consciousness being retained to the end.   They already have full notes of one or more spinal transections for every segment of the cord, with the specimens preserved for future study – a life's work.   Such of the cases as recover sufficiently to be evacuated are sent to Henry Head at the London Hospital, by whom they are subsequently followed." (Cushing, 1936)

Medical enquiry and research, and regular mealtimes, continued in spite of the heavy workload in the casualty stations:

"...Holmes, Sargent and I slip away to have a powwow until midnight over neurological matters" (Cushing, 1936)

Later in 1918, Cushing described a larger, more formal gathering:

"Research meeting continues.   Neuropsychiatry programme under Salmon's guidance – rather disappointing.   Salmon himself suffering from an aphonia, which he explains is not hysterical.   Foster Kennedy – excellent!   Gordon Holmes urges more neurology; and in the afternoon we got it – three more papers by Frenchmen whom no one could understand as they undertook to read in English.   Leri spoke and Babinski; and also Pierre Marie – nice old man!" (Cushing, 1936)

It is very difficult to disentangle where patients with spinal injuries were treated in Britain.   Cushing described many hospitals where these patients were receiving treatment:

"...the Neurological Home Service is all at cross-purposes with patients scattered at Tooting, King George's, Queen Square, Maida Vale, The London Hospital and 200 incurables at the Star & Garter Richmond; also officers in small batches at the Empire, Roehampton, Brighton and elsewhere. I am to see General Goodwin and put the project of organisation and unification before him." (Cushing, 1936)

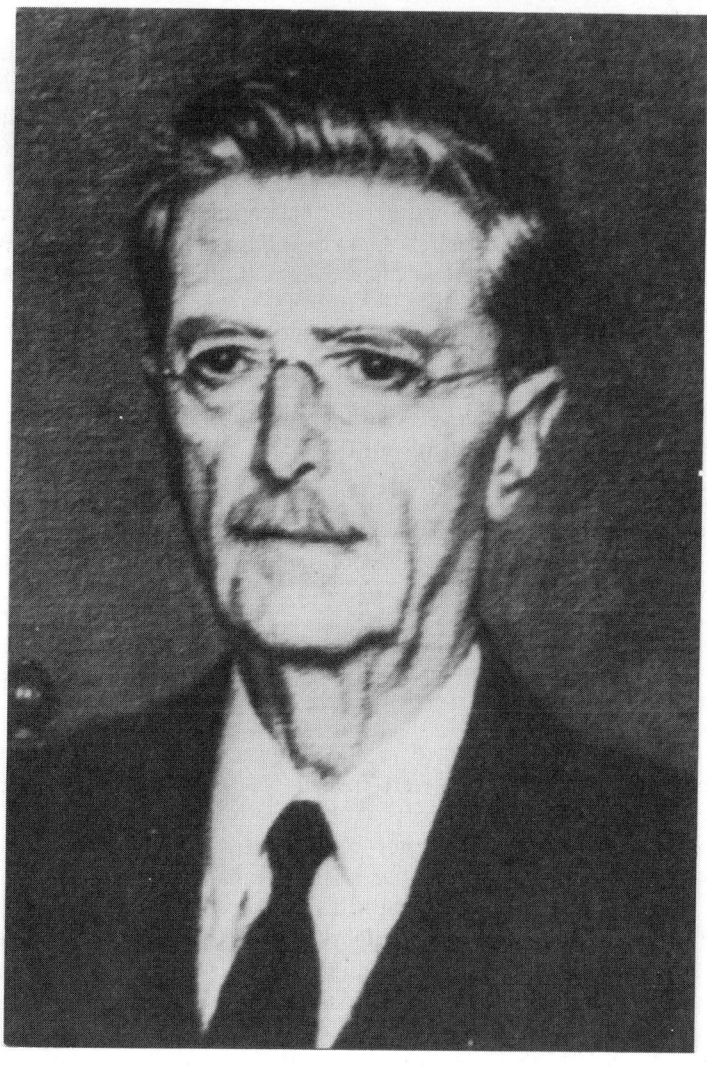

Figure 4. Gordon Holmes (1876-1965) (McHenry, 1969).

Patients were treated at King George V Hospital, the Empire Hospital, Westminster, Netley Hospital and there were individual records in papers from St Thomas's Hospital, the Welsh Hospital, Queen Square, Lonsdale House and The London Hospital. Surviving patients seem to have been congregated at the Royal Star & Garter Home, which was set up by Treves to treat patients with spinal injuries.

Holmes was in overall charge of all neurological cases in France, working at the base hospital, probably No 13. He arranged for patients to be transferred under the care of Head at The London Hospital. Head then arranged their transfer to either the Royal Star & Garter Home or to the Empire Hospital, which was functioning as a spinal unit. When the Army wished to take all army cases away and send them to Bethnal Green Hospital, Head protested and spinal injury patients alone were retained at The London Hospital under his care.

There were only a small number of patients with spinal injuries recorded at Queen Square and it is not known whether they were transferred from there to Lonsdale House, and then eventually to the Royal Star & Garter Home.

The Empire Hospital was a 40-50 bedded private hospital and the building is still in existence as a hotel:

"One of the first purpose built private hospitals...erected in 1912 in Vincent Square." (Richardson, 1998)

The Empire Hospital was not devoted exclusively to patients with spinal injuries, patients with shell shock were also treated there.

In 1918 Riddoch had 40 cases of spinal cord transection at the Empire Hospital. Cushing wrote:

"...dinner with several neurologists and neurosurgeons, among whom there was little agreement about heads, spines and peripheral nerves..." (Cushing, 1936)

Other than this reference to the Empire Hospital, Cushing does not specify where spinal cases were treated. He could have been referring to shell shock patients or patients with other types of neurological injuries.

Arrangements were made for patients to be segregated under specific disabilities but there is no mention at all of spinal patients.

It is unlikely that soldiers that had suffered spinal injury were included in the large statistic of soldiers with shell shock because they were treated differently. Soldiers with spinal injuries were evacuated to hospitals away from the Front while soldiers with shell shock remained nearer the Front, sometimes close enough to hear the sounds of battle. Once back in Britain, from March 1915 they were sent to The Royal Victoria Hospital, Netley and the 4th London General Hospital, Denmark Hill for distribution. Officers were sent to the Maudsley Neurological Clearing Hospital (Denmark Hill, London), the Special Hospital for Officers, Palace Green (Kensington, London), the Red Cross Military Hospital (Maghull, Liverpool), the Officers' Hospital (Nannau, Dolgelly, Ireland), the Neurological Section, King's Lancashire Military Convalescent Hospital (Blackpool) and Craiglockart War Hospital (Edinburgh). Men of other ranks with shell shock went to the Maudsley Hospital, Queen Square, Maida Vale, Welbeck Street, Springfield War Hospital (Wandsworth), Red Cross Military Hospital (Maghull), Abram Peel Hospital (Bradford), Ewell War Hospital (Epsom), Monyhull Section, 1st Southern General Hospital (Birmingham), Glen Lomond War Hospital (Fife), Dunblane War Hospital (Perthshire), Seale Hayne (Newcastle upon Tyne), the Neurological Section, 4th Southern General Hospital (Plymouth), Brinnington Neurological Section, 2nd Western General Hospital (Stockport) and East Preston Military Hospital (Worthing).

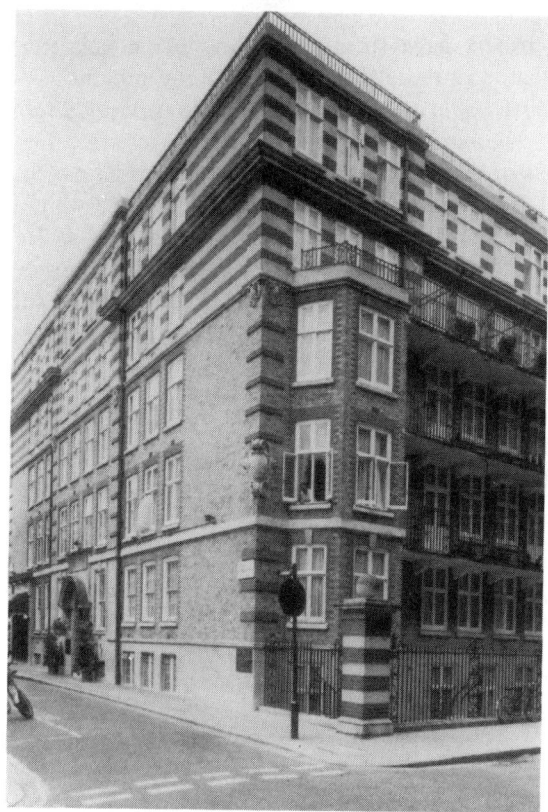

Figure 5. The Empire Hospital, which was not built as a hospital, and is now a private hotel (from Richardson, 1998). Reprinted with permission of English Heritage.

"At the time of the invasion of Poland, 120,000 pensioners had received or were still receiving money from the War Office for psychiatric disability dating from the First World War. The Royal Army Medical Corps had just two psychiatric consultants, one for Britain and one for those troops abroad, and the Ministry of Pensions announced that while it would treat any servicemen found to be suffering from war neurosis, it would not give pensions except in special circumstances." (Holden, 1998)

In his later paper, Thomson-Walker (1937) described how patients arrived at the King George V Hospital about 14 to 21 days after injury. Their stay in hospital was about a month or 8 weeks and they were then sent to permanent institutions such as the Royal Star and Garter Home.

11.2   Patient numbers and level of lesion

Few of the papers gave specific numbers of patients treated and all acknowledged that even these figures were not meaningful. Vellacott and Webb-Johnson listed 66 patients of which 10 had cervical, 28 dorsal and 11 lumbar lesions. Thorburn treated 111 patients plus a further 339 and did not specify the levels of the lesions. Symonds discussed 63 patients of which, 10 had cervical lesions and 53 dorsal lesions. There were 10 cases of cervical injuries from Netley, the Welsh Hospital and Malta. He said cauda equina lesions were common and described 7 cases. Holmes dealt with 13 patients. James Collier described 9 patients, of whom 2 suffered from cervical lesions, 6 from thoracic lesions and 1 was a lumbar lesion.

11.3   Statistics and mortality

11.3.1   Deaths at the Front

Many soldiers died on the battlefield. Thomson-Walker (1917) reported:

"The patient lies exposed for some hours, and in many cases has been inaccessible for two or even more days."

He discussed the delay in getting the patient to medical help, the delay in catheterisation and the practical difficulty of doing sterile catheterisation. Symonds (1917) noted that:

"In the higher lesions and those which are complete about the level of the fourth and fifth cervical vertebrae the patients either are killed outright or die early."

Thorburn and Richardson (1918) said that they did not see serious cases because they died before reaching base hospitals:

"During the last seven months of open warfare in France, we have seen a far larger proportion of injuries to the spinal cord than in the earlier days - a fact due partly, perhaps, to the absence of cover and possibly also to the large proportion of rifle or machine-gun bullet wounds as compared with wounds from shells or bombs. It is at least probable that a great proportion of shell wounds of the spine never reach base hospitals."

Holmes (1915) observed that a proportion of spinal cases died soon after the infliction of the wound of shock or associated injuries to the chest or abdomen. Among those who survived, the greatest danger was from cystitis, pyelonephritis and the development of extensive bedsores. Paraplegic patients who were not evacuated quickly from the battlefield died of hypothermia. Casualties received first aid on the battlefield and were evacuated by stretcher-bearers to the nearest medical post, probably in a dugout.

Patients with cervical injuries were likely to die from a variety of complications but there was an immediate mortality from sepsis of the spinal cord and meningitis and a later mortality from pressure sores and urinary tract infection, which was quite horrendous.

11.3.2   Deaths at the base hospitals in France

Many patients died at the receiving hospitals in France. Vellacott and Webb-Johnson (1919) said:

"During the three months from mid July to mid October last 66 cases of gunshot wound of the spine were admitted into the observation wards at No 14 Stationary Hospital, Boulogne."

While the cases were under observation there were 21 deaths: 2 due to high cervical injury, 2 to direct infection of the meninges, 9 to complicating injuries and diseases, 7 to pyelonephritis and 1 to rupture of the bladder. 14% died of pyelonephritis.

Holmes, who had trained as a pathologist, described the early death rate and carried out post mortems on 9 out of 20 soldiers with cervical lesions.

11.3.3   Deaths in the United Kingdom

The high death rate continued even after soldiers were transferred to the United Kingdom but this death rate was due to ascending infection of the renal tract and pressure sores.

Symonds stated:

"...of those who escape early death, some remain helpless from paraplegia, with incontinence of urine and faeces, and sooner or later die from the effects of renal infection."

At Netley during the last 5 months of 1917, Symonds reported that 65% of the cases admitted died (28 deaths in 43 dorsal and lumbar cases).

Vellacott and Webb-Johnson (1919) reported that 19% of cases died of pyelonephritis during the period of observation.

Thomson-Walker (1917) said:

"Over 90% of cases of spinal injury arriving at the Royal Star and Garter Hospital have a serious infection of the urinary tract, and all cases have at some period passed through a stage of severe infection. Of the total 111 patients 19 have died, all from urinary infection. At the King George Hospital 339 cases of spinal injury have been admitted, 22 were transferred and 160 have died, practically all from urinary infection."

11.4   Treatment

Two aspects of treatment engaged virtually all the doctors to the exclusion of everything else:
a) Management of injury to the paralysed bladder
b) Management of injury to the spine and spinal cord

In the acute stage, associated injuries were the immediate cause of death, followed by overwhelming sepsis from the bladder. The papers give different accounts of sepsis. Meticulous care at the Empire Hospital resulted in better results than at other hospitals and, interestingly, Holmes, Head and Riddoch were carrying out investigations of the function of the bladder.

11.4.1   Management of injury to the paralysed bladder

Many papers were devoted to the crucial problem of management of the bladder.

- There were fundamental physiological investigations of the highest quality carried out by Holmes and Head & Riddoch which delineated the physiological changes following spinal injury.
- There were pathological studies delineating the relationship between infection and morbidity and mortality.
- There were detailed studies of the management of the bladder.

- There were detailed statistical analyses as to how different forms of management of the bladder affected the prognosis.
- Attempts were made to change the management by specific military orders.

There are many accounts which discuss how long the bladder can be left undrained before the patients reach a specialised centre. Thomson-Walker stated that:

"The patient lies exposed for some hours, and in many cases has been inaccessible for two or even more days. In this state the patient, still suffering from profound shock, arrives at the casualty clearing station, where a catheter is passed and the bladder is emptied."

In 46 cases the average time before a catheter was passed was 27 hours. Two patients lay on the battlefield for 4 days and four for 3 days before they could be reached.

Thomson-Walker (1917) stated that the most common, and usually fatal complication in the paralysed bladder was infection. Of 339 patients with spinal injury admitted to the King George V Military Hospital from 1915-1919, 160 (47%) died from urinary infection 8 to 10 weeks after admission. He further reported that 19 cases out of 111 (17%) died later at the Royal Star & Garter Home from urinary infection, 1 to 3 years after injury. In 1937 Thomson-Walker estimated that the total mortality rate due to urinary sepsis in British soldiers with paraplegia in the First World War was 80%. He referred to two types of diseases:

1. Acute cystitis, often haemorrhagic, leading to septic pyelonephritis, "...a peculiarly fatal disease." (Thomson-Walker, 1917)
2. Chronic septic pyelonephritis with recurring acute pyelonephritis.

Vellacott and Webb-Johnson were unique in recognising that in the First World War patients with paraplegia due to gunshot wounds died as a result of catheterisation, and they achieved the best survival rate by avoiding catheterisation whenever possible, leaving the bladder alone so that retention of urine developed. They advised that the bladder should be emptied by retention with overflow and attempts at expression.

A considerable effort was being made to manage the bladder appropriately and this generated considerable controversy.

Thorburn (1922) recognised the danger of retention when patients were being transported and the danger of urinary sepsis:

"In connection with treatment there arose a strong opposition to the regular use of the catheter, this opposition resulting in attempts to evacuate the bladder by pressure alone, in permanent drainage of the bladder by suprapubic cystotomy, and in the use of 'mass reflex' to procure evacuation." "In civil practice and with good nursing the systematic use of the catheter with most careful asepsis of the instruments and of the glans penis, still presents the best method of treating retention of urine..."

Recommendations were made that early suprapubic cystotomy should be carried out. Forbes Fraser (1871-1924), who was working in France, was endeavouring to see this was carried out but not all soldiers were receiving this treatment since Thomson-Walker commented that "the stream of paraplegics dying from catheter infection continued unabated." (Fraser, 1919)

11.4.2   Management of injury to the spine and spinal cord

Seven of the accounts specifically address the management of the spine which was regarded as paramount.

11.4.3   Immediate management at the Front

Only Holmes warned against the danger of moving a soldier with an unstable fracture of the spine whereby movement of such a fracture could cause further damage, advising absolute rest during the first few weeks after injury.

It was recognised that there was a difference between military practice, where bullets had traversed and damaged the spinal cord causing compound wounds, and civilian practice where compound wounds were rare. Discussion hinged on three topics:
– Should a compound wound be debrided like any other compound fracture?
– Should the spinal cord be explored?
– Should the bullet be removed?

There was general agreement that the pathology of cord damage was caused by the immediate injury and not to secondary compression by a haematoma. Great technical skill was needed to operate on the spinal cord and the surgeons who were first in this field such as Cushing or Sargent were very rare. At the meeting of the Medical Society in 1916 both Armour and Sargent were in favour of operative treatment. All acknowledged that laminectomy in the presence of sepsis had a very poor prognosis since incision and closure might lead to meningitis and death.

Laminectomy in an incomplete lesion, where there was no sepsis, was contraindicated. At no stage was there any discussion about closed reduction of fractures. Despite these strictures there was a very high immediate mortality.

11.4.4   Long-term management

Symonds thought an early operation in the hands of Cushing would be beneficial but in the hands of any other doctor would be inadvisable. He considered that incomplete cervical cord lesions should not be operated on and described the risks of laminectomy:

"Excision and closure where sepsis is established lead to wide suppuration and may determine a fatal issue."

He was in favour of operating on the cauda equina to suture nerves.

Thorburn et al (1918) drew attention to the fact that patients sustain multiple fractures of the vertebrae. They said operations were performed in a very limited number of selected cases and were not illustrative of the comparitive frequency of the lesions found. In 1922 Thorburn recommended that surgery should not be performed in the acute stage of sepsis unless there was evidence of meningitis. If the theca was untorn he advocated early removal of the bullet but preferred to wait until the patient's condition had settled down. He discussed the use of investigations such as stereoscopic or combined lateral and sagittal pictures of the spine.

They concluded that operation in the early stage was dangerous and were not in favour of operating on either complete or incomplete cases.

11.5   Early transfer and careful transportation

Those who win a battle and are left in possession of the battlefield can retrieve their casualties; the losers in retreat cannot.

Patients with spinal injuries who were not evacuated quickly from the battlefield would die of intercurrent injuries and hypothermia. Casualties received first aid on the battlefield and were evacuated by stretcher-bearers to the nearest medical post, probably in a dugout. The walking wounded were sent to a collection point or advanced dressing station, the more seriously injured were taken there by field ambulance, hand stretcher or some other form of transport.

At the advanced dressing station, which was as near to the Front as possible, casualties were comforted and had their dressings adjusted before being sent on to the main dressing station, where urgent operations were performed. Dressings were adjusted again and records were made.

Those needing further treatment were taken to the clearing stations by horse-drawn or mechanical transport where skilled surgeons and physicians treated the serious cases before evacuation by ambulance convoy, train or boat to hospitals further down the lines of communication or at base, and then they might be evacuated by train or ship (Mitchell, 1931). When medical transport was insufficient for the number of casualties, they might be evacuated in general transport or utility vehicles (Mitchell, 1931). Although the need for rapid transportation was appreciated, it was also accepted that in wartime the prime consideration was the continuation of hostilities to create further casualties. Priority might be given to transporting provisions of war to the Front rather than removing the injured from the Front.

Vellacott gave 6 case studies seen by him at No 14 Stationary Hospital Boulogne of which one patient fell from a horse, one lay on the battlefield for 24 hours. The cases were under Vellacott's care between 1 day and 4 days after injury.

Holmes described patients arriving at base hospital between two days and five weeks after injury.

Head and Riddoch wrote copious notes on 9 patients who were admitted to the Empire Hospital half an hour, 3, 4, 7, 10, 12, 31, 52 days and 2 years after injury.

It was not just fortuitous that these cases were arriving at specialised centres. Some cases arrived quickly after injury. The dangers of incorrect management in the early stages, with its complications, was well recognised. Considering that some patients were lying on the battlefield and could not be reached, it is very commendable that many of these patients reached specialised centres.

Only Holmes discussed the need to immobilise the spinal column.

11.6   Pressure sores

Pressure sores are a major cause of mortality which can only be prevented by rigorous turning.

Pressure sores are referred to by Thorburn and Richardson, Holmes and Thomson-Walker. They all recognised that pressure sores occurred and could cause adverse effects. The only person to describe treatment, and that indirectly, is Thorburn who advocated massage, tendon transplants, and mobilisation to improve morale and reduce the risk of pressure sores. He also recommended the use of a rudimentary standing frame.

Thomson-Walker described the differential diagnosis between the sepsis caused by pressure sores and the sepsis caused by pyelonephritis. In the case of a pressure sore, the temperature gradually rises, whereas in a urinary tract infection, it spikes, i.e. rigors at intervals.

Riddoch recognised the complications of chest wounds, bedsores and urinary sepsis. He described toxicity producing diarrhoea and vomiting. He discussed venous thrombosis and the complications of pressure sores, which are likely to occur in the stage of spinal shock and became infected. He observed swelling of the legs in patients who sat up in chairs and said that the patients should be encouraged to be in the open air.

Holmes (1915) observed that amongst patients who survived the acute stage the greatest danger was from cystitis, pyelonephritis and the development of extensive bedsores. A large part of the responsibility consequently falls upon the nursing staff.

The prevention of pressure sores is mentioned twice, by Vellacott and by Webb-Johnson who said patients should be concentrated where specialisation could take place. The dangers of catheters and bed sores, which could be lessened by careful nursing, were described (Adams, 1916). However both in the First World War and even in the early 1950s when I was a medical student, pressure sores were rarely discussed. As a student in 1951 I recall one patient covered with bedsores. The consultant did not discuss the sores, pointing out that they were the responsibility of the nurses who had not consulted him. Patients got pressure sores even in teaching hospitals but the consultants did not consider it their role to manage them.

11.7   Specialised staff and facilities

The leading British neurologists before the Second World War recognised the importance of nursing. They were aware of the diagnosis, complications and in particular the relationship of pressure sores to morbidity but the necessity for regular turning and prevention of sores was only hinted at, never described. In patients with spinal injuries fears were expressed that the strain, especially in the early stages, was too great for both patients and nurses. The heavy mortality had a depressing effect on both patients and nursing staff but the advantages of concentration and specialisation was so great as to far outweigh the disadvantages. Most of these men did better in specialised centres than if they had been distributed to various hospitals at the base. Adams reported that the dangers of bedsores had been greatly lessened by better nursing but he queried whether the profession should have handed over cases of spinal cord damage to male nurses for regular catheterisation.

Symonds recognised when he wrote from military hospitals that while experts such as Cushing and Sargent could successfully operate on wounds, less experienced doctors could not.

There was thus a clear recognition that these injured soldiers should be transferred quickly to specialised centres for appropriate care from the surgical, nursing and rehabilitation viewpoint.

11.8 Research

There are superb clinical descriptions of cases by Riddoch, Holmes and Head. The levels of the lesion are discussed, management of the bladder, anuria, hypothermia, the mass reflex, spinal shock and the alternating stepping reflex. The association of autonomic dysreflexia with sweating is described and, although the blood pressure was not recorded, evidence that the blood pressure was raised is provided by the fact that patients experienced throbbing headaches. Some of these case descriptions run into 20 pages and, because they are so detailed, can be used for further research (Silver, 2000).

12. SUMMARY

There are superb pathological descriptions of injuries to the spinal cord, magnificent physiological accounts of spinal cord lesions, spinal cord shock and bladder physiology, and detailed accounts of the complications.

Thorburn (1922) summarising the experience of treating spinal injuries at the battlefront concluded that, in general, patients with spinal injuries should be evacuated to the base hospital as quickly as possible. If there was evidence of thecal injury with meningitis, the only hope was early drainage. If the theca was untorn or if there was a foreign body or other septic mass, this must be removed. If there was sepsis present, the operation should be performed only when the sepsis had ceased since it was unwise to operate in the stage of acute sepsis. He recommended use of a suprapubic catheter to manage the bladder stressing the need for good nursing and asepsis. There is discussion about massage, tendon transfer operations, wheelchairs, getting patients up to prevent pressure sores and improve morale, getting patients back to work and the use of a swimming pool in Tooting for paraplegic patients.

Thus these fundamentals of treatment were recognised:
- Early transfer to a specialised centre where patients can be rehabilitated
- Prevention of complications: pressure sores, urinary tract infections, by meticulous treatment until the fracture has stabilised

The uniformly pessimistic view of treatment is reflected by the fact that Holmes only devoted three paragraphs to the subject in the two Goulstonian lectures he gave in 1915.

There is no one paper devoted entirely to the overall treatment. This had to wait until the MRC publication in 1924.

13.   REHABILITATION

At the time of the First World War physiotherapy was not a recognised speciality as it is today. Nevertheless different forms of treatment, such as electricity, hydrotherapy, massage and manipulation, were used to treat the patients. Massage had a murky history, being associated with quackery and immorality but, by the time the First World War broke out, a Society of Trained Masseurs had been formed.

13.1   Exercise, massage and manipulation

The evolution of systematic exercise as a form of treatment was accredited to Pehr Ling (1776-1839) who was a Swedish practical physiologist.   When he died in 1839, there was a permanent organisation and a devoted band of pupils to carry on his work of remedial gymnastic exercises. This was called the Swedish drill.

Swedish gymnastics were introduced into British schools when the local school boards, following the extension of schooling through the Education Act of 1870, were faced with sickly and undersized children.   Physical education colleges emerged across the country to train the women teachers and most took up the Ling system of educational gymnastics although some authorities preferred the exercises for the re-education of ataxic muscles devised by Professor Ernst von Leyden (1832-1910) and Dr Heinrich Frenkel (1860-1931).

Von Leyden gave priority to flexion and extension movements to improve motor tracts whilst Frenkel concentrated on developing a 'deep sensibility'. Within a few years of Frenkel's first paper (1902 translation), many medical men and masseuses had adopted his repeated and progressive exercises, the majority of which could be done in bed.

In America in the 1870s, a neurologist, Dr Silas Weir Mitchell (1829-1914) developed a completely different type of treatment. This consisted of bed rest, massage, electrotherapy and aggressive feeding.

The Weir Mitchell system became part of a British 'revival in massage', which provided new opportunities for women with the founding of the Society of Trained Masseuses.   A modified Weir Mitchell regime of massage rest and good food was prescribed for 'nerves' which, in Weir Mitchell's view, was seen mainly in women who wore restrictive corsets which were fashionable at the time. Massage after fracture and dislocation became central to the work of members of the Society of Trained Masseuses although it was always a subject of controversy. Indeed, two influential British orthopaedic surgeons of the time, Hugh Owen Thomas (1834-1891) and Robert Jones (1858-1933) were in favour of total rest and believed that 'it was the prerogative of Nature alone to repair'. They would not allow movement or massage on the fracture for at least a month if at all and devised splints to immobilize the affected limb. In contrast, in France Just Marie Marcellin Lucas-Championnière (1843-1913) claimed that immobilizing fractures led to stiff joints and deformity but gentle massage, and passive exercise given within a few days of injury would relieve pain, reduce swelling, build callus and restore function. His disciple in Britain,

Dr James Beaver Mennell (1880-1957) also used the 'early movement' method and the use of Swedish exercises, massage and manipulation by masseuses was much encouraged by Mennell. He recommended that a doctor should supervise massage treatment:

> "When a medical man orders massage he should not try to hand over his responsibility to the masseur. He should consider the prescription of massage treatment in the same light as he would consider that of a potent drug and watch its effects no less closely, varying the dose and the nature of the dose from time to time according to indications." "Manipulation and exercises must often precede, should frequently accompany, and must invariably follow effective work by the surgeon." (Mennell, 1917)

The Incorporated Society of Trained Masseuses (ISTM) grew from 1000 members in 1914 to 3641 in 1918. The Almeric Paget (Military) Massage Corps (APMC) was founded by Almeric Paget M.P. and his wife, an American philanthropist, who within a few weeks of war breaking out recruited 50 skilled and certified masseuses as volunteers. It was a prestigious organization, with its own uniform and only ISTM members were accepted. By the end of October 1914, the APMC employed 110 masseuses (half voluntary) and in November, it opened an outpatient centre in London. A combination of methods, including physiotherapy, massage, remedial gymnastics, electricity and electrotherapy were used to get men back to the Front. Because of the war, people were taught to 'rub the wounded in 12 lessons' and despite efforts by the examination board to maintain standards, this led to many unsuitable candidates qualifying. From the start of the war, massage instruction in the Army and Navy had been given by women and in June 1919, in view of the shortage of male teachers and the strict discipline and close medical supervision in the services, the council reluctantly agreed that this might continue.

The Army Medical Services divided the casualties into first, second and third-class 'matter'. First-class or acute patients were admitted to Territorial Force General Hospitals, of which there were 23, mainly associated with a large teaching hospital; to a separate orthopaedic centre, of which there were 20 by 1918, or to a Red Cross auxiliary hospital, which might be devoted to special cases like head injuries, epilepsy, heart conditions or war neuroses. Second-class patients went to RAMC convalescent camps or hospitals, and the third, who had 'nowhere to go' and were 'too tedious' for the existing services, were sent to command depots. (Barclay, 1994)

Masseuses became adept at manipulations, at restoring sensation to trench feet and badly splinted limbs, and in training amputees to use artificial limbs, about which little had previously been known. In convalescence camps, masseuses and masseurs treated 20-25 patients a day. To get through the work, a masseuse might have four patients under supervision at once, two perhaps on heat treatment, a third on ionisation or interrupted current with a metronome and the fourth being massaged. The masseuses were expected to do dressings, apply strapping and to treat sciatica by painting the whole length of the sciatic nerve with fuming hydrochloric acid. Of the discharged patients 80% were considered fit enough to return to the Front.

Sport was being employed to assist rehabilitation including games of volleyball for amputees (Mayer, 1918).

13.2   Electricity

The therapeutic use of electricity had been recognised since antiquity. Early work had been done by Gottlieb Kratzenstein (1723-1795) and Abbe Nollet (1700-1770). Various textbooks were produced on electricity in the second half of the 18th century but the treatments were appropriated by celebrated charlatans. James Graham (1745-1794) gave lectures, demonstrations and expensive treatments with his "Celestial Bed" and electrical instruments in London, Bristol and Bath As early as 1768 an electrical machine had been installed at the Middlesex Hospital in London.

In 1836 Guy's Hospital set aside rooms for an electrical department and put Golding Bird, the instructor in physics, in charge. Because of his scientific standing he soon had the cooperation of some of the leading clinicians of the time, especially Richard Bright (1789-1858) and Thomas Addison (1793-1860).

Spinal shock was first described by Hall who believed that galvanism could be an important remedy. He questioned whether galvanism had been properly applied. He did not answer the question but Addison tried to in the following year.

Wilfred Harris (1869-1960) wrote about electrical treatment in 1908 but E. Farquhar Buzzard only mentioned it in passing and took the view that electrical treatment and massage probably did more harm than good but by outbreak of the First World War it was being used:

"A hundred men often attend daily and the scene is both sad and amusing; men, two or three at a time with limbs in the radiant heat 'ovens', others having active exercises stretching limbs, with the buzz of vibrators and batteries, an occasional shout from a patient who remonstrated at a strong current and the masseuse all hard at work, made a scene which justified the remark of a big sergeant –'If the Kaiser saw this he might say:- 'The English Army is being tortured to make it go to the front'.'' (Barclay, 1994)

The King's Lancashire Military Convalescent Hospital, Blackpool, which was opened in 1916, had a gymnasium, an electro-massage and hydrotherapy department with whirlpool baths, a room where 'shell shock patients were treated by passing electricity through the brain' and a hot exercise room with machines and heat and light baths to break down adhesions. The workload was huge and in one centre, 20 masseurs were treating 4000 patients. After a year's work, all were discharged and 80% were declared fit to return to some kind of service.

13.3   Hydrotherapy

The use of water as a treatment for therapeutic and recreational purposes dates back to antiquity, to the days of the Assyrians, Babylonians and Ancient Egyptians.

It was the Romans who popularised hot mineral springs and established the first spas in many provinces of their Empire.   Some of these places still flourish as spas.

Hydrotherapy reached its zenith in the early 20th century, a time when physicians could choose from a bigger selection of gadgetry than at any other time before or since.   Cooling baths, subthermal baths: cardiovascular baths, "pool" baths, sedative pool baths; thermal baths, hyperthermal baths, needle baths, douche baths, shower baths, hydro-mechanical and hydro-pneumatic contrivances, reclining baths, upright baths, hot air and vapour baths, manipulation and massage baths, hot air douches, whirlpool baths, sand baths and electric baths.

As methods of administering the waters became more complex, the methods themselves began to adopt more importance than the media.

In the First World War there is an account of paraplegic patients being put in a swimming pool at Tooting Hospital (Buzzard, 1919).

Spinal patients who survived were sent either to The London Hospital, The Empire Hospital or Netley Hospital but then pursued different courses. There was still a high death rate among survivors in the United Kingdom. Some died of pressure sores as the report of Symonds showed.   A few were treated at Queen Square, some went to Lonsdale House but the only spinal patients that we have any details of are those who were treated at the Royal Star & Garter Home and did not go out to workshops.

14. THE ROYAL STAR AND GARTER: THE FIRST SPINAL UNIT IN THE UNITED KINGDOM

In 1915 military hospitals were crowded with wounded sailors and soldiers and it became necessary to make room for new patients by evacuating paralysed patients whose injuries were so serious as to appear incurable.

Sadly, these men would never get better and in 1916, following an appeal in the Times by Sir Frederick Treves (1853-1923), the Red Cross opened the first Royal Star & Garter Home in Richmond for 60 permanently disabled men.

The Royal Star & Garter Home was opened by Queen Mary and the Red Cross on 14th January 1916 for pensioners, paralysed by being shot through the spine or brain, who had been discharged from the Services as: 'totally disabled' (Royal Star & Garter report, 1916). It was the only unit in the world, which functioned as a spinal unit.

It was founded by Her Majesty Queen Mary who expressed the wish that there should be a permanent haven for the young men returning wounded from the battlefield during the First World War. Treves was the driving force and the Women of the Empire funded it after a worldwide appeal. It was a 64-bedded unit, where the paralysed victims of the First World War resided. They were pensioners and were not all spinal injury patients. Some patients suffered from disseminated sclerosis and there were a few hemiplegics. Whilst there is no official history of the Royal Star & Garter Home, annual medical reports, the in house residents magazines and articles by visiting consultants and resident medical staff, provide a detailed picture of the treatment that was being carried out. There is a contrast between the gloomy picture given by the medical consultants who describe patients totally disabled and confined to bed, with persistent urinary tract infections, stones and recurrent pressure sores, and the optimism of the residents who describe being mobilised and discharged home.

In 1920, 43 patients were transferred to Enbrook House at Sandgate (Folkestone) while the Royal Star & Garter Home was demolished and rebuilt. It re-opened as a purpose-built spinal centre in 1924. The Official History of the War does not mention the Royal Star & Garter Home.

14.1 Types of patients admitted and the outcome

At the outset in 1916, there were 112 patients admitted of whom, 92 were paraplegics, and the vast majority doubly incontinent and with bedsores. Nevertheless, as shown in Table 2, a significant number were discharged home.

Initially the importance of segregation, urological management, recreational facilities such as trips on the river and to concerts, visitors, fresh air, specialised nursing, and visiting specialists were recognised at the Royal Star & Garter Home.   There was a hopeful, progressive attitude towards rehabilitating spinal patients. They were very proud of their results:

Table 2. Statistics from The Royal Star and Garter Home Medical Reports

Year	Residents	Admitted	Died	Discharged
1916	112	112	20	23
1917	95	34	17	17
1918	82	21	13	6
1919	91	28	10	19
1920	63	1	5	15
1921	50	7	5	7
1922	44	6	1	3

"18 patients left the Star and Garter 'improved'; while five may be spoken of as immensely improved. Of these 5 – the famous five – the staff never cease to boast without either modesty or moderation; while in the eyes of the patients they are regarded as the great exemplars. At to the achievement that has made them famous it is this:- these five 'totally disabled' men, who were carried into the Star and Garter, have walked out of the front door unaided and have gone home...... One must reluctantly own that nature can do astonishing things in apparently hopeless cases, but it would be useless to present this view to the sister in charge of the Electrical Department or to the masseuses and nurses who had the care of these redoubtable men." (Royal Star and Garter Medical Report, 1916)

The death rate fell steadily as did the number of residents (Table 2). The discharged figure does not include patients sent to other hospitals. In that first year, five residents who were carried into the home were able to walk out after 'continuous and persistent treatment'. Clearly, it was realised that the outcome was not as dire as originally thought.

14.2   Staffing levels

Patients were congregated together under the care of a Medical Superintendent, Major Ronald Stevenson Dickie (1892-1960), and a doctor who deputised in his absence. Other specialists made regular visits. The Matron was experienced in nursing paralysed patients, as was the nurse in charge of the electrical and massage department. The home had an X-ray department and a radiographer.

In the 1916 Annual Medical Report, they discussed the needs of paraplegics:

> "They need many special and costly appliances, the services often of a male nurse as well as of a female nurse, massage, electrical treatment and unremitting medical and surgical attention. This cannot be obtained in a cottage nor even in a cottage hospital."

From the outset, there were 15 nurses, 10 masseurs, 1 electrotherapy/masseuse nurse, 4 occupational therapists and 16 orderlies to care for a total of 64 patients at any one time. Although the nursing staff levels do not appear to have been adequate to look after that number of patients properly, the high number of orderlies would have helped considerably. The nurses and the orderlies made a total of 31 staff looking after 64 patients or a ratio of around 1:2, this compares with current staffing levels of 1.5 staff to each patient at the spinal unit, Stoke Mandeville Hospital but patterns of working and shifts are different today.

The Almeric Paget Massage Corps, formed in the First World War contributed largely to the high number of masseurs and physiotherapists.

14.3   Care

In the early days, the nursing care consisted of turning the patients, evacuating their bowels and getting them up once a week. Of 44 patients on the Upper Ground Floor, only one was able to dress and undress himself and of the remainder, 19 had to be fed at every meal.

14.4   Optimism

As early as 1924 (Royal Star and Garter Annual Medical Report), they realised that the prognosis for paraplegics was not as bleak as it had been 10 years previously.

> "Under modern methods of treatment the important group of cases of paraplegia following wounds of the spine presents a very different picture to that accepted some ten years ago. And it would seem that given scrupulous care and attention to details of surgical cleanliness, etc... there is no reason why a man so afflicted should not continue to live his somewhat restricted life to its normal span". "...Regular massage and exercises, passive and otherwise, maintain the circulation and tone of paralysed muscles, and prevent contractures."

The Royal Star & Garter Home recognised the need to get people near to their homes but they were aware of the difficulties of providing special equipment at the patient's home or local hospital.

14.5   Physiotherapy

When the home opened in 1916, the Almeric Paget Massage Corps, formed in the First World War provided 10 masseuses. By 1930, most of the original 10 masseuses were qualified in electrical treatment and the teaching of medical exercises.

In a report dated 31st December 1917, they quoted: 'by means of electrical treatment, persistent massage and other measures specially suited to particular cases, men have improved so greatly as to permit discharge.' In the 1921 Annual Medical report, they repeated the above statement but added 'special baths ' to the list of treatments. In the exercise room, patients were mobilised and taught to walk with the aid of sticks or elbow crutches. They described the outcome of successful physiotherapy treatment:

> "W.F.R.A. Wear, aged 21 was admitted to the Home on 17th January 1933, suffering from partial paralysis, the result of a fracture dislocation of the fifth cervical vertebra, following a fall on the deck of H.M.S. Rodney in June 1932. On admission he had almost entirely lost the use of his legs, but he was not incontinent. He was wearing a Jury Mast attached to his spinal support, to prevent his head from falling forwards, and to immobilise his cervical vertebrae. This young man has now almost completely recovered; he can walk for considerable distances…..
> The other case is that of G. C. Edwards, admitted to the Home on 14th Dec 1932, suffering from complete paraplegia, which came on in September 1931 after he had undergone considerable hardship on manoeuvres. This young man was not incontinent but he presented all the symptoms of a lesion of the spinal cord about the level of the seventh dorsal vertebra. On his admission it was thought there were great hopes of his recovery, and he is now almost normal. He can walk readily and exhibits no signs at all of paraplegia."

14.6   Specialised equipment

The types of apparatus used in the gym included the Swedish combination, the fixed bicycle, stairs and walking horses. They used appliances to get patients ambulating. However, these were patients with cauda equina lesions who probably had little interference with their bladder. In the Medical Research Council (MRC) report dated 1924, they describe the use of inside iron, outer T-strap or cross strap and toe raising spring from ·front of boot to calf band of instrument. Patients also walked with sticks and elbow crutches. The Home had an electrical department.

In the Annual Medical Report dated 1923, there is a mention of using motor attachments to the wheel chairs subject to the regulations of the Ministry of Pensions. They described one patient who constructed his own motor-wheel in the workshop at Sandgate.

14.7   Rehabilitation

At the Royal Star and Garter Home, rehabilitation was carried out from the outset. In 1916, Lady Slogett organised handicraft, needlework and embroidery classes. Facilities were also provided for shoe making and shoe repairs, toy making, feather work, leatherwork, basketwork, carpentry and pewter work. They also practiced salmon fly dressing, painting, watch making and repairing. In 1944 residents devised a pulley system, which enabled them to carry out engineering work from their wheelchairs.

The idea was that not only could patients return home, they could take up a trade, which would at least in part contribute towards their maintenance and that of their families.

After the First World War, there had been a great emphasis on vocational training. Workshops had been set up for the disabled, but patients at the Royal Star and Garter Home used their own in-house facilities.

14.8   Sport

Apart from providing recreational facilities such as billiards, the Royal Star and Garter Home had a sports club with activities such as tennis and bowling. They organised a sports day or gymkhana for patients and staff. There was an obstacle Zig Zag race in tricycle chairs, chair races and shove ha' penny (Royal Star and Garter Magazine, Sports Day August 1923).

Prior to the Ministry of Pensions, the long-term disabled were at the mercy of their families or charity. The Royal Star & Garter Home had been funded by the Ministry of Pensions since 1917.   This was crucial to the long-term care of paraplegics because the state had a commitment to care for these people for the rest of their lives. The emotional context: these people had been wounded in the service of their country, carried the implication that they had to be looked after by that country.   While long-term provision could be made for them, it had the disadvantage that patients became institutionalised and no thought was given to patients being discharged into the community to become wage earners.

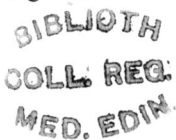

The patients who went to the Royal Star & Garter Home had been sent there as totally incurable and 100% disabled and, in some ways, they lived up to this expectation.   Nevertheless, apart from the five patients admitted totally paralysed who walked out of the home, some patients did leave the home, travelled the World, married and returned to society. They were not encouraged to be independent.   This cannot be entirely attributed to the medical profession.   There was still the influence of the Edwardian era and people were very deferential to their 'betters' whom, they thought, knew best. Because they came from the services, they had been trained to accept discipline. There was no role model for them because spinal patients had not been successfully treated and rehabilitated.   This was compounded by the pension scheme. The state accepted responsibility for these servicemen and patients adopted a passive role.

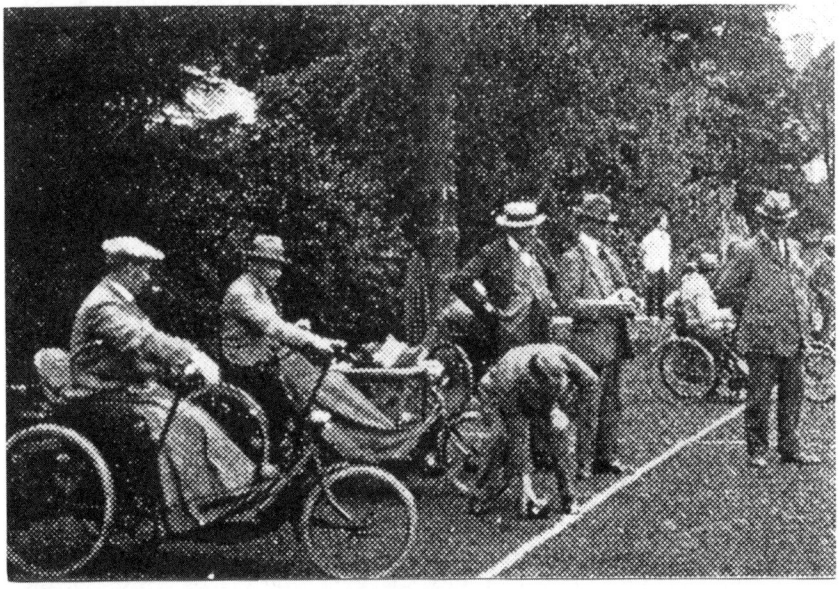

Figure 6: Patients using primitive tricycles at the Royal Star and Garter Home before the Second World War at a bowling tournament (Royal Star & Garter Annual Medical Report, 1923)

14.9   Doom and gloom

A vivid account, which illustrates the flavour of the place, is given by the Medical Superintendent, who looked after 230 paraplegic patients (Gowlland, 1934).   The majority were incontinent and because of the dangers of infection, trained orderlies carried out regular antiseptic bladder washouts. Their bladders were full of calculi. Patients were totally dependent on the orderlies, regimented and addicted to morphine:

"Two or three times a week (except in the case of suprapubic cases) the patient is bathed; this means that he must be lifted from his bed to his ward chair and wheeled into the bathroom, where his pyjamas or night clothes are removed, and he is placed into a very warm bath and washed by an orderly. Regular bathing, in my opinion, is a most important process, relieving the kidneys by stimulating the action of the skin. He must then be lifted from the bath (which is arranged away from the side of the wall so that there may be an orderly on each side), thoroughly dried, clothed, wheeled back, and lifted into his bed.

On the days when he is not bathed he may be given a radiant-heat bath, diathermy, or such other treatment as may be ordered for the very frequent, painful spasms of the legs, thighs, back muscles, and often of the psoas muscles. These painful contractures are a very serious problem in the treatment of such patients. Their general occurrence is undoubted; the pain is often terrible, and the treatment in most cases must be by morphia or the like.

I suppose that there is more morphia, atropine and hyoscine used in the Home which I look after than in any other place of the same size in the country, but when you consider that these patients cannot possibly be cured, it is obvious that the least that can be done is to see that they do not suffer pain. One of the 'snags' is that some of these poor fellows, who really do suffer, and whose pain has been relieved for years by morphia etc. are apt to become addicts; then the complication arises that, as the result of the exhibition of morphia, the digestion deteriorates, and there is the serious discomfort of indigestion as an alternative to pain. It is difficult to explain this vicious circle to these unfortunate patients. They like their morphia with its resulting relief, and they hate their faulty digestion with its concomitant discomfort.

Every day, of course, the ordinary nursing arrangements for the avoidance of trophic ulcers and bed sores are carried out; the patient's back is thoroughly rubbed with methylated spirit; any trophic ulcers are cleaned and dressed...The feet, which are normally plantar flexed, must be propped up with a firm bolster...

It has been found that massage is very useful for the legs, back and abdomen. Passive movements for the joints of paralysed limbs are important in maintaining the circulation. It will be realised that this treatment takes a considerable time, and perhaps at somewhere about 11.30 am the man is dressed and placed in his wheeled chair, and his rubber urinal is adjusted...

These men are persuaded to go to bed fairly early, and, of course again, they must be lifted from their outdoor chairs to their indoor chairs, and again from their indoor chairs to their beds by orderlies. Subsequent toilet of the back is again carried out by a nursing sister.

Not infrequently the patient's bowel has acted, and he is lying in excrement...

It is, of course, realised that most of these patients have lost both sensation and power of movement, so that it is necessary that nursing sisters and orderlies shall be ever on the alert to prevent any mishap. Not that this will mean immediate discomfort to the patient (it would be much better if it did!) but because of the danger of the recurrence of bedsores, or the infection of existing trophic ulcers.

In all these cases the circulation of the skin below the injured area is deficient; the skin will break down under quite minor irritations, and the infection of an existing trophic ulcer or the occurrence of a new bed sore, is a great danger to the patient, because any local infection is liable to be followed by a general infection, cystitis or pyelitis; and pyelitis is almost always the 'end condition' of the paraplegic.

The patients are made to spend one or two days each week entirely in bed; these are called 'enema days'; they are given a slow, steady injection of two or three pints of saline solution into the colon. This injection has not the same effect as on an ordinary patient. The bowel empties itself very gradually, and this necessitates constant attention. After some years of experience it has been found that the use of a large sized air-cushioned bedpan is the only effectual means of dealing with these cases. The patient frequently has to be on the bedpan for two to three hours. Before these air-cushioned bedpans were used, the occurrence of bed sores was frequent because, as will be realised, these men have no sensation, and if they are on the same hard substance, such as the normal porcelain bedpan, their ill nourished parts are apt to break down and become infected, with serious results.

In regard to the treatment of trophic ulcers and of bedsores, I am of opinion that this is comparable with the task of the dermatologist, in that no one line of treatment will cure any given case, even if the diagnosis is certainly correct, so, like the dermatologist, we ring the changes." (Gowlland, 1934)

The account given by Gowlland was of institutionalised patients, addicted to morphia. The pervading message is one of helplessness and hopelessness. His later paper in 1941 showed nothing had changed.
This attitude had not changed in 1944.

"In the spring of 1944 I was called to group headquarters for interview with the group officer, a surgeon of formidable character. 'Allen' he said to me, 'I am sorry to have to inflict this on you, but we have been ordered to open a spinal unit at Leatherhead Hospital and I want you to take charge of it. Of course, as you know, they are hopeless cases – most of them die, but you must do your best for them.' With these words of 'encouragement' I returned home sadly." (Allen 1964/5)

Thus, in 1916, the Royal Star & Garter Home was set up. Initially there was a positive attitude. Patients were not consigned to the scrap heap, but were given work to do. They had a library, games and gramophones, were taught handicraft, taken in the fresh air when possible, on river trips during the summer and entertained with two concerts a week in the winter. There was a feeling of optimism and some patients were discharged. However, as time passed, patients became institutionalised and the staff assumed a custodial role. Patients were seen, particularly by the medical staff as doomed cripples (Guttmann, 1973).

15.   CONCLUSION

My predecessor, Dr Thomas B. Staveley Dick, who wrote his Medical Doctorate thesis in 1949 looked critically at the First World War literature and summarised:

"The literature of this period contains many excellent papers on spinal cord injuries, notably those by Head & Riddoch (1917), Riddoch (1917), Holmes (1915), Frazier & Allen (1918) but they deal with problems of neurophysiology and pathology, neurosurgery and the like and are little or not at all concerned with therapy. Gordon Holmes (1915) in his Goulstonian Lectures on spinal cord injuries devotes one short section only to treatment. Thomson-Walker (1917), Vellacott & Webb-Johnson (1919), Besley (1917), Young (1926), Kidd (1919) and others, did write on the early management of the bladder, but later papers on this aspect serve mainly to stress the enormous mortality from urinary sepsis".

My perusal of the same literature leads me to a different conclusion. I believe the problems were identified and confronted, in particular bladder management, specialised nursing and specialised units, laminectomy and early transfer. Highly competent doctors did try to tackle the problems but were only partially successful. The casualties of the First World War resulted in the setting up of the Royal Star & Garter Home where severely paralysed patients were kept in a state, which I am unfortunately all too familiar with, of being half alive, half dead, but not rehabilitated, aptly described as a "living death". As such, they posed a problem for the medical profession. Riddoch was active in both world wars, and he was responsible for the setting up of spinal units in the Second World War.

Despite the casualty rates in the First World War, the civilian population in the United Kingdom was relatively unaware of the scale of the conflict. There are now very few people with memories of the First World War. My late mother, who was aged 11 at the outbreak of the First World War, relates that she was aware of the number of casualties and the fact that there were a whole generation of women who could never find husbands because they had all been killed. As there was little bombing in the United Kingdom the war was remote. In contrast, the bombing during the Second World War brought the war home to people.

PART 3: BETWEEN THE WARS

16. PENSIONERS

The British Forces sustained 1 676 037 wounded in the First World War (Winter, 1985). The figures are extraordinarily difficult to disentangle. Of 1 331 486 patients discharged from institutional treatment between 1st April 1919 and 31st March 1929, 3531 were paraplegic (Mitchell, 1931). These patients were discharged but we do not know how many were kept in.

It has been estimated that of the casualties admitted to medical units, 82% of the wounded and 93% of the sick and injured were able to return to some form of duty in the Army (Mitchell, 1931).

However, this could not be said of those with serious spinal injuries, the vast majority of whom did not return to any form of useful activity. Apart from the high mortality on the battlefield, many of those admitted to hospitals developed overwhelming renal sepsis and pressure sores. They had a high morbidity and mortality and were unlikely to leave institutional care. Thomson-Walker estimated that there was 80% mortality from renal sepsis.

The whole of the United Kingdom was turned into one vast casualty clearing station to deal with this deluge of casualties, in innumerable hospitals whose names, sadly, can hardly be traced or remembered today.

There were millions of men wounded on active service. Some were rehabilitated in the orthopaedic centres. Others, such as victims of shell shock, remained disabled and sadly it was a familiar sight to see amputees begging on street corners and selling matches.

17.   WHEN THE FIRST WORLD WAR ENDED

When the war ended, the military hospitals were contracted and specialist units closed down. This not only applied to spinal units, but also to the first and outstanding facio-maxillary unit at Sidcup, where Sir Harold Gillies (1882-1960) and Sir Archibald Hector McIndoe (1900-1960) worked, which had over a thousand beds and was responsible for the founding of plastic and jaw surgery. It closed down, its records were dispersed but fortunately two of the surgeons there, Thomas Pomfret Kilner (1890-1964) and Arthur Rainsford Mowlem (1902-1986), moved to other hospitals and plastic surgery was placed on a firm footing between the wars. Kilner set up a professorial unit in plastic surgery at Stoke Mandeville, which was world renowned and worked in cooperation with the spinal unit.

Clinicians returned to their own, chosen fields. Holmes returned to Queen Square, where he continued to investigate diseases of the cerebral cortex and the cerebellum. Head continued to study the cerebral cortex and dermatomes and Riddoch returned to general neurology but he maintained an interest in spinal injury patients, chairing several sessions at the Royal Society of Medicine (RSM) on the subject.

18.   LONG TERM CARE

During the war, those spinal patients who survived the early mortality were transferred to chronic rehabilitation units at Lonsdale House, the Royal Star & Garter and Rookwood, where provision was made to receive serious spinal injuries. The records from Rookwood are incomplete and there are no records from Lonsdale House apart from the annual reports of Queen Square, which describe the transfer of patients there.

19.   RESEARCH

Between the wars, there still remained interest in the management of spinal injuries in the United Kingdom but this was mainly concerned with the management of the spinal fracture from an orthopaedic and a neurosurgical viewpoint.   Spinal patients were not considered to be a priority for medical research.

When D. Denny-Brown (1901-1981) and E. Graeme Robertson (1903-1975) wanted to carry out research on the bladder, they investigated spinal patients at Queen Square in Carmichael's MRC Unit and did not study patients at the Royal Star & Garter Home.   They carried out fundamental work on bowel and bladder function using very elegant pressure studies.

Like Head at The London, Edward Arnold Carmichael (1896-1978) attempted to set up a professorial unit at Queen Square but received no support from his colleagues.   Eventually he departed to the United States of America a very unhappy and bitter man.   There, he received the recognition, which had not been given to him in the Britain, and he carried on research for another few years.

There was no research coming out of the Royal Star & Garter Home, and the consultants who were attached, Samuel Alexander Kinnier Wilson (1878-1937) and Thomson Walker, seem to have been in name only.   One can only assume that, like other honorary consultants in those days, Thomson Walker's responsibility for urological care was honoured in the breach.   Despite being on the staff, there is no reference to spinal injuries in Wilson's standard textbook of neurology (Wilson, 1940).

20.   NEUROSURGERY

There was no neurosurgery being carried out in the UK at this time. Spinal patients were being cared for by physicians and surgeons.   Although Sir William Macewan (1848-1924) and Horsley had carried out operations on the spine, there were no surgeons who were devoting themselves exclusively to this speciality.   Cushing was the first modern neurosurgeon in the world.   He trained all the neurosurgeons in the world at this time.   Dott worked for him initially.   Neurosurgery was not recognised as a speciality until Cairns, who was trained by Cushing in 1926-27, was stimulated by Riddoch to start neurosurgery at the London Hospital, taking over from James Sherren who had had an interest in neurosurgery.   Later Cairns was backed by Riddoch and was appointed to Queen Square but never operated there as he considered there were inadequate staff to look after his patients.

There were eventually a small number of neurosurgeons in the United Kingdom, directly trained by Cushing: Cairns at the London Hospital and Dott in Edinburgh. They did not have their own departments and when they did have beds, they were of such a small number that patients had to be admitted under the neurologists, transferred to the neurosurgeons for a short spell while they were operated on, and discharged back to the care of the neurologists. Jefferson was not trained by Cushing but he acknowledged his debt to Cushing.

Patients with spinal injuries need long-term care so although the neurosurgeons were dealing with these cases in the first instance, because they could not keep them under their care, they were unable to pursue a rehabilitation programme.

These three neurosurgeons took a keen interest in the management of spinal injuries and it is significant that all the spinal units that were set up at the outbreak of the Second World War were under the care of these three. When the war broke out Cairns had moved to Oxford but Jefferson had remained in Manchester. Responsibility for neurosurgery in the United Kingdom was split up between Cairns and Jefferson. Dott looked after the patients in Scotland and when Cairns became neurosurgeon to the army, Jefferson was responsible for neurosurgery in the whole of the United Kingdom.

21. MANAGEMENT OF THE FRACTURED VERTEBRA

The only fresh development between the wars was that attention was being directed to the management of the fractured vertebra. Until this era, the fracture had largely been ignored although it was recognised that undue movement could cause deterioration in neural function but the actual mechanics of vertebral fracture had not been addressed.

Two surgeons, Sir Geoffrey Jefferson (1886-1961) and Sir Reginald Watson-Jones (1902-1972), wrote a series of papers on the mechanics of injury, how it could cause a fracture and be treated.

21.1 Sir Geoffrey Jefferson (1886-1961)

Jefferson worked as a houseman at Manchester Royal Infirmary where his interest in the nervous system may have been stimulated by watching Professor Thorburn operate and by attending his lectures.

Jefferson went to Canada as his wife was Canadian but he returned to serve as neurosurgical specialist. In 1918 Jefferson took over from Cushing as the neurosurgeon in charge of the 14th General Base Hospital in France where he dealt with head injuries but he did not contribute to the literature until later. Jefferson returned from France at the end of January 1919 and finally succeeded in meeting Cushing.

Jefferson was a strong advocate of specialisation. He worked at a small hospital, Salford Royal Hospital, where the administrators allowed him to specialise and he set up a neurosurgical unit just as Harry Platt (1886-1986) had established a segregated fracture service under orthopaedic control at Ancoats, as opposed to the London tradition (Cooter, 1993). In these units patients were congregated together and this work led the way.

He managed to travel to the United States, observed Cushing's methods and incorporated them into his practice. Eventually he was appointed to Manchester Royal Infirmary where he took a great interest in spinal work.

In 1924 Jefferson attended a BMA meeting and took part in a discussion on paraplegia, but considered he had little experience on the subject. (Schurr, 1997)

In 1927 Jefferson pointed out that direct violence is a rare cause of vertebral disruption. He said spinal injuries were usually caused by force being transmitted through the skull or buttocks. He illustrated this with the case of a young man who was:

"...Struck on top and right side of the head by a falling cotton bale at the docks and was admitted to hospital, unconscious, with a scalp wound on the right parietal bone. When he recovered he complained of pain in the neck and of paralysis of the right arm. Those attending him believed him to have had a contrecoup contusion of the left motor cortex, until we were able to demonstrate a dislocation of the fifth cervical vertebra with injury to the upper cord of the brachial plexus." (Jefferson 1927).

He described a Jefferson fracture:

"We know that in rare instances, the head may be 'mushroomed' down on to the spine, which drives a ring of bone around the foramen magnum up into the skull."

He reviewed the literature and showed that there were two peaks of injury, one at the 5/6 cervical vertebrae and the other at the first lumbar vertebra.

He was a profound thinker and pointed out that a dislocation of the vertebra could not take place unless the vertebral disc was also torn, an observation that had been lost sight of until Bohlman's observation for his M.D. thesis.

He described the case of a woman who dislocated her neck while combing her hair. A similar case was seen at the spinal unit, Stoke

Mandeville Hospital when a nightclub dancer put a huge headdress on and dislocated her spine while dancing.

In 1933 Jefferson discussed 50 cases at Salford Hospital '...23 were uncomplicated by cord damage'. Presumably, 27 had cord damage. He considered that laminectomy had:

> "...a very limited place in the treatment of injury, and none at all during the early stages. The patient with a spinal injury is best served by reduction of the damaged bones without special reference to cord injury" (Jefferson, 1933).

Jefferson's whole approach was thoroughly modern. He addressed issues, which are still being addressed today: the benefits of manipulation under anaesthetic of cervical dislocation, postural reduction and traction in cases of cervical fracture. He described halter traction, that is the application of a halter to the chin for management of a cervical fracture. He said that once the fracture was reduced, over 72 hours, the patient should be put into traction for 6 to 8 weeks. He discussed the Watson-Jones method of reducing mid-thoracic fractures by the two-table method. He recommended that non paralysed patients could be got out of bed within a week and paralysed patients should be treated in plaster beds. He recognised that the outlook for spinal patients was poor and they had a diminished life expectancy:

> "Although the prognosis in some of these patients is bad, it is always worthwhile to begin treatment in an optimistic spirit, the most hopeless cases being those with complete transection of the cord in the upper and middle reaches of the thoracic region. Fortunately injury is not so common at these levels as it is lower down, where the prognosis is decidedly better" (Jefferson, 1933).

By 1936 Jefferson was able to discuss the pathology of 75 cases of cord or root injuries. He said that in a Jefferson fracture (a fracture of the arch of the atlas) there is space for the cord (Jefferson, 1936).

He took a holistic approach and discussed all the complications of spinal injuries including the interesting complication of hypothermia when he referred back to the observations of Holmes. He mentioned oliguria, which was also noted by Holmes. Jefferson described patients who survived with cervical injuries and quoted the work of Denny-Brown and Robertson on the reflex action of the bladder. He delineated the pathology of closed injuries and showed how they should be treated but it is clear that the prognosis was still very poor from the complications of urinary sepsis and pressure sores. The advocacy of plaster beds could only have caused pressure sores.

Jefferson was the outstanding figure in neurosurgery and, along with Cairns, was responsible for the development of neurosurgery in the United Kingdom. Jefferson was appointed as neurosurgeon at the same time as Cairns, to Queen Square but unfortunately the neurologists at Queen Square did not follow the Cushing approach which Cairns and Jefferson followed and they would not allow them to have beds, or investigate the patients. As a consequence, Cairns would not operate on patients at Queen Square. Jefferson remained in Manchester. He was appointed to the Honorary Staff at Queen Square where he operated once a fortnight arriving on the overnight sleeper.

Jefferson served on the EMS Advisory Committee on Peripheral Nerve Injury. In 1940 he became a member of the Brain Injuries Committee along with Cairns, Dott, Riddoch, Charles Symonds, Joseph Godwin Greenfield (1884-1958), Carmichael and A.J. Lewis. Of these only three were neurosurgeons. Jefferson and Cairns were among the very few neurosurgeons in Britain who were still available and who had First World War experience.

At the end of 1940 when the No 1 (Canadian) Neurological Hospital arrived in Britain, Jefferson helped to locate a unit for it at Hackwood Park, Basingstoke. Hackwood became the central neurological, neurosurgical and psychiatric hospital for the Canadian army and Jefferson later arranged for its use as a head and spine centre in the British EMS system.

In 1941 he was too busy to revise a paper he had written, saying:

"Geo Riddoch and I are too fully occupied with 'Rehabilitation' to allow time to think of anything else" (Schurr, 1997).

He was already involved in rehabilitation was responsible for supervising the spinal unit at Winwick.

21.2   Sir Reginald Watson-Jones (1902-1972)

By contrast, Watson-Jones was an excellent and practical communicator, whose book on fractures was the standard text in the United Kingdom after the Second World War until the 1960s. He was the first lecturer in orthopaedics in Liverpool and set up an outstanding fracture unit there. He eventually moved to London to be in charge of the fracture unit at the London Hospital.

In a series of papers between 1930 and 1936 he described the pathology of fractures of the spine using the two-table method, without general anaesthesia. He recommended a quarter grain injection of morphine as the maximum amount of local anaesthetic. The patient was laid on two tables, in the prone position, so that his spine sagged to the normal limit of hyperextension. The method reduced gross displacements without exerting undue force, and without the risk of over-reduction, which could cause further spinal cord damage. The patient was put into a plaster jacket while on the tables. The whole procedure took only 10 to 15 minutes. The patient was subsequently able to sit up wearing the jacket, which facilitated nursing.

Watson-Jones was of the opinion that general anaesthesia was unnecessary. He considered that the reduction was painless (possibly for the surgeon but certainly not for the patient) and the required position could best be maintained in conscious patients. He thought that anaesthesia aggravated the early complications of spinal fracture: shock and pneumonia.

He discussed the method of treatment in cervical and lumbar fractures. Unfortunately, he gave no follow up of the X-rays. He described 80 cases of lumbar fractures, of which 57 were treated personally and 23, who were treated by other surgeons. Amongst these there were 21 fracture dislocations with paraplegia, 9 of whom died. He recognised that the cord was transected. He was opposed to laminectomy, either early or late. He considered it to be a useless procedure because he realised that the pressure was in front of the cord. He believed that immediate reduction of the displacement by hyperextension relieved further compression and allowed revascularisation of the injured area. He postulated that his treatment made the difference between permanent paralysis and complete recovery. He advocated face down transportation.

There were no controls, no statistical analysis, and this was largely speculation but, despite the unscientific nature of his regime, such was the force of his personality and the clarity of his exposition, that it had considerable influence on contemporary medical practice (Watson-Jones, 1934).

22. THE OUTBREAK OF THE SECOND WORLD WAR

With the outbreak of the Second World War, large numbers of casualties were anticipated, so much so, that paper coffins were ordered and a series of papers were produced to instruct first-aiders and doctors on how to cope with emergencies.

Amongst these were two papers produced by Douglas McAlpine (1890-1981) and Geoffrey Cureton Knight (1906-1994) prior to the opening of spinal units to instruct the uninitiated on the practical care of patients who had suffered spinal injuries.

McAlpine was a formidable neurologist, the first to be appointed to the Middlesex Hospital, who wrote a textbook on multiple sclerosis. He was a man of considerable presence and independent spirit, a keen teacher who had time for research as he was from the McAlpine building family. The neurological wards were built by generous donation from Sir Robert McAlpine.

McAlpine's summary of treatment followed the recommendations of Watson-Jones and Jefferson. He recommended immediate reduction of the fracture and immobilisation in plaster beds. He drew attention to the effects of regular turning and advocated intermittent catheterisation and the tidal drainage of Munro, modified by Lawrie & Nathan (1939).

"A simple modification of such an apparatus, originally described by Munro, has recently been made by Lawrie and Nathan (1939); it has been used with success in the Neurological Ward of the Middlesex Hospital" (McAlpine, 1940).

It should be noted that the cases he was referring to at the Middlesex Hospital were not traumatic paraplegics but patients with multiple sclerosis. Peter Nathan has confirmed this in a personal communication.

Knight said:

"The immediate treatment of spinal injuries will therefore consist of efforts to limit the amount of cord injury resulting from the displacement of closed fractures..." (Knight, 1938).

He describes how the patient should be carried to avoid movement. He discusses how to deal with an open wound, reduction and immobilisation, spasms, and different methods of bladder management, which he does not seem to know much about.

23.   CONCLUSION

The treatment of spinal injuries between the wars is a sad reflection on the practice of medicine at the time. As a result of the First World War, recommendations had been made in the MRC monograph (Medical Research Council, 1924), which set out a satisfactory method of treatment. This incorporated the outstanding work of Holmes, Head, and Riddoch.

The fundamentals of treatment had been delineated. It was recognised that patients with spinal injuries should be segregated in specialised centres but Cairns did not operate at Queen Square because the neurologists there did not follow the Cushing approach and denied him facilities. The deleterious effects of plaster beds was not appreciated and only lip service was paid to the prevention of complications because patients had pressure sores and urinary tract infections. Attention was concentrated on the management of the fracture by conservative means. The need for rehabilitation was recognised but was not implemented.

The development of neurosurgery was tardy in the United Kingdom. It can largely be attributed to the work of Cairns at The London Hospital. He trained Joseph Buford Pennybacker (1907-1983) who went with him to Oxford where he set up a comprehensive training programme for neurosurgeons. Jefferson, whose work centred in Manchester, trained Rowbotham. Dott, another of Cushing's pupils, was responsible for Scotland. These three outstanding neurosurgeons, in a small world, split up the work between them during the war. They served on committees with Riddoch at the outbreak of the Second World War and took over responsibility for setting up spinal injury units.

The comparison with shell shock is instructive. The work done and the reports produced at the time were progressive with excellent accounts of aetiology, prognosis and treatment (Rows, 1923, Holden, 1998). As a result special units were set up close to the battlefront and the recognition of psychological symptoms with psychotherapy as a method of treatment was accepted. Psychotherapy became an integral part of medical practice between the wars and when the Second World War broke out, a coherent and intelligent programme of treatment for aircrews and other victims of shell shock, was in place.

In contrast, the chapter on spinal injuries in the Official History is poor (Thorburn, 1922). After the First World War specialist units were closed. The same attitude of hopelessness and helplessness pervaded as had pertained prior to the opening of the units in the First World War. Lessons had not been learnt and at the outbreak of the Second World War, even after specialist units had been opened at the recommendation of Riddoch, patients were developing the same hideous complications as they had in the First World War with the same high mortality. These units were not properly staffed, not properly led and as a result, patients with spinal injuries were not being treated much better than they had been in the First World War. Dick, in his MD thesis (1949), described the appalling conditions at Winwick Spinal unit.

PART 4: THE SECOND WORLD WAR

24. INTRODUCTION

The study until this point was based on study of the literature with evaluation of treatment in terms of modern practice. I began working at

Stoke Mandeville 50 years ago in 1956 and was witness to the practice there at the time which was strongly based on wartime experience.

Lady Liddell Hart (1971) drew attention in the foreword to her husband's book, *History of the Second World War*, to his first book, *The other side of the Hill*, in which Liddell Hart had understood how valuable it was for generals to know what was happening on the other side of the battle. Under the Freedom of Information act, a study was carried out of the Public Record Office Archives and Ministry of Health's plans for spinal units in the United Kingdom, both at Stoke Mandeville Hospital and Liverpool where I worked from 1965-1970. This material, 539 pages of letters and memoranda, gives an immediate insight into the obstacles encountered in setting up spinal units. Interviews with surviving medical and nursing staff, secretarial staff and patients have also provided first hand knowledge, which differs from the sanitised glamorised versions, published subsequently.

25. THE SOCIO-POLITICAL BACKGROUND

As Hitler's aggression spread across Europe, a resumption of hostilities was inevitable. Unlike the First World War, when casualties had all been servicemen, many civilian casualties were anticipated because of bombing.

Before the war, the medical services consisted of Voluntary Hospitals, County Council Hospitals and a few Ministry of Pensions Hospitals (for First World War pensioners). In 1939, when the Second World War began, these Ministry of Pensions hospitals were used as treatment centres but they could not fulfil the large demand for beds (Dunn, 1952-1953).

26. CASUALTIES

In 1926, the Royal Air Force estimated that for each ton of bombs dropped, there would be about 17 killed and 33 wounded and 1000 tons of bombs would be dropped on the first day of the attack. This provided a figure of 33 000 wounded which was expected to decline to about half that number by the third day and remain at that level on each of the days of the following month and then gradually continue to fall so that an additional 36 000 beds would be needed. By the outbreak of the war, and drawing on the experience of the Spanish Civil War, the Royal Air Force estimated that a million beds would be required, on the basis of a 30 days' average stay in hospital. Half the contingent of doctors available would be needed to treat the civilian casualties alone (Dunn, 1952-1953).

27. HOSPITAL PROVISION FOR CASUALTIES

27.1 The deficiency of beds

There was a shortage of 353 000 beds and this was compounded by the difficulty in providing medical and nursing staff commensurate with the number of beds. On the War Office scale of 17 doctors to a base hospital of 600 beds, 24 225 doctors would be required for the civilian hospital services alone out of 45 000 doctors available in the whole country. Such a number was so vast as to be entirely beyond the capacity of the medical and nursing personnel force. Despite the scaling down of the number, more beds would be required. The majority of hospitals were in towns and cities where the centre of population were congregated and in turn likely to be bombed and destroyed thus exacerbating the shortfall of beds.

27.2 How were beds to be provided?

1. Using the existing beds in Voluntary Hospitals
2. Using the existing beds in Local Authority Hospitals
3. Using Mental Hospitals and Institutions
4. Building hutted or tented hospitals
5. Expanding Ministry of Pensions Hospitals
6. Adapting schools

Bombing of the metropolis meant that casualties would have to be transported 40 to 50 miles away. In the event of an invasion, some of the hospital accommodation would be lost to the invading forces (Dunn, 1952-1953).

27.3 Financial arrangements

There was no health service. Financial arrangements were fragmented. Up to June 1938, local authorities as part of their air raid precautions schemes were responsible for the provision of Casualty Clearing Hospitals in the event of war. The cost of providing base hospitals was to be borne solely by the Exchequer. At the beginning of June 1938, the Ministry of Health assumed responsibility for the organisation of the Emergency Medical Service (EMS). This was set up for the reception and treatment of large numbers of military and civilian casualties in England and Wales.

27.4   Hospitals: The Emergency Medical Service (EMS)

EMS hospitals were primarily provided for the treatment for civilian and service casualties due to enemy action (air raids). But later, other patients were being admitted until by the end of the hostilities, civilian patients of all categories, for whom the best treatment was considered essential, were included. In the early days of the EMS, the authorities did not wish to have surplus fully staffed military hospitals, which would lie empty for long periods of time. Instead, hutted hospitals would be set up to treat civilian patients and be available to service patients if required.

"...*The proposals for New Constructions.* It will be observed that in these calculations no provision could be made for concentrated enemy attacks on a limited number of places as this would mean a further considerable increase in the demands for beds accommodation. It was therefore decided to recommend as a short-term policy the provision of 40 000 beds in huts at the earliest possible date and a provisional allotment to each Region was drawn up. This allotment provided hospital accommodation where it was normally most required, in non-vulnerable areas so that local authorities could use the beds pending the outbreak of an emergency, on terms to be agreed. Thus some return for the capital expenditure might be obtained..."(Dunn, 1952-1953)

Despite these hospitals being erected on a temporary basis, with a lifespan of 21 years, they still give very good service today and considerably less trouble than the flat roofed post war hospitals (the Oxford Plan).

27.5   Plan for surrender of accommodation to the Emergency Medical Services

During the early months of 1938, the Board of Control undertook, at the request of the Ministry of Health, a survey of the accommodation in mental hospitals and mental deficiency institutions in England and Wales with a view to estimating the numbers of beds, which could be made available for civilian casualties in the event of a war. This resulted in a proposal to evacuate and surrender to the EMS 16 of the 101 mental hospitals.

27.6   Administration of the hospitals

The medical superintendent remained in administrative charge of the whole hospital, including the EMS part. Generally, medical officers of the EMS were appointed to the EMS wards, but in some hospitals it was found more convenient for hospital staff to undertake the care of the EMS patients in addition to their normal duties. All larger EMS units had a surgeon or physician of high professional status appointed as the medical or surgical director of the unit (Dunn, 1952-1953).

27.7 Relationship between the EMS (Emergency Medical Service) and the Services

Initially, it was suggested that hospitals should be under the control of the army but the Ministry of War declined this offer.

"It was therefore suggested in the interests of economy of personnel and uniformity of administration that the additional hospital accommodation required should be under one central authority, which would permit fully equipped units to be handed over, if and when required to the Services. This proposal had the merit of keeping medical and nursing personnel employed to the best advantage and avoided their immobilisation in Service institutions where they might not be immediately required at a time when the civilian hospitals were expected to be subjected to their severest strain. A further advantage would be effected in the use of consultant advisers who otherwise would be appointed separately for each service" (Dunn, 1952-1953).

PART 5: THE FIRST SPINAL UNITS

28. INTRODUCTION

In the First World War, 65% of injuries involved the locomotor system and under Robert Jones's influence, a series of specialised orthopaedic hospitals were set up to deal treat those casualties. After the war, these were closed. The pattern was followed in the Second World War and specialised orthopaedic units to treat many types of trauma were set up many using the original First World War buildings. A survey of hospital facilities was completed by the beginning of 1938. Mental hospitals were warned of the need to surrender their beds. By June 1938 these efforts were being coordinated under the Emergency Medical Service (EMS), with responsibility to the Ministry of Health. The EMS was in charge of all civilian medical and ancillary facilities and it controlled all Voluntary and Local Authority Hospitals. In 1938/1939 arrangements were made to evacuate the Neurosurgical Department of Queen Square to Hurstwood Park Hospital, Hayward's Heath, Sussex. The evacuation of other London hospitals and any considered endangered took place on the declaration of war in September 1939. In Scotland, Dott was to work at Bangour Hospital.

Jefferson and Cairns, as Consultant Advisers to the Ministries of Health and Pensions, were made jointly responsible for the organisation of neurosurgery throughout the country until Cairns joined the Royal Army Medical Corps in 1940 and all responsibility fell to Jefferson (Schurr, 1997).

It was appreciated that peripheral nerve and spinal injuries were special cases. In 1939, Riddoch was appointed consultant neurologist to the army with the rank of brigadier. More significantly, he was chairman of the MRC committee on peripheral nerve injury, with responsibility for setting up spinal injury units. He, like other doctors such as Jefferson, remembered his experience from the First World War. Just as second lieutenants in the infantry had returned to the Second World War as generals, determined that there should be a different type of war with the abolition of trench warfare and conservation of the soldiers' lives, so Riddoch was determined that provision would be made for servicemen with spinal injuries. It is to Guttmann's credit that he always acknowledged Riddoch's role and he dedicated his book to him as "pioneer advocate of specialized units for the treatment of sufferers from spinal cord lesions" (Guttmann, 1973).

A distinction was made between acute spinal trauma (where the patient was suffering from major intercurrent trauma) and long-term incurable patients.

The former would require resuscitation, bone and spinal cord surgery, access to pathology and radiography departments and all the facilities of a properly appointed neurosurgical and orthopaedic unit.

29.   PATIENTS WITH AN ACUTE SPINAL INJURY

In 1940, four units were designated to receive acute casualties.
- Agnes Hunt and Robert Jones Hospital at Oswestry, serving the Midlands
- Royal National Orthopaedic Hospital Stanmore, serving London
- EMS Hospital Winwick, Warrington, serving the North West
- Bangour Hospital, serving the whole of Scotland

The situation was reviewed regularly and by 1944, the acute spinal units comprised Oswestry, Winwick, Haywards Heath and Basingstoke, the No 1 Canadian military hospital, which served both Canadian military personnel and civilians (Public Record Office documents, 1940-1944).

30.   PATIENTS WITH A CHRONIC SPINAL INJURY

By contrast, 'incurable' patients would be transferred to long-term units (conveniently situated in isolated mental hospitals) so as not to demoralise acute spinal injury patients. These units, where the patients were largely abandoned, were to be like the Royal Star and Garter.

"Gradually, 12 spinal injury units were set up in various parts of the country,.where most of the 700 odd casualties with spinal cord injuries were collected (Winwick, Warrington; Barnsley Hall; Park Prewett, Basingstoke [No 1 Canadian military hospital]; Wharncliffe, Sheffield; Chapel Allerton, Leeds; Ronkswood, Worcester; Dunstan Hill, Newcastle; Rookwood, Cardiff; Llandrindod Wells; Stanmore, London; Leatherhead, Surrey; and Bangour, Edinburgh" (Guttmann, 1973).

The care in the chronic units was fragmented. Patients were admitted late in a debilitated state or not at all. Despite directives, up to half of spinal injury patients (out of a total estimate of 970 for the whole country) never reached a spinal facility and were cared for at home or in various hospitals around the country (Campbell Munro, 1945).

Spinal injury units were due to open in 1940. The South of England unit, originally planned to be at the Wingfield Morris Hospital at Oxford, was not opened until 1944 because of administrative wrangles with the director Sir Herbert John Seddon (1903-1977), who refused to release orthopaedic beds for a spinal unit, which resulted in a change of location to Stoke Mandeville. This may have been serendipity because lessons could be learned (Public Record Office documents, 1942-1944) and the mistakes made in the early spinal units could be avoided and certainly not repeated.

31.   THE FIRST FOUR SPINAL UNITS

Four units are described in detail, primarily in the period from 1940 to 1944.

31.1   Sources

See Table 3 on next page.

Table 3: Sources of Information about the first spinal units

Name	Information
Public Record Office archives	Information on all the UK units
Thesis by T. Dick	Worked at Winwick 1940-1941 and as Guttmann's assistant
Interview with Mrs E. Goddard	Secretary at Wharncliffe in 1941
Interview with Joan Scruton	Secretary to Guttmann who worked at Stoke Mandeville in 1940 before the unit was set up
Interview with Gwen Buck	Patient who was treated at Stoke Mandeville in 1948
Interview with Philip Harris	A house surgeon who worked at Bangour in 1944
Discussion with D.N. Baron	Information on Stoke Mandeville before the unit was opened
Book by S. Goodman	Based on Sir Ludwig's unfinished autobiography & tapes recorded for the Imperial War museum
Discussion with Peter Nathan	Information on Riddoch & Guttmann
Letter from Jack Colover	Information on Riddoch & Guttmann
Discussion with Ruth Bowden	Information on Riddoch & Guttmann

31.1.1   Winwick

Dick, wrote an MD thesis entitled *Rehabilitation in Chronic Traumatic Paraplegia* (1949) describing his experience whilst a medical officer on the neurosurgical ward at Winwick, during the war (1940-1941). He visited Stoke Mandeville Hospital (1946) at Jefferson's instigation and worked as Guttmann's assistant. He had first hand experience of the treatment at Winwick and Guttmann's methods. He worked closely with Alan Sutcliffe Kerr (1909-1977), Neurosurgeon, who was later to become consultant in charge of the Liverpool Regional Spinal Centre situated at Southport from 1948-1965 until I was appointed in 1965.

31.1.2   Stoke Mandeville

I have personal experience of Guttmann's early days at Stoke Mandeville Hospital, having worked there in 1956. I have reviewed his scientific papers and books. Guttmann's experiences are also recorded in a biography by Susan Goodman (1986) based on Guttmann's unfinished autobiography and tapes recorded for the Imperial War Museum.

I have interviewed Joan Scruton, Guttmann's secretary, who was at Stoke Mandeville Hospital before the unit was set up (1940), and Gwen Buck, a patient who was treated at Stoke Mandeville in 1948 (personal communications, 2000).

There are numerous accounts in the Public Record Office Archives of official visits to Stoke Mandeville Hospital in the period 1940 to 1950. Dick gives a testimony in his thesis (1949).

31.1.3 Wharncliffe

E.A. Nicoll's report on Traumatic Paraplegia in Miners (Nicoll November 1948) for the Miners' Welfare Commission provides a detailed description of the unit. In addition, I interviewed Mrs Goddard who was a secretary at the unit in 1941 (personal communication, 1999).

31.1.4 Bangour

There are no written records but Phillip Harris a house surgeon in 1944 has sent me a detailed account of the spinal unit (personal communication, 1999).

31.1.5 Other units

The situation in the other units was quite comparable to that of Winwick. In his thesis, Dick observed:

"From the observation of the cases admitted to Winwick from other spinal centres in different parts of the country it seemed likely that conditions prevailing there were similar to those at Winwick, with the exception of Stoke Mandeville Hospital" (Dick, 1949).

A visit to the Newcastle unit by the Ministry of Health described demoralised staff. They were very pessimistic about treating paraplegic patients believing that they had no future other than life in an institution. The staff did not think that they ought to keep them alive (Campbell Munro, 1945).

A meta-analysis of the treatment in these units gives an overall picture of spinal injury management in Britain during and after the Second World War.

31.2   The Hospitals

31.2.1   Hospital situation

All the units were EMS hutted hospitals (because of the national shortage of bricks). Winwick, Wharncliffe and Bangour were attached to mental hospitals. Set in large grounds, they were isolated on the basis that mental patients and paralysed patients with brain injury should be kept away from society (Dunn, 1952-1953).

Stoke Mandeville was a Ministry of Pensions hospital which served two purposes: as a naval hospital with a nominal naval commander, with its own Resident Surgical Officer and naval consultants. It was also a sector civilian hospital under the aegis of the Middlesex Hospital. Resident staff had moved down from the Middlesex. Stoke Mandeville was supervised by visiting consultants who treated local civilians and waiting-list patients from London. Medical students came down and lived in Aylesbury as part of their clinical training (Personal communication D.N. Baron, 1999). The spinal unit was a new facility on a site which already housed a fever hospital.

Bangour comprised of acute general medicine, acute general surgery, plastic surgery, and Ear Nose and Throat (ENT) surgery. The non-EMS general psychiatric hospital was set apart.

31.2.2   Hospital facilities

Stoke Mandeville, Bangour and Winwick had excellent facilities with operating theatres, radiology departments, physiotherapy and occupational therapy facilities, pathology laboratories, and visiting consultants.

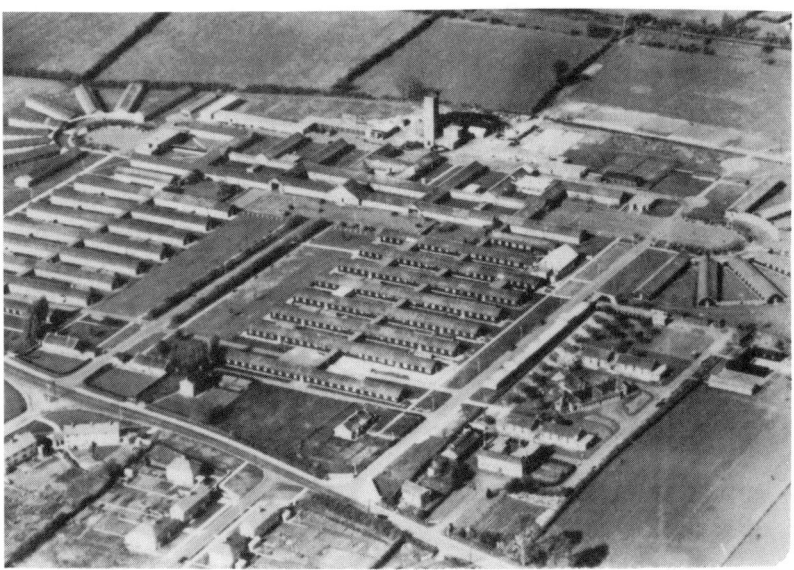

Figure 7. Aerial view of Stoke Mandeville General Hospital with the National Spinal Injuries Centre. This is a standard EMS hutted hospital. (Stoke Mandeville Hospital postcard)

Winwick and Bangour had neuro-trauma units with research and teaching facilities. There was a plastic and maxillary facial unit at Stoke Mandeville, under the direction of Professor Kilner.

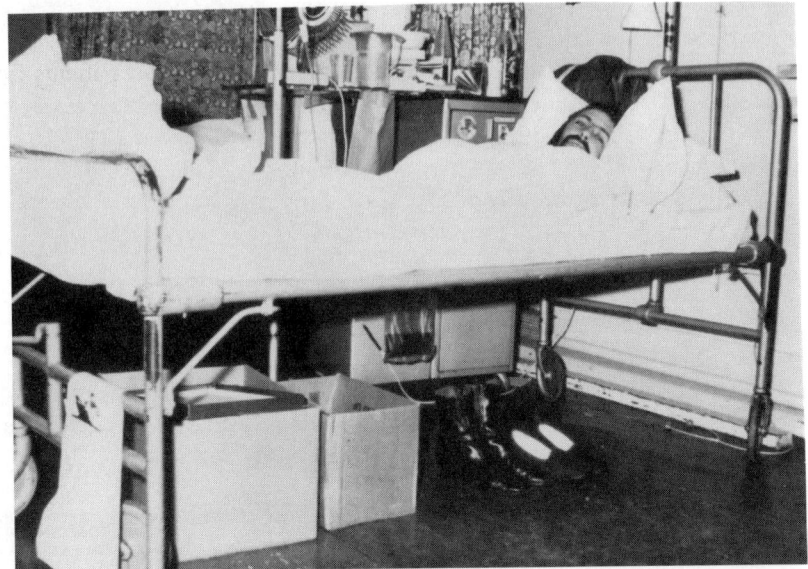

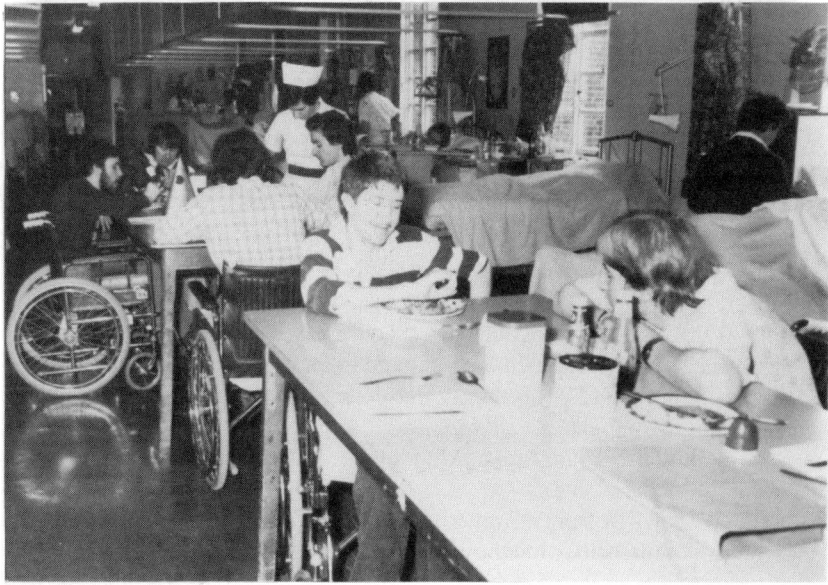

Figures 8,9. Photographs of the Spinal Unit at Stoke Mandeville Hospital showing the lack of space and privacy. Patients ate their meals in the middle of the ward. There was no storage space. (Personal photographs)

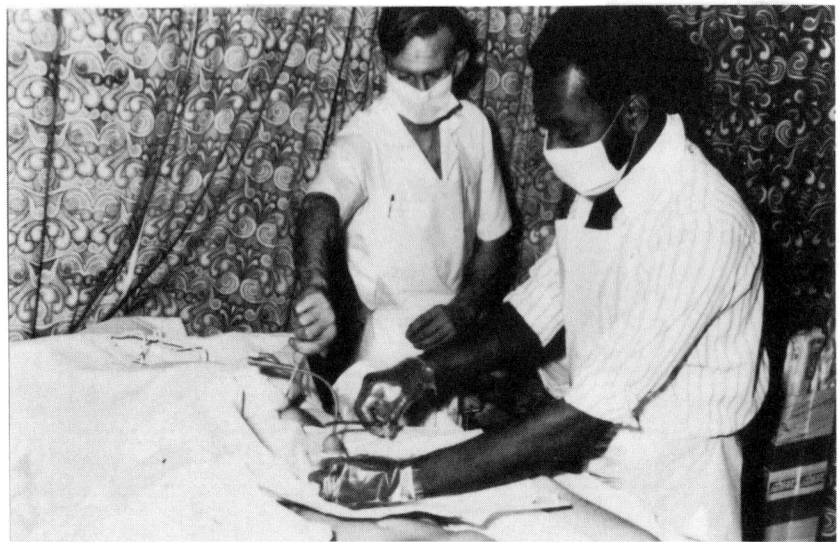

Figure 10. Intermittent catheterisation was carried out on the patient's bed. The trailing curtain makes asepsis questionable. Despite these limitations, magnificent work was done which pioneered the modern treatment of spinal injuries. (Personal photograph)

By contrast, facilities at Wharncliffe were inadequate and impractical. Operating theatres, orthopaedic facilities, radiography and pathology services were far away from the ward and patients had to be conveyed by ambulance.

31.3   Where patients were treated

At Winwick and Bangour, patients were treated under the care of a neurosurgeon on a combined cerebral and trauma service. They were sent to many different wards together with other orthopaedic, neurosurgical or general surgery patients.

At Wharncliffe and Stoke Mandeville, patients were congregated in specially designated units.

The Wharncliffe spinal unit was housed in 'the bungalow', previously a tuberculosis sanatorium for the asylum. Whilst it was a neurology ward, it was referred to as the "paraplegia ward" although some patients suffered from other neurological and psychological conditions. It became known as a spinal unit only when the unit moved to Lodge Moor in 1954.

When Guttmann arrived at Stoke Mandeville Hospital, there was a designated ward for spinal injury servicemen. Service women were scattered around the hospital. In the early days, non-traumatic cases such as polio (6%), transverse myelitis (6%) and other conditions such as thrombosis of spinal artery, haematomyelia, tuberculosis, tumours, syphilis, etc (21%) were also treated at the spinal unit (Guttmann, 1962).

31.4 Specialised facilities for treating spinal injury patients

Facilities were uniformly inadequate. Wharncliffe had no physiotherapy or occupational therapy department on the unit. Wheelchairs were insufficient (Winner, 1949). At Stoke Mandeville there were metal bedpans, no wheel chairs, no specialised mattresses or beds. Guttmann had no office, his secretary worked in a bathroom off one of the other wards and the radiography cabinet (for the storage of X-rays) was a wooden cupboard laid flat on its back (Goodman, 1986). The situation at Winwick was identical, with inadequate physiotherapy and occupational therapy. A very small proportion of patients with cord or cauda equina lesions were able to sit out of bed in a chair, and initially, the hospital did not possess a single padded wheel chair. Plaster beds were still being used. Bangour was the only unit with adequate facilities.

31.5 Specialised staff

31.5.1 Medical staff: The consultants

Guttmann at Stoke Mandeville was the only full time resident officer until Dick assumed responsibility for Winwick in 1944; neither were consultants. The other units had visiting consultants, Dott at Bangour, Kerr at Winwick (neurosurgeons), and Holdsworth at Wharncliffe (orthopaedic surgeon).

Orthopaedics, neurosurgery (there were only four neurosurgeons in the United Kingdom at the outbreak of war), and neurology were not well-recognised specialities then and the setting up of spinal units, in particular at Stoke Mandeville, were delayed because of the difficulty in appointing visiting orthopaedic surgeons. There was a shortage of orthopaedic surgeons, who numbered only 98 in 1940, and even these were not fully trained. Their numbers rose to 227 in 1949 (Cooter, 1993). Gathorne Robert Girdlestone (1881-1950) initially fulfilled the role of orthopaedic surgeon to Stoke Mandeville. Because Seddon would not travel to Stoke Mandeville, Pennybacker agreed to look after neurosurgery but the distance from Oxford made hands on care impossible. Riches, an urologist at the Middlesex, who had served in the First World War, visited once a month. He remained urologist to the spinal centre at Stoke Mandeville and developed the suprapubic catheter. Visiting consultants had other commitments and caring for spinal injury patients came well down on their list of priorities. When the opening of the spinal unit in the south of England was held up because of lack of a neurological consultant, in desperation, and despite his numerous commitments, Riddoch, the neurologist for the army, offered to undertake the neurological care at Stoke Mandeville (Murchie, 1943).

31.5.2   The nursing staff

Staffing problems were universal. Nurses were insufficient in numbers, untrained, and of poor quality. In Guttmann's words "the medical and paramedical staff delegated to the unit, were clearly unprepared and untrained for this purpose." (Guttmann, 1973). The shortage of nursing staff was addressed by seconding untrained army orderlies to the wards. Complex administrative arrangements meant that if they returned to their units immediately after the war, they would be discharged. If they stayed at the hospital, they had to remain in the forces, a point of view that the senior officers sympathised with and accepted. This led to mutiny and exacerbated the already critical staff situation (Medical Superintendent 1945). Stoke Mandeville had eight medical orderlies seconded from the army. When Guttmann enquired of one of these first orderlies what his medical experience in the Army had been, back came the cheerful answer 'shovelling coal sir...' However, he found that despite their total lack of experience, these strong young men could be satisfactorily trained (Goodman, 1986).

At Winwick, the nursing staff had to provide a variety of care and frequently moved to other wards. The number of trained staff was so inadequate, that many dressings were performed by untrained nurses. There were at that time only five male orderlies for the whole hospital (750 beds). The inadequacy of the staff is well illustrated at Winwick where in November 1944, one large ward with 94 patients including 11 spinal injuries and 20 fractured femurs, had 19 nurses, including one sister, three trained nurses, one male orderly and one male nurse. There was always a proportion of these nurses off duty, and a part-time nurse, a male nurse, a male orderly, and three untrained female nurses were the entire staff allocated to attend to 11 patients with spinal injuries as well as 17 other general surgical cases (Dick, 1949).

31.6   Types of patients

The units' first responsibility was to servicemen and servicewomen but if beds were available, civilians were also admitted. Initially, female patients were not admitted to spinal units but they were treated in the same hospital. Bangour and Wharncliffe also treated miners.

31.7   Early transfer

Despite official directives, patients were not being transferred early. With the exception of a few acute patients, these invariably arrived late with pressure sores and gross bladder sepsis.

Wharncliffe patients were treated in the first instance at the Royal Infirmary, Sheffield where Holdsworth had his orthopaedic unit. It was recognised that cases transferred early were less likely to get pressure sores. Very few cases came in to Stoke Mandeville Hospital on the day of their injury and this did take place consistently until about 1956.

At Winwick, it was not uncommon for patients to be received several months after injury, and rare for them to be received in the first two or three weeks. They came from military and civilian hospitals, and occasionally from other spinal centres, to be nearer to their homes. Similarly, the desire to be near home often led to re-transfer of cases after only a few weeks or months (Dick, 1949). This delay in transferring the patients to specialised facilities was universal and not restricted to patients with spinal injuries.

31.8   Pressure sores

Pressure sores seemed inevitable despite regular turning in all the units (assuming this was rigorously implemented which is doubtful). At Winwick and Bangour, pressure sores were exacerbated by the use of anterior and posterior plaster beds. These were used to facilitate turning of the patients in view of the nursing shortage. Whilst both Wharncliffe and Stoke Mandeville used Sorbo mattresses, healing pressure sores were only seen at Stoke Mandeville where turning of the patients took place two hourly day and night. Mrs Goddard commented that pressure sores improved dramatically when the Wharncliffe unit was moved to Lodge Moor because of the improved facilities and earlier transfer of patients (personal communication, 1999).

31.8.1   Surgical treatment of sores

Surgical treatment was variable. At Stoke Mandeville it consisted of excision of the slough and skin grafts when appropriate. The other units were more ambitious but in no unit was there primary excision closure of the pressure sores as practised in the United States (White & Hamm, 1946). Winwick was the only unit where plastic surgery on sores was not performed (Dick, 1949).

31.9   Bladder management

All the patients had chronic urinary infections and their bladders required constant attention. Therapy consisted of daily washouts, the administration of urinary acidifying agents and tidal drainage although the latter was only practiced at Stoke Mandeville and Bangour.

Almost every patient had a suprapubic catheter at Winwick and Bangour. By contrast, indwelling catheterisation was used at Wharncliffe and Stoke Mandeville (in the early days, Guttmann meticulously attended to the catheters himself). This later changed to intermittent catheterisation. It is very striking that patients who survived from the First World War were all soldiers who had minimum interference with their bladder (Frankel, 1971) and the one patient we saw, Gwen Buck, who survived for a year in a non specialised hospital, had never had a catheter placed in her bladder. This reveals the role of the catheter in inducing infection.

31.10   Frequent staff supervision and one doctor responsible for all aspects of care

Guttmann at Stoke Mandeville and Dick at Winwick were the only doctors working full time with sole responsibility for spinal patients. An early advocate of 'total care', Guttmann believed it essential that each unit had its own experienced physician. He insisted that he was the doctor responsible. He excluded the orthopaedic surgeon, the urologist and the neurologist from the spinal unit and fulfilled the role of the psychologist himself (Goodman, 1986).

31.11   Specialist rehabilitation facilities

Rehabilitation facilities were universally inadequate. In Britain rehabilitation was in its infancy (inadequate physiotherapists and occupational therapists) and the equipment was insufficient and impractical. Despite these shortcomings, the benefits of physiotherapy were recognised by all. Guttmann in particular was convinced that work and recreation of all kinds greatly improved the mental and physical rehabilitation of spinal injury patients. He devised a programme of 'purposeful management' to replace the outdated traditional passive massage approach. Despite their initial reluctance, physiotherapists, after teaching patients to walk, became most anxious to work entirely for paraplegics and tetraplegics, and thus became most important members of the team (Goodman, 1986).

31.12 Physiotherapy

Whilst all the units attempted physiotherapy, due to shortage of staff, it was largely only a gesture. At Wharncliffe, physiotherapists were originally called remedial gymnasts and there was an occupational therapy department. At Winwick, only two physiotherapists were available to treat sixty cases of which half had spinal cord injuries. At Stoke Mandeville, physiotherapy was carried out in the middle of the ward. Miss Hobson, who worked on the unit in 1944, remembers particularly "all those things we tried out *for the first time*...because there was no pattern of treatment for the physiotherapist to follow." There was a new dynamic approach. Patients were made to stand and walk to relieve spasms. Physiotherapists were struggling to attain recognition and in those days they were called masseurs. The massage school of the Middlesex Hospital used Stoke Mandeville as a training centre to the mutual benefit of both (Goodman, 1986). Stoke Mandeville's physiotherapy department pioneered rehabilitation of paraplegics.

31.13 Vocational training and reintegration

Vocational training was in place at Stoke Mandeville, Winwick, Wharncliffe, and Leatherhead. At Stoke Mandeville, pre-vocational training was started while the patient was still confined to bed; it included leatherwork, watch repairing, precision engineering and correspondence courses in commerce, economics, banking, accountancy and law. In Aylesbury, a radio-manufacturing firm employed six paralysed and rehabilitated soldiers still being treated at Stoke Mandeville (Goodman, 1986). This successful experiment resulted in Industrial Rehabilitation Centres being set up by the Ministry of Labour in different parts of the country.

At Winwick, they learnt clock repairing and cobbling. The West Street Labour Exchange District Rehabilitation officer helped Wharncliffe patients to work at the Remploy factory at Handsworth. At Leatherhead, patients attended part-time courses at The Queen Elizabeth's Training College (Sector Hospital Officer, 1945). The Ministry of Pensions later established a training centre near London for patients with chronic paraplegia.

A few patients with low or incomplete lesions were sent home provided there were family members to look after them. The others went to long-term residential accommodation such as the Royal Star and Garter in Richmond.

31.13.1 Servicemen and women

Once home, service patients were entitled to a 'constant attendance allowance' (the scale of which was controversial) and an inspector of wheelchairs visited them. They were equipped with hand-propelled chairs such as the 'Travaux' chair, suitable around the home; and for journeying, the hand propelled tricycle. Some were fortunate enough to own a motorcar and the Ministry of Pensions would provide a grant for the adaptation of the hand controls. There were also motor wheelchairs but because of petrol rationing after the war, these had their limitations. The Ministry of Pensions would supply specialised equipment such as beds, mattresses, sterilising equipment, bedpans, etc. Unfortunately, in practice, this was not straightforward and there was a long wait for replacement of equipment.

31.13.2 Civilians

Prior to the formation of the NHS, very little provision was made for civilians until Section 28 of the National Health Service Act of 1946, which required that paraplegic patients discharged home be provided by the local authority with nursing equipment required for their condition. Unfortunately, this resulted in endless wrangles between the hospital authority, the local authority, the regional health authority and the Ministry of Health (who delegated the supply of equipment to the Ministry of Pensions) as to what the equipment entailed. It was suggested that callipers, splints, and any personal or fitting appliance should be provided by the hospital on departure. The Ministry of Pensions, after a request by the hospital, would supply Travaux or motor chairs. The bed, Dunlopillo mattress, bed pulleys and nursing equipment were the responsibility of the NHS and the hospital was advised to contact the local health authority in good time to request these. Because these were not considered to be medical or surgical appliances, it was left at the discretion of the local authority to charge the patient. Often, the equipment would not be available in time and the hospital had to provide it on loan, or an appeal was made to the Red Cross or the Ministry of Pensions. Linen and bedding were not covered under the terms of the Health act. There was no universal policy and wide discrepancies occurred from one local authority to another, causing resentment and a feeling of injustice. Unlike servicemen, civilians could not receive grants to adapt a house to the needs of a paraplegic. Consequently their case was referred to the housing authority (Public Record Office documents 1945-1959).

31.14   Maintenance of nutrition

The importance of blood transfusion and good nutrition was recognised.

31.15 Surgery, position to early laminectomy and postural reduction of the fracture

All the units performed operations on the injured spine although Wharncliffe and Stoke Mandeville did not do laminectomies.

31.16 Research, fundamental and applied

There was no fundamental research in any of the units and the only publications were from Stoke Mandeville. Riddoch attempted to stimulate interest and issued forms and examination guidelines to all the spinal units (Riddoch, 1943). When appointed at Stoke Mandeville as Medical Officer in charge of the spinal unit, Guttmann insisted that his contract should include 3 half days a week (1 and ½ days) for research work. He had initiated research on sweating in Germany with Foerster. He continued this work at Oxford and developed it into a seminal study on autonomic dysreflexia at the spinal unit, Stoke Mandeville Hospital (Murchie, 1943, Silver, 2000).

31.17 Statistics, mortality

Mortality varied greatly, ranging from 60% at Wharncliffe (mainly miners), 12% at Winwick and 7% at Stoke Mandeville. Mortality rates are not available for Bangour. This variation is interesting but not meaningful because patient populations were not comparable, whether in numbers of patients, types of lesions or time span used to calculate the death rate (for example, mortality at Wharncliffe was 25% in the first 3 weeks after injury and went up to 60% after two years). Nicoll was nevertheless appalled at the high mortality rate of miners with spinal injury at Wharncliffe compared with the excellent results obtained both in the United States and at the spinal unit, Stoke Mandeville Hospital. Mrs Goddard commented on the high death rated among the high, complete cervical lesion patients.

31.18 Recreational facilities

Recreational facilities were not available in acute units but open-air outings and sport took place in long-term rest homes such as the Royal Star and Garter Home (Royal Star and Garter Medical Reports, 1916-1940). At the spinal unit, Stoke Mandeville Hospital, patients could see a film once a fortnight, concerts occasionally and use the library weekly.

31.19   Overall view of the care of the patient

At Winwick, Dick commented 'the mental attitude of both patients and staff was one of stoic apathy' (Dick, 1969-70). Nothing had been learned and nothing had changed since the First World War. It was just a continuation of misery and apathy. Spinal injury patients inevitably suffered from pressure sores and urinary tract sepsis. It was acknowledged that congregating spinal injury patients would improve the standard of treatment but until Guttmann set up the spinal unit at Stoke Mandeville, there was no integrated treatment programme. These views were echoed by McAlpine, a senior neurologist who had already written on the management of spinal injury at the beginning of the war:

"We began the Second World War with a much better knowledge of traumatic paraplegia as a result of the classical work of Head and Riddoch. However, the ultimate outlook for these patients seemed no brighter than it had been following the First World War until the Peripheral Nerve Injuries Committee, with Dr George Riddoch as chairman, recommended setting up Spinal Injuries Centres in this country, of which that run by the Ministry of Pensions at Stoke Mandeville Hospital became the best known. Dr Guttmann has shown us that not only has the expectation of life of these patients been materially improved, but that with appropriate methods of treatment and rehabilitation, a degree of functional recovery may be achieved that a few years ago would not have seemed possible" (McAlpine, 1947).

Chapter 3

Sir Ludwig Guttman (1899-1980) & the National Spinal Injuries Centre

Guttmann is regarded by many as the founder of the modern treatment of spinal injuries in the United Kingdom and because of his dominant role a separate chapter has been allocated to evaluate his contribution.

1. INTRODUCTION

Ludwig Guttmann was born in Silesia in 1899. He finished his schooling in 1918 and as part of his military service he was recruited as a medical orderly, working at the Accident Hospital for Coalminers (Knappschafts-Lazarett) in his hometown of Königshütte, where Wagner had treated spinal injury patients twenty years previously. He had his first contact with a spinal injury patient, a miner, who he was told would be dead within a few weeks from pressure sores. When the First World War ended, he trained as a doctor, qualified in 1923 and after a short spell in general medicine, he applied for a job in paediatrics but was unsuccessful (Goodman, 1986). This was a turning point in his career as he opted instead to work for Foerster in Breslau. Foerster was to have a major influence on Guttmann's approach and philosophy towards spinal injury treatment.

Having worked successfully as first assistant to Foerster, Guttmann was expelled from his university appointment and his job in 1933 under the Nuremberg Laws and his title changed to Krankenbehandler (one who treats the sick). He was only allowed to treat Jewish patients at the Jewish Hospital in total isolation from the universities and academic medicine. The German Neurological Association was dissolved in 1934. Guttmann escaped to England with his family in 1939 and began work almost immediately as a research fellow at the Nuffield Department of Neurosurgery in Oxford. There too, he was not allowed to treat patients, as his neurosurgical operative skill (he was trained in the European and not the Cushing tradition) was not recognised (Goodman, 1986). The Cushing tradition meant that the neurosurgeon should make the diagnosis, determine the management, and operate with extreme care and gentleness, stopping the bleeding with electrocoagulation. Although Guttmann had already developed his research on peripheral nerve injury and sweating in spinal injury patients, in five years at Oxford, he published only six papers. Whilst Riddoch was impressed with his research (Riddoch, 1945), Cairns, whom he was attached to at Oxford, was not. Guttmann did not fit in well into Cairn's teams and they were relieved to see him go. In reality, he was a most unhappy man, thirsting to teach and treat patients, even contemplating going into general practice.

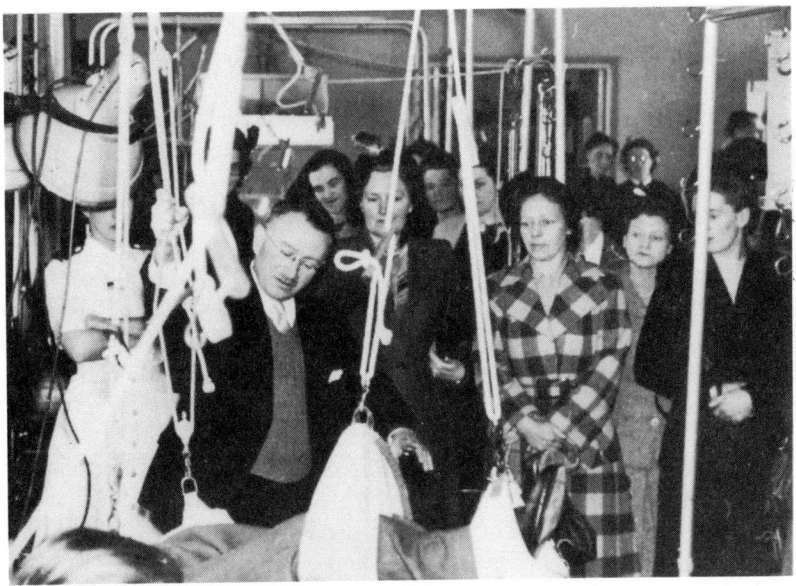

Figure 11. Guttmann at his happiest, teaching in the Physiotherapy Department at Stoke Mandeville Hospital (personal photograph).

When Guttmann came to Stoke Mandeville in February 1944, to set up the spinal unit, he was already armed with well-established ideas on spinal cord physiology, neurosurgical techniques and rehabilitation. Despite being single-handed, he insisted on having three research sessions to continue his work on sweating (Silver, 2000). His ideas on rehabilitation can be seen in his presentation on the rehabilitation of peripheral nerve injuries at the Royal

Society of Medicine (Guttmann, 1941). His plan was prophetic and it is striking that he used these ideas for the rehabilitation of spinal injury patients:

- The need for several specialised peripheral nerve injury centres
- Continuous treatment
- After-treatment and after-care
- The need for a nerve specialist to see the patient immediately
- Thorough records of all treatment with proper documentation
- Supervision of patients immediately after injury
- Late supervision
- Availability of public health service
- Co-operation of health service with Ministry of Pensions and employer
- Rehabilitation/work
- Not to leave the patient alone in the reconditioning period.

Guttmann's methods of treatment are detailed in many publications and are set out in Table 4. How he achieved these results has not been analysed and is discussed below. It is also based on working directly for him for four years and close contact with him for fifteen years after his retirement. "Retirement" was not a word that Guttmann recognised.

2. GUTTMANN'S ROLE AND PHILOSOPHY FOR THE REHABILITATION OF SPINAL INJURY PATIENTS

Guttmann adapted these principles for the treatment of peripheral nerve injuries and used them as the foundation of his treatment of patients with spinal injuries. These ideas are still relevant today. His attitude was quite different to that prevalent in the London teaching hospitals where consultants were honorary and part time, devoting their energies and making their living in private practice (Cooter, 1993).

Guttmann was reared in the German tradition of medicine where there were full-time professors at University hospitals and doctors devoted themselves exclusively to the treatment of hospital patients and carried out clinical and applied research. Guttmann believed that unless he was committed full-time, all efforts would be fragmented and uncoordinated and would only have minor effects. The ward was his workshop. He saw every patient when they came in and taught on them subsequently. He would not be excluded from the wards as in the teaching hospitals when there were only limited time slots when patients could be examined. Thus the whole unit had dynamism because the patient came first.

Table 4. Guttman's methods of treatment

TREATMENT IDEAS	Winner Report 1948/9	S. Goodman 1986	Medical Times 1945	Sandifer & Guttmann 1944
Careful transportation		√	√ (by air)	√
Immediate transfer to specialised centre		√	√	√
Use of pillow packs		√	√	
Opposition to plaster beds, use of Sorbo and air mattresses	√	√	√	
Regular turning of the patient	√	√	√	
Removal of pressure sore sloughs (surgery and measurement of sores)	√	√	√	√
Regular dressings and inspection of sores	√		√	
Closure of suprapublic catheter (start of intermittent catheterisation?)	√	√	√	
High output of acid urine from clean bladder				√
Tidal drainage			√	
Use of antibiotics	√		√	
Regular cytoscopy	√			
Reduction of the fracture	√			
Tendon lengthening for contractures	√			
Importance of nutrition and blood transfusion	√		√	
Trained specialised staff/extra staff	√		√	
Teaching of staff	√			
Physiotherapy (walking)	√		√	
Wheelchair sport	√		√	
Occupational therapy	√		√	
Discharge patients home	√			
Motivation of patients		√	√	
Monkey pole				√
"Total care" by one doctor		√		
Research facilities (both fundamental and applied)		√	√	
Psychological care		√	√	
Special equipment		√	√	
Overcoming the indoctrinated prejudice		√	√	
Careful patient supervision by the doctor in charge		√		
Supervising the staff		√		
Preparing statistics		√	√	
Social and vocational rehabilitation		√	√	
Concern for the fate of the patients		√	√	
Self progress reports by the patients		√		
Electrotherapy			√	√
Musical band			√	√
Massage		√		

These ideas are taken mostly from early papers and reflect the situation at the very start of the spinal unit at Stoke Mandeville Hospital. (√ = agrees)

2.1 Determination

Guttmann refused to accept that patients who were the hopeless and helpless should be cast on the human scrap heap (Guttmann, 1945).

2.2 Inspiration and motivation

He was a very inspiring man and he uplifted the patients and the staff and made them feel wanted and worthwhile. He motivated other people and his enthusiasm was infectious. He inspired people to believe that they were part of something bigger than themselves, so staff and patient cooperated fully. I have experienced this personally. He had been made to feel worthless while in Germany and in Oxford, so he had great empathy, sympathy and charisma to motivate people to do the work.

2.3 Leadership

Guttmann recognised that leadership is an essential ingredient for success in the search for excellence. He stressed that he should be totally responsible for every aspect of the patients' care. He did not accept that physiotherapists and nursing staff were independent professionals; His philosophy was that the unit must be impregnated with enthusiasm to inspire the patient to cooperate to the full.

"This positive proof of recuperation is invaluable in convincing the man that hope is not lost. Indifference, anxiety and resentment, as well as the over-cheerfulness and self-deception which some of the cases show, also need attention in later stages, as all these psychological reactions may impede successful training or impair the patients' working efficiency" (Guttmann, 1945).

2.4 Monitoring

Because of the force of his personality, Guttmann saw that things were done. At the outset and much to the staff's annoyance, he gave the order that all patients should be turned supine and prone or from one side to another, every two hours, night and day, waking or sleeping. To ensure that his orders were being carried out, he began appearing on the ward unexpectedly, at all hours. He bullied patients and staff and established a series of checks and monitors. He would prescribe a treatment and closely supervise and measure the results, monitor the performance of patients and staff, inspecting the sores numerous times and measuring them with X-ray films. He made everyone feel important by praising them when they did well but criticizing them when they didn't. Guttmann always sought to blame someone else if anything went wrong with a patient's treatment. Whilst it was very unjust on some occasions and encouraged lying and prevarication by the weaker minded spirits, it did concentrate one's mind to see if things could be done better. He always took the credit if things went right. Cushing was a similar hard task master and also claimed primacy for discoveries and was loathe to acknowledge other opinions (Fraenkel, 1991, Fulton, 1946, Jefferson, 1960, Symonds, 1970, Thomson, 1950).

2.5   Teaching

Guttmann taught everyone. He taught doctors, physiotherapists and nurses at the bedside, he taught at formal lectures at the Royal Colleges, and the most vital aspect is that he taught the patients how to look after themselves. Practical and applied research was an integral part of his teaching. He set up and ran the unit on the basis of a German academic institute with case presentations, tutorials and lectures. Initially, every new case admitted to the unit was brought to the examination room, the case presented and the treatment discussed at a weekly teaching session that lasted well into the night. Everyone was physically exhausted but mentally stimulated and thoroughly bullied and humiliated. He was a superb neurologist. All the patients were presented to all the doctors in the unit on a weekly basis at a teaching session so that in a 200 bed unit, there was a unique experience not only of all types of spinal injuries but also all forms of neurological diseases affecting the spinal cord (since it was the only unit of its kind in the South of England).

2.6   Research

Guttmann instituted research at all levels. He insisted on meticulous note taking so that these could be used as a database for future studies. Physiotherapists dressed the sores and applied ultra violet light to see if it helped healing and as a control, the nursing staff dressed the sores without ultra violet light. He instituted measurements of the size of the sores by means of X-ray transparencies as he had done in Germany. He carried out basic clinical research on patients at the bedside.

In 1956, whilst carrying out a cystogram under x ray control, I found initially that in some views the cystogram showed no reflux. But when the patient's bladder contracted, the reflux went right up to the kidneys. Guttmann got very excited and said we should take photographic records and write a paper on the subject. When exercising a patient who was recovering from spinal injury, he made me do very detailed measurements of the timing.

He made us feel as though practical research was important. It was not some arcane subject that could only be carried out in laboratories by specialised people in some very esoteric way but it was something that was within everyone's grasp. He did research on sweating and the control of the autonomic nervous system. He carried out practical research on wheelchairs and the result of treatment.

I wrote 5 papers in collaboration with Guttmann and his ideas provided a stimulus for numerous others.

2.7   Physiotherapy

Guttmann's views on physiotherapy were revolutionary in the United Kingdom. No doubt he learned them from Foerster but he was anxious to put them into practice. He set out a systematic programme for the physiotherapists to follow. Immediately a patient was paralysed, he prevented contractures and atrophy of the joints, muscles and skin by correct positioning of the limbs. He was a believer in electrotherapy to prevent the denervated muscles atrophying and to promote better circulation. He reduced intractable spasticity by passive movement, and directed compensatory training towards the over development of the trunk and abdominal muscles. Special attention was paid, particularly in the early stages, to develop those muscles which have a synergetic action with the paralysed muscles, thereby compensating for their loss, and helping to improve the balance and mobility of the trunk. Combined operation of these muscle groups would restore the walking capability of the paraplegic patient in parallel bars or on crutches by pelvic tilting. He followed Frenkel's ideas on restoration and re-orientation whereby the patient compensates for the loss of postural sense in the paralysed part of the body, particularly hip joints, by using the eyes. He pioneered the idea of restoration of independence by teaching the patient to dress and to walk with the use of appliances. This was the beginning of rehabilitation in the United Kingdom. Unfortunately, because the spinal units were isolated, whilst rehabilitation progressed in the spinal units, such programmes did not permeate through to other hospitals and disciplines.

2.8   Sport

At an early stage Guttmann incorporated sport into his rehabilitation programme in the form of wheelchair polo and archery. Sport is of great value in rehabilitation because the patient can become fit by exercising and having fun. Sport had already been used in Germany by the amputees and the blind and in the United Kingdom at the Royal Star and Garter home (Royal Star and Garter Medical Reports, 1916-1940).

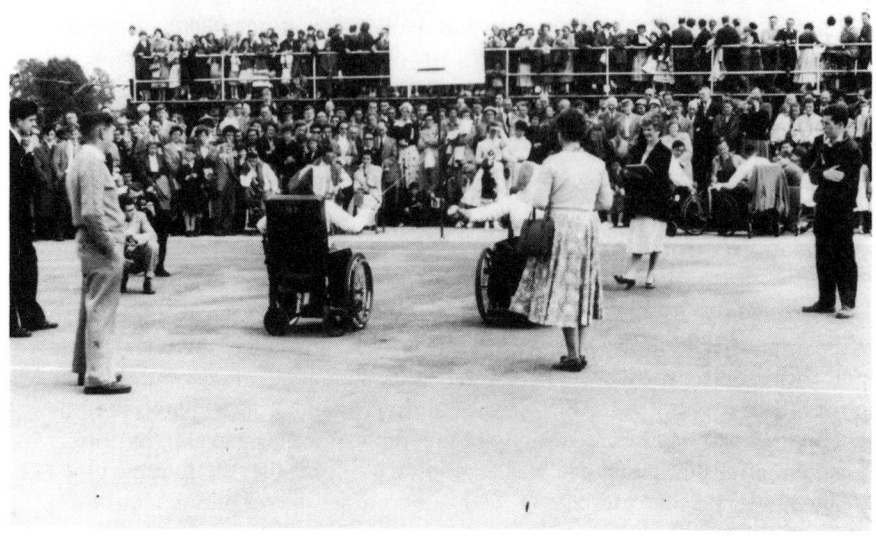

Figure 12. Wheelchair sports (personal photograph).

3.   GUTTMANN'S CONTRIBUTION

Guttmann was well trained in neurology, neurosurgery, research and rehabilitation. His reputation stands and falls by the results he achieved and all could see the effect of his expertise. This was a new field, his methods were innovative and he showed that something could be done for spinal injury patients.

His early work at Stoke Mandeville is described in the following references:

Dick, 1949

Goodman, 1986 (Guttmann's dictated tapes)

Guttmann, November 1945

Sandifer & Guttmann, December 1944

Winner, 1949

3.1   Achievements

In the early days, Guttmann acknowledged the work of others in the development of the treatment of spinal injuries but as time passed and he became more confident, he claimed priority for himself. In his private moments, he said that other people had developed individual aspects of treatment but he had put it all together (Scruton, 1999 personal communication). His unique achievement was to bring together existing ideas and develop an integrated programme of treatment. He personally supervised the implementation of the treatment and would not rely on the staff to do things in their own way, which might well conflict with other treatment plans.

3.2   Recognition

The views of doctors, administrators and patients at the time provide a valuable insight (Table 5). They had no preconceived notions, and saw Stoke Mandeville Hospital as it was, a rudimentary hutted hospital. Their comments were not for Guttmann's benefit, but confidential for the Ministry of Health in the form of reports and letters. They are contemporaneous and carry more weight than the glamorised image of Stoke Mandeville today, which was built on Guttmanns' worldwide reputation and media exposure engendered by high profile patients such as Arias (husband of Margot Fonteyn), Mrs Tebbit, eminent visitors such as the Royal Family, successive Prime Ministers, visiting Heads of State and glamorous visitors such as Christopher Reeve. In addition, Jimmy Savile, the well-known personality raised money to build the new unit and ensured it was always in the public eye.

Within six months of opening the unit at Stoke Mandeville had already acquired a reputation for clinical excellence, despite the fact that it was wartime when communications were poor and there was censorship. The work of the unit was recognised by patients who had been treated there, by doctors who worked in a comparable unit and by colleagues such as Seddon and Riddoch. Mortality was reduced. If a treatment is effective, such as the use of penicillin, its value is rapidly recognised. Within months the recognition of the Spinal Cord Centre at Stoke Mandeville Hospital was such that there was a waiting list and patients were being turned away.

When addressing staffing of a spinal unit at Park Prewett, Fraser wrote 'if Brigadier Riddoch can supply a resident officer with experience such as Dr Guttmann, that would be the best plan...' (Fraser, 1943, MH76/142). This implies that Guttmann was already regarded as knowledgeable in that field.

In her report, Dr A. Winner wrote:

"As far as I have been able to ascertain, there are only four centres functioning today, which have any pretensions to the title of paraplegic or spinal centres. Of these, only the Ministry of Pensions Hospital at Stoke Mandeville can be regarded as really satisfactory"

"Its high reputation is causing an embarrassingly large number of applications for admission. Its slow turnover, together with the inevitable ruling of the Ministry of Pensions that serving, ex-service and pensions cases have absolute priority, make its long civilian waiting list a pure fiction unless more beds can be opened for civilians" (Winner, 1949, MH58/653 Appendix A).

3.3   Contemporary accounts

George E. Gask (1875-1951) had been chief assistant to the orthopaedic department at St Bartholomew's Hospital. He was a man of considerable varied experience since he had served as one of Cushing's assistants for 12 months. He was later director of the professorial surgical unit at St Bartholomew's. An opponent of specialisation in orthopaedics, he visited the Spinal Cord Centre at Stoke Mandeville Hospital in 1945 and was very supportive. In a letter to Fraser, he wrote: 'the resident there is Guttmann, I should guess an Austrian, he spends the whole of his time, his life in attending to the patients and he is very good' (Gask, 1944, MH76/142).

Dr Ferguson was a chief medical officer at the Ministry of Health who visited the Spinal Cord Centre at Stoke Mandeville Hospital at Riddoch's request in 1944 (Commissioner of Medical Services Scotland Region, 1944).

Dick, a junior resident in neurology, had seen the appalling condition of the patients at Winwick after three years of treatment. He went to the Spinal Cord Centre at Stoke Mandeville Hospital and learned Guttmann's methods and later came back to Winwick. He is the only one to write contemporaneously about the treatment of spinal injuries in his MD thesis (1949), and subsequently in various papers, where he describes Guttmann's methods and the spirit of hope and achievement that there was at Stoke Mandeville. He had hands on experience, and was well aware of the difficulty of treating spinal injury patients.

Riddoch had treated spinal injury patients in the First World War, had done outstanding research work on the management and neurophysiology of the bladder and was instrumental in the setting up of spinal units. His criticisms and evaluations are invaluable. He first described the mass reflex and encouraged Guttmann in his research on sweating and on the bladder (Riddoch, 1945). Jack Colover (houseman to Riddoch in 1939) told me that Riddoch had the highest opinion of Guttmann's work (Colover, 1999 personal communication).

Mr Sykes was a doctor requesting permission to visit Stoke Mandeville (Campbell Munro, 1945).

Nicoll was a general surgeon who after passing his FRCSE and a Cambridge MD was appointed honorary consultant surgeon to the Mansfield General Hospital, with particular responsibility for trauma cases (Cooter,

1993). He did some interesting and innovative work setting up rehabilitation units for coal miners and fundamental work on spinal stability. Watson-Jones also sat on the coal board and worked on spinal injury as well as writing a standard textbook Fractures and Joint Injuries (Watson-Jones, 1955). Nicoll was anxious to set up a spinal injury service for the miners. Following a tour of North American units in 1948, he wrote a report that gives a critical account of the facilities available in the United States and Great Britain at the time (Nicoll, 1948). Professor Roaf and Professor McKibbin both commented that they thought Nicoll was the instigator of the ideas on spinal stability although Holdsworth received recognition (personal communication, 1999). Nicoll was an informed expert orthopaedic surgeon and his comments as an outsider striving to set up a spinal service in the North of England are particularly relevant.

Seddon was an orthopaedic surgeon who set up peripheral nerve injury units at the Nuffield Hospital, Oxford and then became the director and professor at Stanmore. Whilst he did not personally like Guttmann, he recognised his abilities.

Dr Winner was an administrator from the Ministry of Health responsible for all the spinal injury units. She visited every spinal unit in the country and was able to compare and contrast them so her opinion is of great value.

Watson-Jones was the dominant figure in orthopaedics in the United Kingdom after Robert Jones, and came from Liverpool to London to set up a fracture unit at the London Hospital. He then became consultant adviser on orthopaedics to the Royal Air Force (RAF). It was in this capacity, independent of the Ministry of Health that he created the country's first comprehensive rehabilitation service by organising and integrating the sixteen RAF orthopaedic centres with its four major rehabilitation centres. In 1949, Watson-Jones who was a member of the Miners Welfare Committee, wrote in confidence to the Ministry of Health:

"There was at present in this country no suitable hospital service to cover the acute period of say 24 hours after the accident up to 3 weeks. As a result of this, 60% of our civilian patients were dead within 3 years as against 6% of service cases in America.

It has to be admitted that there was a general lack of facilities and that patients even in teaching hospitals were in a deplorable condition. The discrepancy between what was possible and what was generally available in treatment was sensational" (Watson-Jones, 1949, MH58/653).

The Executive Committee of the Miners' Rehabilitation Committee thought that facilities were inadequate. In reviewing the different sites, there was no mention of Stoke Mandeville. We can assume that Stoke Mandeville Hospital was considered a chronic rehabilitation unit.

In contrast, by 1955 Watson-Jones changed his views and said that acute treatment was available at Sheffield and that Stoke Mandeville was doing remarkable work:

"Remarkable results have been gained by Guttmann at the Stoke Mandeville Hospital near London. Not only has he cured neglected decubitus ulcers, contractures of joints, and spasms of the lower limbs in patients with traumatic paraplegia of long standing, but above all, he has inspired them with a new faith and new hope. Only those who have visited and stayed at this centre for paraplegics can understand how great has been his success in restoring a spirit of confidence and self-dependence. Visitors come away humbled but inspired " (Watson-Jones, 1955).

The doctors who commented on Guttmann's results were all experts in the field of spinal injury; they had tried to treat patients themselves and failed.

The administrators from the Ministry of Health came to visit Stoke Mandeville and sent doctors from the Ministry. These said that Stoke was the only unit doing good work in the field of spinal injury. The nurses and the physiotherapists were not enamoured with his methods initially but once they saw how successful his treatment was, they became his keenest supporters as illustrated in these quotes from Susan Goodman's book (1986), The Spirit of Stoke Mandeville:

"From the very beginning of his directorship, Guttmann gave the order that all patients at the Spinal Injuries Unit were to be turned prone to supine and back, or from one side to another, every two hours, night and day, waking or sleeping. At first, this aspect of his treatment was greeted sceptically by staff quick to resent extra heavy work and extremely doubtful of value. He had made his point, both to his staff and to his patients, many of whom had arrived at the unit in an almost putrefying state. Turning became and has remained a byword at Stoke Mandeville."

"To get one physiotherapist to treat only paraplegia in those early days was asking too much, for no physiotherapist worth her salt could ever be expected to treat only 'those chronic cripples'. In the end, physiotherapists became anxious to work entirely for paraplegics and tetraplegics, and thus became most important members of my team."

Other contemporaneous comments are very striking and pay tribute to Guttmann's work as early as 1949.

Table 5. Contemporary views on Guttmann

DATE	NAME	D/P/A	COMMENT (Quotes are from Public Record Office documentation)
15/07/44	George Cask	D	Impressed by the spirit of self-help and cheerfulness. First mention of Guttmann "Guttmann very good. Astonished to hear that patient can be returned to the workplace."
29/11/44	Ferguson	D	Chief Medical Officer at the Ministry of Health who visited Stoke and was much impressed with what he saw.
01/01/45	Dick	D	Came to Stoke Mandeville Hospital in 1945 and commented on the new methods being tried out, much better staffing but most important, there was an attitude of hope.
15/03/45	Riddoch	D	"I am personally satisfied that the work he has been doing is good. The other work is excellent, in fact his is the best spinal injury centre we have got."
15/03/45	Cyril Lee	P	Requested a consultation with Guttmann. Spoke of wonderful work done by G. and his assistant at SMH.
01/04/45	Ministry of Health	A	It was recommended that all medical superintendents and some sisters should be sent to Stoke Mandeville Hospital.
13/04/45	Doctor from Chapel Allerton	D	Describes Stoke Mandeville Hospital as " a wonderful show, he is of course madly enthusiastic and recommends that it be made THE centre for ALL paraplegics. He comments on very generous staff and limitless physiotherapy trainees."
18/07/45	Sykes	D	Desirous to visit Stoke Mandeville Hospital to see the work of the spinal injuries centre.
01/01/47	Nicoll	D	Commented on how "appalling death rates were at Wharncliffe compared with USA and Stoke Mandeville Hospital."
08/12/48	Seddon	D	"A very able German refugee, LG a pupil of Foerster has established a remarkable centre at the Ministry of Pensions Hospital Stoke Mandeville, for the treatment of patients with paraplegia. No one in this country has ever made a comparable contribution to the treatment of these dreadful cases. He has a waiting list of 80 and needs more facilities."
18/03/49	Winner	D	"Only the Ministry of Pensions hospital can be regarded as satisfactory. He runs his unit very autocratically, he is a good showman. There is no question however that he has completely changed the face of the world for the paraplegic pensioner, that his single minded enthusiasm has moved mountains and that his patients are almost passionately grateful to him, his results speak for themselves and the difference in the atmosphere between Stoke and the other spinal centres is remarkable. Incredible as it sounds, a patient walks with his shoulder girdle and upper trunk muscles. Exercises including definite drills designed to render patients independent eg. dressing, putting on callipers and getting from bed to chair is 7 minutes!"

DATE	NAME	D/P/A	COMMENT
			(Quotes are from Public Record Office documentation)
23/11/49	Ministry of Health	A	"A very efficient institution; two other units, Sheffield (Wharncliffe) and Liverpool (Winwick) are not up to Stoke Mandeville's standard."
27/03/50	Seddon	D	They are requesting that a doctor be sent over to Stoke for training before going to Stanmore together with two ward sisters and physiotherapists."
30/03/50	Seddon	D	"Dr Guttmann's experience must now be unique."
01/01/48	A patient	P	Patient account in The Cord 1947-1952. "The hospital has come to be the principal spinal unit of the Ministry of Pensions and one of the largest spinal injury centres in Europe."
01/02/44	Miss Joan Scruton	A	"Many think that his main achievement was sport."
01/01/48	Mrs Gwen Buck	P	"Guttmann was cruel to be kind. He timed us when we got dressed. We were always busy and doing physio, he came in the ward to check up on us. When I came to Stoke, my life changed and I looked to the future. Guttmann gave us confidence. Rehabilitation was physical as well as psychological."

A: Administrative directive; D: Doctor; P: Patient

3.4   Recollections

The recollections of Miss Joan Scruton and Mrs Gwen Buck are valuable but they are recorded 55 years later and are inevitably clouded. Nevertheless, they provide another interesting insight. Guttmann commented to Joan Scruton: 'Other people might have done sections of the treatment but they did not do the whole thing'. He called this 'comprehensive care' (Scruton, personal communication, 2000).

As I have tried to show, other people had ideas and carried out the treatment, particularly Wagner, Kocher, Holmes and Munro, but it was Guttmann that put it altogether and did it all and his remark shows that he did have insight.

Chapter 4

United States

1. INTRODUCTION

In the United States the role of Donald Munro was paramount. Munro's work, starting in 1936 at the Boston City Hospital, and his publications, were the beginning of the effective treatment of patients with spinal injuries.

Until the First World War, European medicine and the burgeoning speciality of neurology, especially in Germany, led the world. The giant figures of Jean Martin Charcot (1825-1893), Charles Edouard Brown-Séquard (1817-1894), Hermann Oppenheim (1858-1919) and John Hughlings Jackson (1835-1911), dominated the field. Doctors from the United States, if they wished to further their knowledge, had to travel to Europe.

2. THE AMERICAN CIVIL WAR

In the American Civil War, as in other major conflicts, the large number of injuries made it difficult to produce accurate casualty figures. The editor stated in the introduction to Medical and Surgical History of the War of the Rebellion (1861-65) that the surgical statistics of the war were absolutely worthless (Barnes, 1875). A figure of some 408 072 wounded and 37 531 deaths between May 1st 1861 and June 30th 1865 was produced. Spinal injuries were discussed in a section of some 66 pages. There were 642 cases of gunshot injuries to the vertebra, of whom 349 died, a mortality of

55.5%. The majority of patients who survived did not have spinal cord involvement.

There are a large number of individual case reports but the presentation of them was not systematic and it is not possible to tell whether the bladder was paralysed or how it was drained, nor was there a description of the nursing regime.

The cases were analysed according to whether the vertebra was injured and according to the level at which the cord was involved. When a bullet damaged the great cavities leading to severe intercurrent injuries of the chest or abdomen, and the cord was damaged, the outcome was very poor.

There were 76 soldiers with spinal injuries, the majority of which had only mild cord involvement. Only 2 died, 39 returned to duty, 27 were discharged, 3 were transferred to the reserves and 5 left the army. The complications of bedsores, tetanus, pyaemia, dyspnoea, dysphagia and priapism were recorded. Treatment was discussed only cursorily with little mention of bladder management or skin care. The only discussion on treatment was whether a laminectomy should be performed. The patients were not segregated in a special hospital.

3.   SILAS WEIR MITCHELL (1829-1914)

Mitchell was the outstanding American neurologist whose reputation had reached Europe. Although he was treating wounded soldiers during the war, and was already recognised as an authority on nervous disorders, it was purely in the context of peripheral nerve injury not spinal injury patients. His wartime experiences of dealing with the wasted, nervous condition of Civil War soldiers made him develop a regime of bed rest, massage, electrotherapy and 'aggressive feeding'. This formed the cornerstone of the treatment regime in the United States. After the war Weir Mitchell described building patients up in 6-12 weeks with the help of nurse-masseuses who should be young, refined and cheerful, gentle but firm, intelligent enough to converse with her patient on matters of the day and able to write a good letter (Mitchell, 1877). Weir Mitchell demanded absolute obedience; isolated his patients from outside influences and allowed them little effort of mind. Although he had his successes, his instructions to a writer to have no more than 2 hours 'intellectual life' a day and never touch 'pen, brush or pencil as long as you live' nearly brought her to disaster (Barclay, 1994).

4. JOHN KEARSLEY MITCHELL

In 1895 Silas Weir Mitchell's son, reviewed patients with spinal injuries from the Civil War in a long-term follow up 30 years later. He made the point that you could not tell from the initial examination, what the long-term effects would be:

> "In considering all of these cases together, one deduction is at once apparent. With no matter what care we may study and examine spinal wounds, but one judge can decide their future course, and that is time himself. No completeness of recovery, no seemingly perfect return to health, even though it should have lasted years, will bar out the possibility of late sclerotic or other change." (Mitchell, 1895).

He described the signs and symptoms and speculated on their causation. With hindsight, it is possible to recognise their significance. He seemed to be aware of polyuria as a symptom of spinal injury, which may have been indicative of chronic pyelonephritis. Some patients deteriorated after a long period of time, possibly due to post-traumatic syringomyelia; several patients who were severely paralysed at the outset, recovered and then deteriorated 26 or 27 years later. He described excessive sweating, possibly due to autonomic dysreflexia, and treating pressure sores with heat and cold as recommended by Brown-Séquard.

In the 30 years up to 1895 there had been advances in the management of paraplegia. Some of the fundamentals of treatment were appreciated but this could not be described as systematic treatment. The significance of the hospital and the need for specialised treatment had been noted. Prolonged bed rest had been recognised as a cause of contractures and bedsores. An Army hospital patient survived because he had to follow orders and be exercised and mobilised; in a civilian hospital he would have died due to inanition. Several patients were discharged home; one practiced as a lawyer in Richmond.

5. HERBERT LESLIE BURRELL (1856-1910)

Burrell made a detailed study of 244 cases of fractures of the spine treated at Boston City Hospital between 1864 and 1905 in a series of papers with extensive statistical analyses. He drew attention to the high mortality of 78% reported in the early paper and compared it with the mortality of 37.5% found in his latter series of cases, the difference being that in the latter series the cord was not necessarily involved.

He presented the clinical findings of fractures at different levels and discussed the management of spinal injuries without marked cord symptoms.

Burrell believed in reduction of the fracture followed by fixation in a plaster jacket. Many of these patients were fit enough to be discharged home.

He described conservative treatment of a patient who was admitted with tenderness over the cervical spine but who was not paralysed, emphasising the dangers of moving a patient with an unstable fracture:

> "...patient was put to bed and cautioned not to sit up or to roll in bed, because there was an injury to his back, which might be, more than was then apparent. Four days after injury, however, when unattended, he sat up in bed and immediately complained of numbness of the limbs and body. Examination then showed a paresis of all the skeletal muscles from the neck down and diminished cutaneous sensation from the clavicle downward. Reflexes increased. Abdomen somewhat distended." (Burrell, 1905)

He believed that immediate surgery offered '...a hope, unfortunately, and nothing more'. He carried out a detailed review of all the patients who had had surgery and concluded that cord involvement was the critical factor and that treatment could only be carried out on an individual basis. As John Mitchell had recognised, the degree of severity of the injury could only be assessed by observation. Any pressure on the cord should be relieved once spinal shock had subsided.

6.   HARVEY WILLIAM CUSHING (1869-1939)

In contrast to the European powers, who had been involved in the First World War for three years, the American experience leaves us with few written accounts of spinal injuries. The dominant figure was Cushing. During the first 3 years of the war, before the United States became a belligerent, Cushing was seconded as neurosurgeon to the British Forces and produced comprehensive papers on the management of cerebral trauma but little on spinal injuries. Cushing dominated neurosurgery from well before the war until the 1940s and trained almost every neurosurgeon in the world. He founded the modern tradition of neurosurgery, that the neurosurgeon should make the diagnosis, determine the management and operate with extreme care and gentleness, stopping the bleeding with electrocoagulation (Fraenkel, 1991). Apart from being an outstanding neurosurgeon, he was an excellent writer whose accounts of contemporary treatment are gripping and can be read like a novel. He subsequently won the Pulitzer Prize for his biography of Sir William Osler (1849-1919) published in 1926. Cushing's book, *A Surgeon's Journal* (1936) gives a profound insight into the management of casualties and treatment of spinal injuries by Gordon Holmes.

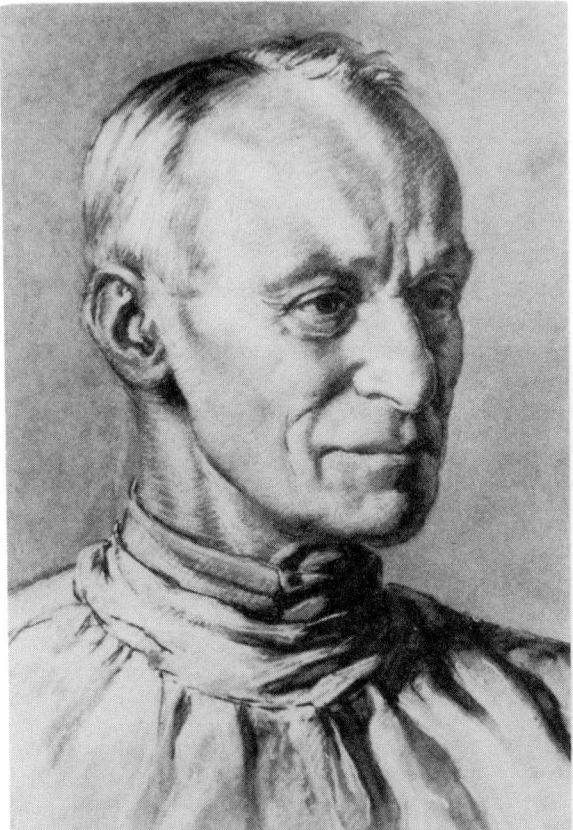

Figure 13. Harvey Cushing (1869-1939) (Thomson, 1950)

7.   THE FIRST WORLD WAR

The United States entered the First World War on 10th April 1917. They had the greatest difficulty in organising, training and equipping an army to serve in France.   Within 18 months they transformed a force of 127 000 men from the backwoods and garrison duty into an army of 4 000 000 men. They had to rely on France and Britain for the supply of artillery, planes and machine guns.   Army medical services were not nearly as well organised from the hospital point of view as those of the European allies.   Cushing repeatedly praised the well-organised services of the French units and the fact that spinal injury patients could not receive better treatment than in the Empire Hospital in London.

In the later stages of the conflict, the United States had its own army under its own commanders with its own hospitals and medical services. When they launched an offensive in the Argonne, neurosurgical teams were set up to deal specifically with trauma to the central nervous system but such was the weight of casualties that they were forced into doing other emergency surgical procedures. The spinal and cerebral cases, which took longer to operate on, were neglected.

As in other wars, the only survivors of lesions of the spinal cord were those with partial lesions. Those with serious chest or abdominal injuries died. 80% died in the first few weeks from infections, bedsores and catheterisation. The unfortunate survivors did not obtain the treatment that their condition required. There were no specialist hospitals, no waterbeds and insufficient staff. Little had changed since the Civil War. The Medical Department of the United States Army in the World War records the following counsel of despair:

> "War wounds of the spine were particularly distressing. These injuries were so frequently associated with chest and abdominal wounds of a serious nature that one scarcely knew where to begin, if to begin at all." (Cushing, 1927)

Spinal cases, if transportable, were evacuated early and many died soon after evacuation to the rear.

> "...it was rather common to have men with spinal cord injuries arrive dead or dying. Injuries of the spine, perhaps formed a much larger group than those computed from hospital records would lead one to think, as the serious wounds involving the chest and abdomen in which death occurred at the front, were undoubtedly in many instances, complicated by spinal injuries." (Cushing, 1927)

The patients were clearly abandoned.

7.1   Bladder management

In common with the British experience, management of the bladder was not resolved. Argument continued as to whether permanent or intermittent catheterisation or non-intervention was the best form of treatment.

Reviewing the situation in 1926, Young wrote:

> "On this account Murphy, Besley, and others strongly recommended a course of non-intervention as to the bladder in such cases, and in the Manual of Military Urology the surgeons of the AEF (American Emergency Forces) were urgently requested to follow this plan if

possible. We have been unable to obtain accurate statistics as to how successful this was." (Young, 1926)

7.2   Operative management of the spine

There was some brief discussion as to whether wounds to the spine should be treated. Where the dura was not opened, the external wound was excised and where the cord was compressed, decompression was performed. The results of surgery were appalling with a high mortality. Cushing reported:

"Of 32 injuries of the cord, 7 were cervical, 2 were thoracic, 8 were lumbar and 15 were not specified. Eight were inoperable and there were 23 deaths, or a mortality of 71.8%; 24 were operated on with 15 deaths, or an operative mortality of 62.5%." (Cushing, 1927)

Of those who survived, only a few reached the United States:

"Figures, which have been quoted from armed service records, indicate that there were some 400 cases of traumatic spinal paralysis as a result of World War I. Only a few of these patients were alive, two years after the receipt of their injury." (Munro, 1952)

It is extremely puzzling when there were so many casualties and so many neurosurgical consultants that there was virtually no literature on the subject of the management of spinal injuries. This paucity of publications may be because, although the war produced a large number of paraplegic patients, few of them survived. American servicemen rendered paraplegic in Europe were unlikely to survive the initial treatment or the long sea journey back to the United States.

7.3   The Official History

Charles Harrison Frazier (1870-1936) edited the section on neurosurgery. He was in charge of the Army Medical School of Instruction in Philadelphia and subsequently General Hospital No 11 New Jersey, where he was chief of neurological services. The New Jersey Hospital received patients from the war zones with peripheral nerve, skull, brain and spinal cord injuries. In the case of peripheral nerve injuries, it was hoped to draw conclusions from long-term study of the medical records. This proved impossible due to wide dispersal of patients in France where they were not segregated in specialist hospitals. There seems to be no records in the USA of these patients. The reason for this is obscure, maybe they died in transit. In neither place were there sufficient doctors with the skills required for the task. The same problems would apply to patients with spinal injuries. The contributions to the Official History (Hays, 1959) were very sparse. It had been hoped to produce a separate volume on surgery in cases of spinal injury but statistical information was insufficient, probably, for the reasons given above. One can only speculate on how Frazier found sufficient information for his own book on the subject (Frazier and Allen, 1918).

7.4   Spinal injury monographs

Despite the war, two monographs dealing with spinal conditions were published by Charles Albert Elsberg (1871-1948) from New York (1916) and Frazier, professors of neurosurgery and surgery respectively. These books were the cornerstones of the management of spinal injuries after the First World War, until Munro published his paper in 1936.

7.4.1   Charles Elsberg (1871-1948)

Elsberg's book (1916) is slighter. In his early career he had trained as a pathologist and is said to have slept by the incubators, such was his motivation. He became Professor of Surgery at New York University and Bellevue Hospital Medical College and subsequently Professor of Neurosurgery at the College of Physicians and Surgeons of Columbia University. He wrote on surgery from personal experience. Elsberg said damage to the cord did not correlate with the severity of the bony injury. He evaluated the importance of an operation to improve the patient's condition and described reduction of a thoracic fracture by counter traction on the patient's neck and legs. If this failed, he recommended open reduction.

Elsberg discussed treatment in detail. He recognised the vulnerability of the cord immediately after injury and the risk of further deterioration. He valued the role of the nursing staff and considered that waterbeds, pneumatic rings and rubbing with alcohol were useful in the prevention of pressure sores. He advocated that intermittent followed by suprapubic catheterisation should be carried out with extreme care. Although he recognised the bad prognosis of pressure sores and paralysis of the bladder, he claimed that with careful nursing patients could remain alive for several months or years but sooner or later would die from ascending infection. He recommended treatment with electricity and passive movements for lumbar lesions. Even so, the mortality rate was more than 50% in the first week and 70% due to remote effects:

> "The patient should be disturbed as little as possible in order to avoid any increase of the cord injury. Very often it is inadvisable to palpate the back in order to feel for any irregularity of the spinous processes, because

the necessary change in the position of the patient might increase the injury to the cord." (Elsberg, 1916)

"Nursing is of paramount importance, especially the prevention of cystitis and of bedsores." (Elsberg, 1916)

Elsberg discussed a progressive ascending lesion which would appear to be an early description of post traumatic syringomyelia. He quoted Burrell's 1905 work from the City Hospital with a mortality of 85%. He described remote complications and incomplete lesions.

In an acute injury, he recommended incision into the cord, to relieve the pressure, and discussed the indications. Death often occurred in the middle of the third week after injury. Of the patients who recovered, few returned to complete health.

He considered the early appearance of bedsores to carry a bad prognosis,

'with careful nursing, an individual who has a transverse lesion of the cord may remain alive for many months or years. Sooner or later, however, cystitis occurs followed by ascending infections of both kidneys' (Elsberg, 1916).

Elsberg gave an early description of acquired spinal stenosis. He documented progressive symptoms due to excessive callus formation around the injury, which could produce a later compressive lesion.

7.4.2 Charles Harrison Frazier (1870-1936)

Born in -1870, he studied in Philadelphia 'and spent a year in Berlin working with Rudolph Virchow (1821-1902) and Ernst von Bergmann (1836-1907). He became Professor of Clinical Surgery in Philadelphia and, as a result of working with von Bergmann, started a neurosurgical unit. He was strongly influenced by Weir Mitchell and, by all accounts, was a tyrant, like Cushing, Otfrid Foerster (1873-1941) and Guttmann.

His book contains chapters on neuroradiology, trauma and gunshot wounds. Frazier devoted 172 pages to spinal injuries, including a section on gunshot wounds of the spine in which he described his experience, and that of others, of treating such wounds in France (Frazier & Allen, 1918).

The book is not just an historic document, it is a major textbook. It is not clear how many of these patients Frazier treated, whether they were in separate neurosurgical beds, in general wards or on a spinal unit. His comprehensive survey quoted not only his own cases, but also a total of 717 cases of spinal injuries from the world literature. The work involved in translating German and French papers (he quotes Wilhelm Wagner (1848-1900) in four different sections), and the detailed statistical analysis on results of surgery, prognosis, life expectancy, discharge home and work, make this a formidable source of information and very humbling.   He presented a carefully prepared statistical analysis:

"From this array of figures, it is evident that while the mortality was high both with and without operations, the percentage of recoveries or improvement was larger in the operative than in the non-operative cases.

Bearing upon this question it may not be amiss to call attention to the fact that, with the addition of measures of safety in recent years, the mortality of operations upon the spinal cord has been materially reduced."(Frazier & Allen, 1918)

As knowledge increased, mortality fell.   Before 1911, 68% died; between 1911 and 1915 only 27% died.

Frazier described dislocations of the cervical and lumbar spine and correlated them with the mechanism of injury. He felt that the cervical spine was more likely to be injured because of its greater mobility and if there was a total dislocation, death would occur in a few days.   He pointed out that dislocation could occur without the cord being damaged. Dislocation of the thoracic spine could not be distinguished from a fracture. He thought that the higher the lesion, the worse the prognosis.   He discussed the merits of open and closed reduction and believed that immediate reduction was ideal.

"The general dictum is made, however, with certain reservations. The propriety, for example of attempting reduction of a cervical dislocation when there is little or no involvement of the cord might well be questioned because of the possibility of sudden death or of cord pressure during the attempt at reduction. On the other hand, while the persistence of the deformity is not inconsistent with life and activity, there is always the risk of the consequences of gradual or sudden displacement. Immediate reduction is of course desirable, and yet there are on record cases in which there has been restoration of function when reduction was not accomplished for from one to eight weeks after the accident. No doubt, in many instances, irreparable damage to the cord has been inflicted at the time of the accident, and though reduction has been successfully accomplished, the cord symptoms persist." (Frazier & Allen, 1918)

This approach is thoroughly modern. The only unresolved question today is whether one should carry out an open or a closed reduction and that one should warn the relatives of the risks.   Frazier said that if proper facilities were not available, the closed reduction method was safer, and produced figures to support this. He described isolated fractures and made an elegant statistical analysis of 228 cases of fractures and 86 fracture dislocations.   Out of a total of 228 cases of fractures (not necessarily all servicemen or under his care), 75 patients were discharged and when he followed them up, 1 in 4 were well, 1 in 2.5 were partially incapacitated and 1 in 9 died later.

Frazier gave the following prognosis: 'To recapitulate, ten years after the accident, 1 in 9 entirely recovered, about 1 in 3 was partially self supporting and 1 in 7 was entirely incapacitated' (Frazier & Allen, 1918). In the book, there is a section on concussion of the spine and a critical and valuable account of Railway Spine (whiplash injury in 1917). Frazier trained Munro.

7.4.3   Alfred Reginald Allen (1876-1918)

The experimental work of Alfred Reginald Allen described the effect of traumatising the spine by dropping a weight of 30 grams upon it and then carrying out a laminectomy. This is still the recognised way of producing controlled trauma to the spinal cord to see if different forms of treatment can affect the outcome. Like Elsberg, Allen wished to determine if this could be relieved, by making a longitudinal incision in the cord. He discussed the secondary effects of oedema and haemorrhage and whether this could be relieved in the same way. He considered mortality depended on the level of lesion and its completeness. The worst prognosis, in common with current findings, was a high, complete cervical lesion. Allen suggested:

"Based upon these experimental observations we may say that in all cases of contusion of the spinal cord we are always confronted with the impossibility of a definite prognosis immediately after the trauma, as the symptoms in this early stage may be just as severe for a mild lesion as for a very severe crush. Unfortunately we cannot escape from the feeling that more harm is done by the expectant treatment in these cases than in an exploratory laminectomy." (Frazier & Allen, 1918)

He was particularly concerned about the possibility of performing a laminectomy on a slightly injured patient, or, on the other hand, waiting until the intractable condition became hopeless.

The questions Allen raised and his evaluation of them are still pertinent today with various experimental modes of altering spinal cord function, such as the use of hyperbaric oxygen and corticosteroids.

"It is not enough that we are confronted with statements that there has been a return of sensation or that paralysis of muscles innervated from segments below the level of injury has given way to restoration of function. The burden of proof is so overwhelmingly on the operator that any such statements may well be set aside unless there be a detailed description of his technique and findings in the examination for muscular function and the various types of sensation. Likewise, the bald statement that there is a disappearance of the paralysis of the bladder and rectum is not sufficient unless it be made perfectly clear that the restoration is restoration with complete voluntary control of the viscus in question. The implantation of a segment of a peripheral nerve or a section of spinal cord from a lower animal does not deserve consideration." (Frazier & Allen, 1918)

His approach, like that of Sir Charles Bell, and his strictures, are thoroughly sound. Unfortunately, his critical evaluation was not maintained in the section on physical care, which was dismissed in a page and a half. It is not clear what his input was or where the patients were treated: a neurosurgical unit, a spinal unit or in general wards.

"It is a comparatively simple matter to say off-hand that the prognosis in injuries of the spinal cord, with or without fracture, is always grave; but, when we attempt a more critical analysis of the results we are confronted with much difficulty...the quotations as to this large group must be discounted because many a case reported as improved at the time of the published record subsequently died as a direct or indirect consequence of the injury." (Frazier & Allen, 1918)

There is a distinction between civilian and military practice 'In military practice, the selection of the time for operation depends upon considerations which would not affect the civilian surgeon' (Frazier & Allen, 1918).

In conclusion, there was argument about the best form of treatment for the bladder and they did not have the benefit of equipment such as plastic catheters. The importance of nursing, the value of water beds and careful catheterisation were recognised by Elsberg. Frazier produced a statistical analysis of the results of surgery, prognosis, life expectancy, discharge home and work. Whilst the need for segregation was recognised, it is not clear whether patients with spinal injuries were, in fact, segregated. Just as in the United Kingdom, the fundamentals of treatment were recognised but they probably were not being carried out.

8.   BETWEEN THE WARS

The situation for patients with spinal injuries after the First World War was regarded as hopeless. The interest in spinal injury management was directed to two aspects, the management of the spine and the evaluation of the bladder.

Just as in the UK with Jefferson and Watson-Jones, the emphasis of Burrell's work was on manipulative reduction and plaster fixation and there was a great advance in the treatment of vertebral dislocation. It was recognised that in some cases reduction could not be maintained. Traction was found to aid maintaining apposition in cases of cervical fracture dislocations (Taylor, 1929). Consequently he employed a halter, which fitted about the mandibles and occiput and to which constant traction could be applied. This method proved to be a distinct advance in the treatment of this special type of injury. Crutchfield (28.9.1900-) devised a pair of self-tightening tongs, which could be fixed into the calvarium and to which measured traction could be applied (Crutchfield, 1933). The results were so encouraging that Crutchfield devised a better pair of cranial tongs (Crutchfield, 1937, 1938). McKenzie in 1935, unaware of Crutchfield's experience, applied a pair of ordinary ice-tongs to the skull for traction. William Cone (1897-1959) in 1937, after trephining the skull in the parietal region of both sides, passed a strong wire between the dura mater and bone through the two openings and attached to it a movable pulley at the head of the bed. Cone reported that he had used skull tongs which were similar to those of Crutchfield (Barton, 1938). For better fixation, they wired or fused the cervical vertebrae with a bone graft.

In 1934, Byron Polk Stookey (1887-1966) described a method used by him in the treatment of incomplete cervical fracture-dislocations with spinal cord injury, and which did not require the use of skeletal traction. The patient was placed on an air-cushion mattress of special design with a blanket roll between the mattress and the bed at the level of the shoulders. The head was allowed to hang over the end of the mattress, producing hyperextension and gravitational traction.

Frederick Christopher (1889-1967) presented 100 patients with fractured spines without cord involvement (1930). He described the value of reducing the fracture and the use of skull traction. He was the first to describe the meticulous management of the bladder, acidifying the urine and follow-up of progress by the use of intravenous pyelograms and cystograms (Cumming, 1932). One of these patients, who had survived from the war, was discharged home.

There was a paper by John Fox Connors (1873-1935) *et al.* (1934) from Harlem Hospital which described bladder management and recommended non-interference of the bladder, with an appalling mortality of 57%.

9.   DONALD MUNRO (1889-1973) & THE HARVARD MEDICAL TRADITION

Donald Munro was a pioneer in the modern treatment of spinal injuries and it was acknowledged by his contemporaries that he was the father of paraplegia.

Munro set up the first effective treatment centre for spinal injuries in the United States at the City Hospital in Boston. He qualified at Harvard and served for a year and a half at Boston City Hospital where he became the first surgical resident in genito-urinary surgery under Dr Paul Thorndike (1863-1939). In 1916 he became Frazier's assistant at the Augustana Hospital, Chicago. During the First World War he was stationed in France with the United States Army Medical Department. In 1919 he returned to Boston and was appointed to the Boston City Hospital general surgical staff. He was primarily occupied in administering anaesthesia to other surgeons' private patients. In those days surgical training was not as circumscribed as it is today and people pursued a rather eclectic course. In 1929 he took charge of the surgical part of the neurological unit in conjunction with Dr Abraham Myerson (1881-1948) and Dr Stanley Cobb (1887-1968). That service expanded.

Boston City Hospital was under the shadow of a superb neurosurgical service rendered by Cushing at the neighbouring Peter Bent Brigham Hospital.

Specialisation had already been developed in the United States. At the Massachusetts General Hospital, the orthopaedic outpatient department was staffed by 16 salaried surgeons, and in 1911 America's first inpatient ward for orthopaedics in a general teaching hospital was created. By 1923 there were over 300 full time orthopaedic specialists in America (Cooter, 1993) and in 1924, 8 – 10 neurosurgeons (Schurr, 1997).

Harvard Medical School serviced three hospitals: Massachusetts General, Peter Bent Brigham and the City Hospital. At that stage, the feeling at Harvard was that they should set up an academic unit. All this work was being done by the neurosurgeons and neurology had not got the same standing as neurosurgery.

"The Harvard Neurological Unit at the Boston City Hospital was deliberately founded to fill this assumed gap. It was started with a grant from the Rockefeller Foundation, which provided not only the salary of a director but funds for teaching and research. The Unit was built clearly as a research-orientated department with a staff primarily of full-time academicians. Dr Stanley Cobb was chosen to the its first Director." (Beecher, 1977)

Cobb was a neurologist who was interested in psychiatry and, at that stage, the Rockefeller Foundation's chief administrator, Alan Gregg, was particularly interested in sponsoring research into psychiatry and the neurosciences. The Rockefeller Foundation had contributed to Queen Square where they built the MRC Unit. They sponsored Foerster's unit at Breslau and funded the unit at the City Hospital, Boston. The Rockefeller Foundation also funded Guttmann's research on the autonomic nervous system when he was in Oxford and in more recent times the epidemiology unit at Yale where the controlled trial of steroids for the treatment of spinal injuries was carried out.

Cobb was professor of neurology and Donald Munro was professor of neurosurgery. Cobb and Myerson were particularly interested in epilepsy and encephalography. Cobb only stayed a short while but he was replaced by Professor Denny-Brown who had worked on the neurogenic bladder in 1936 at Queen Square and was recognised as the greatest neurologist in the world. In the 1960s, all the young neurologists in London made a pilgrimage to study with Denny-Brown. It is hardly surprising that in such an atmosphere, with the first neurological unit in the city, the finest neurologist and neurosurgeon in the world, and the link with Harvard University, that ideas must have been generated, in the same way as they were in Florence in the Renaissance and in Cambridge in the time of William Harvey (1578-1657). Innovative and original research and treatment were developed in Boston, which had a long tradition of doctors working together. Munro pursued his own studies and researches on traumatic injuries of the brain and spinal cord. He realised that more than half of the neurosurgical admissions were the result of trauma. This could have been because the City Hospital was paid for by public taxes and trauma cases were admitted indiscriminately. Treatment was consumer driven.

Stimulated by the teaching of Frazier, Munro set up an experimental unit for the treatment of spinal cord injuries, funded by the Rockefeller Foundation. He was the first to show and prove that spinal cord injury was not fatal but could be treated. He published extensively from 1936 onwards. His paper written in 1943 laid the foundation for the modern treatment of spinal injuries. His views are dogmatic and forceful. He maintained that by meticulous care of the patient and prevention of pressure sores, if the patient had a good pair of arms, he or she could be returned to a useful, independent existence.

9.1   Munro's doctrine

The Munro doctrine is the cornerstone of modern treatment of spinal injuries:

> "...no matter how extensive the paralysis may be in such a patient and provided only that he has full use of his hands, arms and shoulders, ambulation, with infallible 24 hour control of bladder and bowel (without the need of a urinal or other artificial aid) – as well as that degree of overall rehabilitation that comes only with the ability to lead a normal social and work life within the limits imposed by the necessary use of braces and crutches – is well within the possibilities of present-day treatment." (Munro, 1952)

9.2   Munro's tidal drainage

Munro recognised that care of the bladder was paramount.   It was no good performing the most intricate operations on the spine if the patient died from overwhelming renal sepsis or pressure sores.   He stressed this and would not countenance genito-urinary sepsis in his service.   Regardless of any other causes of death, kidneys, ureters, and bladders removed at autopsy should show no more than a very superficial cystitis.

It is striking that he achieved this in 1936 before the development of antibiotics.   This is reinforced by the work of another pioneer, Bors, who understood that the bladder emptying mechanism and the prevention of sepsis are critical and that the role of antibiotics is marginal (Munro, 1936, Bors, 1971).

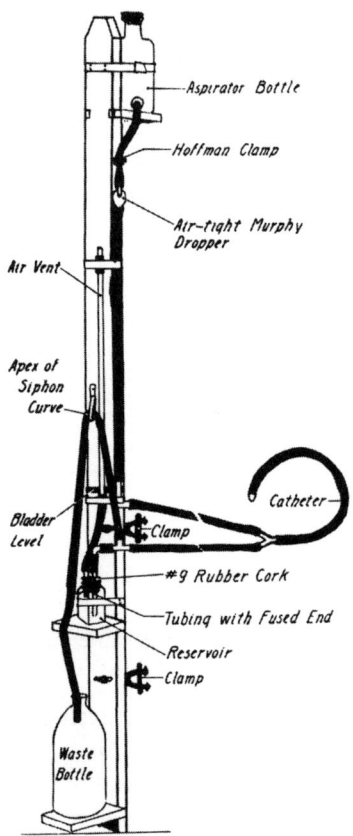

Figure 14. Tidal drainage apparatus designed by Munro, the idea being that the bladder should fill up from the reservoir and then when it contracts, expels the fluid, and then refills, there being continual re-irrigation of the bladder. Reprinted from *The Treatment of Injuries to the Nervous System*, Munro, p.84, Copyright 1952 with permission from Elsevier.

Possibly due to his training under Thorndike, he developed the Munro method of tidal drainage (a method for giving continuous bladder washouts with antiseptic solution), which had been tried at Guy's Hospital. This resulted in a lessening of the frequency and severity of infection. This was the first time paraplegic patients were not riddled with sepsis so they could survive long enough to have other forms of rehabilitation and learn to cope with the problems of living. Munro showed that patients did not need to die of urinary sepsis and they could be returned successfully to a useful life in the community.

9.3   Pressure sores

Munro recognised, in a forthright dogmatic way, that the patient's skin had to be protected from developing pressure sores. He said pressure sores always antedated bedsores. The former developed because of prolonged weight bearing on bony prominences and of maceration of the horny layers of the skin. The latter followed because of interference with the skin-vascular reflexes. According to Munro the best treatment of bedsores was prevention and this should be accomplished by keeping patients constantly dry and never allowing them to lie in a wet bed for even as little as 15 minutes and turning patients every two hours day and night as long as they were bedridden. Serum protein levels must be maintained. He thought it best not to carry out surgery on the bed sore but that the sore should be dressed only once a day by sterile dressing and did not recommend the application of Plaster of Paris beds in paraplegic patients. Regular turning was considered essential:

> "My experience thus indicates that the only therapeutic essentials to prevent the development of bed sores are to move these patients on an exact hourly time schedule: to avoid, except as described above, all forms of external artificial splinting or support to the spinal column so long as the patient is bedridden; to prevent the development of any serious sepsis or exhaustion; and to keep the patient constantly and completely dry – a desideratum that can be accomplished only by the use of a properly adjusted tidal-drainage apparatus. Tincture of benzoin is the only worthwhile local application, and sponge-rubber mattresses appear to be desirable and useful in thoracic-cord injuries. Active surgery and wet dressings are contra-indicated." (Munro, 1940)

9.4   Operative management of the spine

Munro believed that the treatment of the patient's spine was of only secondary importance, and that no effort should be made to reduce a fracture by operation, but that gentle traction should be used to replace the vertebrae. He recommended that constant X-ray checks should be made of the bone injury until such time as the physician was certain that it was completely healed and capable of bearing body weight without the aid of a splint. He was not in favour of decompressive laminectomy, stating that it should not be undertaken lightly. He showed a drop of 30% in the mortality of cervical cases after laminectomies were abandoned.

Munro was the first in the field. His work and extensive publications on the management of the spine, prevention of pressure sores, prevention of urinary tract infections, and his insistence on non-operative treatment, led the field for many years. He was a true pioneer.

9.5   Overall management

Munro took a holistic approach to the overall management of the spinal injury patient. He recognised the virtues of physiotherapy in mobilising patients, was willing to carry out rhizotomies to eliminate spasms and was a strenuous advocate of returning patients home to a wheelchair life.

By 1937 Munro had treated 90 spinal cases. In 1943 he wrote:

"Nothing less than an active self-supporting wheelchair life is to be considered for a moment as an end result, and ambulatory activity with the aid of splints should be the eventual goal if at all possible. Time must not be allowed to be a factor, and physician, the patient and his relatives should all constantly be striving toward that end." (Munro, 1943)

In October 1945 he described rhizotomy to eliminate spasms and thereby enabling patients to walk. His teaching was pragmatic, direct and forceful. He did not restrict himself to purely describing the mechanics and pathophysiology and method of treating the bladder. He went further and discussed the doctor's responsibility for training the nursing staff and junior staff, seeing that patients were transferred to a specialised hospital, and when people's performances did not match up to his expectations, whether they were administrators or doctors, he recommended their dismissal. Munro said:

"The institutions in this country that are equipped (outside of the veterans' and certain armed services hospitals) to properly care for such invalids (spinal injury patients) can be counted on the fingers of one hand. The number of such patients in need of such institutional care as a necessary prerequisite to rehabilitation otherwise unattainable to them is in the many thousands. These patients require a long hospitalisation; they and their families frequently either do not have or shortly run out of enough money to pay hospital bills; they tie up hospital beds that the staff wants to use for more fluid surgical or medical cases; their care requires a meticulous attention to detail which the surgeon in charge is not only unwilling to learn how to give, but will not provide even if he does know how, because of the time it takes; finally, those civilian centres that are willing and able to cope with this problem are already badly over crowded and have waiting lists. What more natural then, than for the community hospital that has had this incubus dumped in its lap, and for the general surgeon who is not really interested in the problem and who is being subjected to constant pressure from the superintendent to free the bed for better-paying, less troublesome and more fluid patients, to arrange for the transfer of this unwanted member of their professional family to the county hospital, the poorhouse or to some nursing home, even in the light of certain knowledge that this but signs his death warrant after subjecting him to a lingering, painful illness complicated by bed sores, kidney and bladder stones, renal infections, a constantly wet or soiled bed, spasms and deformity. Who can blame the family or the patient for believing that death cannot come too soon under such circumstances and that when it does come it is a merciful release to all concerned? This particular problem is so big that it is not only a matter for the attention for the trustees and staffs of small hospitals but should be the active concern of the big hospitals and the communities as well. The key to its solution still remains with the general surgeon, however. He can prevent the invalidism by increasing his knowledge of how to handle such injuries and he can make the community see that failure to provide means for the rehabilitation of these patients is not only short-sighted and uneconomic but, worst of all, is uncharitable and an evasion of proper responsibility as well." (Munro, 1952)

The texts that are quoted show what a superb, forceful, inspirational writer Munro was, a teacher and a prophet. His graphic descriptions of how the administration, nursing and medical staff should behave were very influential shown by the fact that Guttmann made 25 underlinings in his copy of Munro's book and quoted Munro's work ten times in a monograph (Guttmann, 1953). In his early publications Guttmann quoted Munro literally. Munro's views were widely adopted in the treatment of American servicemen during and after the Second World War. Munro's contribution to the treatment of spinal injuries was acknowledged in a review of the experience of the American Forces which stated that most of the diagnostic and therapeutic procedures employed in Army hospitals had previously been tested in civilian clinics. Considerable space was devoted to Munro's methods of tidal drainage. The Second World War simply supplied the opportunity for their trial on a mass scale (Prather, 1947).

Unfortunately this was only being achieved in service hospitals. Munro tried to demonstrate that it was possible to treat and rehabilitate civilians from his unit and in 1954 an end-result study was published of 445 cases cared for from January 1930 to July 1953. With the exception of 15 veterans they were all the victims of civilian accidents. The corrected overall mortality was 28%. There was a decrease in mortality from 47% during the ten years from 1930 to 1940 to 20% from 1950. Munro stressed that:

> "It is this improved therapy that is still usually not available in large numbers of these invalids. For it to be available and effective requires community interest and co-operation, enthusiasm and knowledge on the part of the local medical profession and, most important of all, education of the public so that they, as individual patients, will insist on their right to these essentials. The 27 additional lives that will be saved out of every 100 such injuries justify the effort." (Munro, 1954)

He described a patient who was doing mouth painting. 81% of patients were 100% self-caring. 85% of 212 patients lead a fully (61%) or partially (24%) active social life. Some stayed away from home overnight and visited their friends freely. One hundred and thirty five (46%) of 291 patients were fully or partially self-supporting and either owned their business or worked on a salary. 27% were unemployable because of their disabilities. 18% were employable but not working. Many patients had allowed their bladder training to decline. One hundred and forty seven of 316 patients (46%) walked normally or had no paralysis, 27% walked only about their home or place of work and 25% did not walk. Thirty-eight were bedridden and 56 used a wheelchair. Fifty one per cent had normal sexual activity. Late complications included bedsores, bladder infections and genito-urinary tract calculi associated with infection. Munro said psychological problems were virtually non-existent in this group of cases. Only 16 patients felt bitter. Treatment of the bone injury played virtually no part in the rehabilitation of these patients. Plaster of Paris casts were never used.

Munro acknowledged how expensive it was to treat spinal patients and described how the problem had been overcome by funding from the Liberty Mutual Insurance Company of Boston who had arranged to concentrate those patients they were responsible for at the Neurosurgical Unit at Boston City Hospital. Patients were seen by nurse counsellors and were treated by genito-urinary consultants, all paid for by the insurance company. They had access to widespread facilities. The staff of the Medford Ambulation Centre provided corrective therapy at their own Rehabilitation Centre. Families were kept indoctrinated, patients were encouraged and opportunities for job training provided. When the patient was ready, arrangements were made for employment.

Rehabilitation led to healthy patients who could care for themselves, were able to lead active social and work lives and had regained their self-respect. For the insurance company, rehabilitation of spinal patients led to financial benefits in the long term because of a reduced need for care:

> "The initial cost of rehabilitation is high, but any money properly spent initially is more than returned in later individual, community and governmental savings. For an expenditure of $223,089 on 26 spinal paralytics there was a net saving of $1,222,911, or 600%, on the investment." (Munro, 1954)

Munro concluded that the setting up of such a programme presented no problem, the humanitarian benefits were indisputable and the financial savings made it virtually mandatory.

10. THE TREATMENT OF SPINAL INJURY PATIENTS IN RECEIVING HOSPITALS OUTSIDE THE UNITED STATES

The Second World War served, just as in other countries, as a great stimulus for the treatment of servicemen with spinal injuries. The service hospitals were well organised. In contrast to the First World War, the treatment of these patients was well documented and in the Official History some 200 pages are devoted to the management of these patients whereas in the First World War only 5 pages are devoted to spinal injuries.

Barnes Woodhall, in his introduction to the Official History of the Second World War, acknowledged the paucity of information on spinal injury patients in the First World War.

In the Second World War a comprehensive and extremely detailed manual was issued on the treatment of spinal patients. There was discussion on how spinal patients should be transported and what efforts should be made to prevent pressure sores. Under wartime conditions in busy wards, tidal drainage was not considered useful, although it gave good results once the patient had been transferred to a better-staffed unit. There was no established plan regarding management of the bladder. Some favoured tidal drainage, others suprapubic catheterisation. They had the greatest difficulty, evacuating patients to the forward hospital. Plaster body casts were thought inadvisable. Patients were instructed, before departure, about their needs, particularly about turning, so that they could remind their attendants if necessary.

Treatment was reviewed in the different zones. In the European theatre and the Tunisian zone they thought that the spine should be operated on immediately under local anaesthetic. 479 operations were carried out in 1260 cases of wounds of the spinal cord, some patients experienced improvement in 48 hours.

Barnes Woodhall admitted that during the early months of the Second World War casualties with spinal injuries had very little encouragement offered to them. This was due to the feeling of hopelessness inherited from the First World War and the fact that the administrative policy was that these patients should be passed through the Army General Hospital system as rapidly as possible and then discharged to the VA (Veterans' Administration). In 1945, there was a change of policy that paraplegic casualties should be retained in the Army General Hospital system until maximum benefit had been achieved and they should not be transferred to the care of the VA until their progress appeared to have levelled off, i.e. the patient should have no bedsores, they should have an automatic bladder, and they should be able to walk if they were paraplegics. Only when these requirements had been met was a patient discharged to the care of the VA.

As early as 1945 it was recognised that paraplegic patients should be taught to walk with braces and crutches and that practically all paraplegics could achieve self-support by means of some sedentary occupation. This was regarded as the ultimate objective of all rehabilitation. Before discharge, paraplegic patients should have achieved a degree of rehabilitation "essential for the preservation of morale and human dignity." (Woodhall, 1959)

11.   TREATMENT IN THE UNITED STATES

The policy was to evacuate paraplegic patients to the United States where they were concentrated into Neurosurgical Centres in army hospitals such as Newton D Baker and McCaw. The plan was that the VA would take over these hospitals thus ensuring continuity of care. The hospitals selected were Birmingham General Hospital, Vaughan General Hospital, Cushing General Hospital, McGuire General Hospital and Kennedy General Hospital. In spite of the serious condition of many paraplegics, few patients died.

The need for teamwork was recognised. At the inception of the programme in each hospital, it was considered useful to assemble the ward personnel, including nurses, nurses' aides, ward masters and ward attendants, and explain to them in detail the objectives and techniques of the programme. The explanations covered the methods employed in the restoration of bladder and bowel function, the care of pressure sores, the importance of adequate nutrition, and the other clinical responsibilities, which ward personnel would assume. The explanation also included the mental and somatic approach to these patients and the extreme importance of the psychological encouragement, which those who cared for them could best supply.

As in the United Kingdom, trained staff were in short supply. There was general agreement that staff should be a select group, who were intelligent, well trained, enthusiastic and interested.

While patients were admitted under the neurosurgeons they received treatment from specialists in urology, orthopaedics, general surgery, medicine, laboratory and neuro-psychiatry. The efficiency of care was proportional to the teamwork shown and the ambition of the officer in charge (Kennedy, 1946).

Many patients arrived with suprapubic catheters. The policy was to get rid of these as quickly as possible. Tidal drainage was recommended. The urine was to be kept acid. Any patient with low haemoglobin was given blood transfusions. The dangers of recumbence causing calculosis of the renal tract were recognised and there was an aggressive attitude towards pressure sores which were treated as abscesses and by primary closure (White & Hamm, 1946). Every effort was made to encourage patients to walk. Patients were fitted with braces and undertook a graduated programme of physiotherapy treatment. Surgical division of the nerve roots and cordotomy were carried out to alleviate pain. Intrathecal alcohol block was considered for the treatment of spasms.

In December 1945 a survey of paraplegic patients showed that there were approximately 1500 paraplegic patients in Army Hospitals in the United States at the end of the Second World War. Of the 1389 paraplegics still to receive maximum improvement, 440 were to be discharged home and 949 would require continuing indefinite care. The majority of these patients were completely paralysed. It was thought that four out of ten would walk. It was recognised that some patients' families could not care for them and they would have to be institutionalised.

In contrast to the British, the Americans were much more aggressive and systematic in monitoring the status of their renal tracts by intravenous pyelography and cystography. They acknowledged that they had no experience with female patients. They described skin grafting and primary excision and closure of sores. The problems of calcium metabolism, protein deficiency, correcting dietary defects, managing the bowels, personal hygiene, and psychiatric and emotional considerations were explored.

Physical treatment included hydrotherapy. Paraplegics on Stryker frames were assigned to the same ward under the care of a physical reconditioning officer. Patients were turned a minimum of 6 times a day and a programme of exercises was followed including group exercises. Progress reports were made. The exercises were designed to increase the strength of the muscles of the shoulders, arms, hands, back and trunk so that they could achieve ambulation with braces. Patients were encouraged to leave hospital and return to society (even though they had pressure sores), to work and to continue their education. The most successful results from the standpoint of occupational therapy and training were accomplished in work that existed and was not created. In one centre, several paraplegics worked 4 hours a day, 2 hours in the morning and 2 hours in the afternoon, carrying out precision work in a nearby factory. They were paid by the hour, punched the time clock, and lost pay if they were absent or late. Their interest in what they were doing was amazing. One of these men, his ward officer stated, did more to help the morale of the other patients than anybody else, not excluding the Red Cross workers and the Gray Ladies. He gave a practical demonstration that a man with paralysed legs could still lead a useful life and hold down a paying job, and his determination and cheerfulness did more good to the other patients than any medical care. The objective of the training phase of the paraplegic programme was to provide patients with complete economic security. Before they were discharged from hospital they had to be provided with a way to make a living in a dignified occupation in a line of work where they would be given business on their merits and not just because of their paraplegia.

Teaching and training of doctors took a high priority in the United States and a large conference was organised in June 1945 when doctors and surgeons from all the Neurosurgical Centres met at Newton D Baker General Hospital to discuss treatment of spinal injury patients. (When I was carrying out my National Service in 1956 which is not long after this, although I was in the Orthopaedic Division, I had not attended a single training meeting until I went to a neighbouring United States Air Force Hospital where they had a postgraduate teaching session.)

The policies of closure of the suprapubic and primary closure of pressure sores were reiterated. They were very pleased with the attitude engendered towards rehabilitation. The days when the patient who had received a spinal cord injury with resulting paralysis was treated as a troublesome and hopeless invalid were definitely over. The men of the Army Medical Corps were considered proud to have led the way in bringing about such a complete reversal of attitude and had met the issue with all the resources of the medical profession. The importance of specialised staff was recognised. The early admission of spinal injury was stressed. When patients came in late covered with pressure sores, they were demoralised. When they came in early, their morale was better than in any other ward in the hospital (Woodhall, 1959).

Kennedy stressed that rehabilitation should be carried out with imagination as well as competence. Otherwise he said, quoting Douglas Thom, they will be "merely living memorials to the skill of medical officers during World War II, but to no good purpose. They must be given something beside just the privilege of staying alive." (Woodhall, 1959)

12. VETERANS' HOSPITALS

In order that there should be continuity of care, paraplegic patients were congregated together in 19 hospitals. Patients were then transferred en masse to the Veterans' Hospitals. A predominant figure in the Veterans' Hospitals was Ernest Bors.

Bors said that with only the three publications of Munro's work in the early 1930s to guide him, he proceeded to develop the first unitary, comprehensive, continuing, multidisciplinary spinal cord injury treatment and rehabilitation programme in the United States as opposed to the small 10 bedded experimental unit of Munro (Comarr, 1983).

The role of Bors in the development of spinal services is critical. He was a Jewish refugee doctor from Czechoslovakia who went to the United States. Following training in Prague, he held research and faculty positions at Universities in Zurich, Switzerland and Germany. He was a young professor in Freiburg when the Nazis took control of Germany. He returned to Prague and then to the United States where he enlisted in the Army Medical Corps.

As a result of the Second World War, many servicemen were rendered paraplegic. The policy of the Americans was that these patients should be treated in military hospitals. When no more could be done for them they were transferred to a Veterans' Hospital.

During the war, Bors was stationed at the Hammond Army Hospital in Modesto, California where he was managing urological problems of paraplegic patients. He requested that he be given a ward and all the paraplegic patients were moved there. He sought complete administrative, medical and professional control over the programme that he was to develop. He obtained adequate staffing from all disciplines, specialties and support services in the hospital.

In the summer of 1945, Bors had in place all of the most essential elements that are available in most modern spinal cord injury centres today and word was spreading to military hospitals throughout the services of his work. Teams were sent to Modesto to observe and then return to their units to establish similar programmes to care for their severely ill, dying and sometimes, woefully neglected spinal cord injury patients.

By the spring of 1946 the Second World War was over and plans were made to transfer patients who were not ready for discharge to Veterans' Administration Hospitals. It was thus that Bors, together with his remaining patients, was transferred from Modesto to Birmingham Army Hospital, Van

Nuys, California, with plans to turn the hospital and patients and those staff who wished, over to the Veterans Administration. A 205 beds spinal cord unit service was established with Bors as chief and spinal cord injury patients were transferred there from throughout the West of the United States. In the spring of 1946, Bors gave his forceful support to his patients' efforts to form the California Paralysed Veterans' Association in a military installation.

In 1950 the entire Birmingham VA Hospital was moved to the former Naval Hospital in Long Beach, California. Bors wrote about the development of the Spinal Cord Injury Centre at Long Beach:

"Historically, the development of the present unit can be traced to its humble beginnings in the Army in 1944 and 1945. Patients with spinal cord injury during World War II were then housed in a large neurosurgical section of the Hammond General Hospital at Modesto in Central California, where I served as a member of the urology staff. Since urology undoubtedly is one discipline, which deals with the most common complications of these patients, it was decided to transfer these patients from the neurosurgical to the urological wards in order to facilitate their care. Approximately 70 patients belonged to that unit. At the end of 1945, all patients from our own and three other hospitals with neurosurgical units, within the 9th Service Command, were transferred to the Birmingham General Hospital in Van Nuys, California, close to Los Angeles. That Army Spinal Cord Injury Center started with 180 patients, but their numbers swelled quickly to approximately 220 after the Veterans Administration had taken over from the Army in the spring of 1946. The Veterans Administration was very generous in supporting the project of a Spinal Cord Injury Centre and created not only the foundation for the present facilities but also that policy which made the unit quite autonomous. In June of 1950 the entire complex in Birmingham General Hospital, patients, personnel and a great deal of equipment and supplies, were transferred to what until then was the Navy Hospital in Long Beach, California, about 30 miles south-east of Los Angeles". (Bors, 1967-1968)

Facilities were inadequate so a new centre was constructed. In 1958 the spinal cord injury service moved into the first purpose built spinal injury centre in the United States. Throughout the 1950s and 1960s this centre was host to a stream of professionals, administrators, and dignitaries from throughout who came to observe and learn from Bors and his long-term colleague and successor, Dr A. Estin Comarr (1915-1996).

Bors is remembered for originating the concept of the comprehensive, co-ordinated, multidisciplinary, continuous, from-injury-to-death spinal cord injury treatment centre. He made a monumental contribution to urological treatment, which is documented in his classic text *Neurological Urology'* (1971). As treatment improved and the population of quadriplegics was surviving to become more than half the population of spinal cord injuries, Bors initiated studies on mortality and morbidity and showed that life expectancy was much better than commonly thought.

Munro, in his lifetime, recognised Bors' contribution. While Munro had worked on a small scale in an experimental unit, Bors had worked on a large scale. He achieved for American paraplegics what Guttmann accomplished for paraplegics in the United Kingdom.

13.   POLITICS AND MEDICAL CARE FOR VETERANS

Despite a unified approach in the Veterans' Hospitals, there were still problems. They only admitted servicemen and patients did not always co-operate because they were on drugs and alcohol. They felt that as they had a pension they had a right to custodial care. Rehabilitation did not proceed universally well. It has to be recognised that the Veterans' Hospitals did not attract the best of the American medical profession.

Despite Munro's efforts to rehabilitate civilians by getting the insurance companies to fund treatment in a separate spinal unit, treatment outside spinal units was virtually non-existent.

Munro was a visionary. In a small neurosurgical unit with 10 beds, he successfully rehabilitated spinal injury patients. By 1954 Guttmann in the United Kingdom and Harry Botterell (1906-1997) in Canada had showed that a lifetime's commitment was needed to spinal patients and that their treatment did not just finish when they left hospital. Munro recognised this and he sought to obtain financial continuity by getting insurance companies to fund care. He kept in touch with the progress of his patients after they left hospital by postal survey.

After Munro's death, Alain Rossier, a Swiss national, was appointed Professor in Charge of the Veterans' Spinal Unit at West Roxborough between 1973 and 1984. He told me that he was the only person treating civilians with spinal injuries at a Veterans' Hospital. After his departure, no further civilian patients were treated.

It can thus be seen that the Veterans' Hospitals were first in the field in the setting up of a comprehensive rehabilitation programme but this was only available to ex-servicemen, and this module remained circumscribed and did not enter mainstream American practice.

14.   OUTSIDE THE VETERANS' HOSPITALS

Until now the review of the American experience has concentrated on the role of spinal units. Until these were opened, patients died rapidly. However, where there is a very high standard of medical care, it is possible to keep patients alive outside spinal centres and in Scandinavia, which has the highest standard of medical care, they were tardy in developing spinal centres because care was so good in general hospitals. Similarly, in the United States, for different reasons, specialised spinal centres were not available for civilians. By contrast with the United Kingdom, there were significant contributions to spinal injury management in the United States from outside spinal units.

In the United States, unlike Europe, the role of the rehabilitation doctor was recognised largely owing to the work of Howard Rusk (1901-1989) who in 1941 established an Institute of Rehabilitation Medicine. In a few short years, this institute was acclaimed for providing the best possible treatment for the disabled, for developing new and improved treatments through its research laboratories, and for training outstanding physicians in the newly-emerged speciality of rehabilitation medicine. A large number of American physicians studied in Rusk's institute.

15.   REHABILITATION

The American approach to rehabilitation was much more scientific. Arthur S. Abramson (1912-1982), in particular, recognised that significant osteoporosis could take place in bones through disuse. He showed that calcium output in the urine increased steadily and could give rise to calculosis within the renal tract. He also recognised that ossification could take place in the muscles and advocated standing patients up to avoid this complication (Abramson, 1948).

Abramson worked with Henry Kessler (1896-1978) and they wrote a joint paper on the rehabilitation of the paraplegic, which was presented to the 143rd Annual Meeting of the Medical Society of the State of New York (Kessler & Abramson, 1950). The completely rehabilitated paraplegic patient was regarded as someone who was able to care for his daily needs without assistance, ambulate with braces and crutches and who was reintegrated into society to such an extent that he could hold down a job. They recognised that a close-knit team of specialists were required to look after spinal patients. Plaster casts were not used because of the risk of patients developing pressure sores. As soon as it was medically possible, patients were set up on braces and crutches and taught to walk. Occupational therapists provided patients with activities to occupy them and psychologists were considered to be useful in evaluating the patient's mental capabilities. Patients were tested to assess their suitability for work at a watch repair bench, radio repair unit, or at a typewriter. It was not their intention to turn the hospital into a workshop or classroom but "rather to apply the available facilities in a manner which will be truly therapeutic in nature". They said:

> "In this way, the approach of the doctor and therapist can be truly psychotherapeutic in nature, and the patient will be encouraged and stimulated to expend the vast amount of energy to be required in the months and, perhaps, years of training which lie ahead. It must always be remembered that it is the patient who does most of the work – it is his program – and without his full understanding and cooperation it will be doomed to failure." (Kessler & Abramson, 1950)

Early physiotherapy treatment of patients was stressed by Captain J E Cameron in 1945 and Kennedy in 1946. At a meeting held in the United States Captain Cameron reported on treatment at Newton D Baker Army Hospital:

> "In the treatment of paraplegia we define ambulation as the ability to get about by means of braces and crutches proficiently enough to care for oneself at home; to carry out the necessities of ordinary life without help." (Cameron, 1945).

The programme at the Newton D Baker General Hospital included exercises to strengthen the muscles of the upper extremities used in crutch walking, braces, a standard army walker with crutch type arm support and crutches. They recognised the virtue of getting rid of spasms:

> "Early initiation of a program of ambulation for paraplegic patients raises their morale. Physical therapy may overcome clonus and mass movements in partial lesions and improve the nutritional state and vasomotor tone. Such a program consists of exercises for the upper extremities, the early fitting or braces and supervised instruction in paralytic ambulation, starting in a walker and progressing to crutches." (Cameron, 1945)

The most important member of the treatment team was considered to be the hospital corpsman or ward attendant who was given special training in the handling and care of spinal patients. Their duties were mainly concerned with care of the bladder and bowel, changes in position of the patient and assistance with ambulation. Cameron suggested that the Army should create a rehabilitation centre for paraplegics to return patients to society but this was never done.

The name, George Deaver, is never mentioned now but his contribution was acknowledged at the time to be fundamental. He was medical director of the Institute for the Crippled and Disabled at Bellevue Hospital, New York University and worked with Rusk.

Deaver (19.7.1890-?) systematically described in a series of papers how those patients with crutches or walking sticks could carry out bed or mat exercises, wheelchair exercises, transferring from wheelchair to mat, standing exercises with support, walking exercises with support other than crutches and standing exercises with crutches. He discussed in detail the methods used to walk backwards, sidewards, to turn round, open and close doors, sit down and get up from chairs, ascend and descend ramps, stairs and curbs, get up and down from the floor, how to fall, clear obstacles, and pick up and carry objects (Deaver, 1945-1946). The measurement of Activities of Daily Living was developed as a baseline assessment required of all patients and was not restricted to those with spinal cord injury but the methodology could be adapted for spinal injury patients.

In 1945 Deaver was using a scale rating the physical demands of daily life which was expanded to include 82 activities. Once a daily activity inventory was taken, a programme was devised and methods of performing activities taught to the patient. Many patients were surprised by what they managed to achieve. Disabled patients were encouraged to undertake daily activity rehabilitation over a trial period of at least six months and then decide whether or not to continue.

The American attitude at this time was to assume that all activities were possible until demonstrated to be impossible (and the latter was rare). Exercise was thought to be psychologically beneficial, increasing certainty, confidence and speed in activities To keep up their motivation patients were encouraged to keep graphs of their own progress recording small milestones in their progress.

The emotional and therapeutic benefits of recreation were recognised:

"It is just as important to teach the crutch-walker social and sports activities best suited to his disability as it is to teach him to travel and care for his daily needs." (Deaver & Brown, 1946)

Severely disabled patients were encouraged to play games such as basketball, quoits, bag punching, shuffleboard, table tennis and billiards.

Deaver recognised that in choosing a job for a disabled person his disabilities must come first and interests, satisfactions and need have second place and vocational counsellors were available to assist with the choice of vocation.

"Thus the greatest and most fundamental need in the rehabilitation of disabled persons is the evaluation by objective testing of their physical capacity to perform the activities essential for daily life and work. It is the right of every disabled person to have an inventory of his abilities and disabilities. To help the disabled person make the most of himself is the goal of rehabilitation." (Deaver & Brown, 1946)

15.1 Munro's debt to Deaver

Munro modelled his rehabilitation programme on Deaver. Munro described dealing with contractures by surgery but was totally opposed to amputation of the legs. He emphasized that physiotherapy should commenced immediately the patient was injured and he devoted a whole chapter to braces and splinting. He discussed rehabilitation of the bowel. He was in favour of splinting to prevent undue movement but stressed that the use of splints is not to support the weight of the body but to maintain a normal posture. He wrote:

"While the patients are being gradually mobilized within the limits imposed by the degree of healing of the bone injury, steps should be taken to provide splints that will permit ambulation. This is particularly necessary for the quadriplegic, quadriparetic, paraplegic and paraparetic invalids. Rehabilitation in its final form depends on the patient's learning such mobilization as will guarantee him the ability to care for himself and, if there is no physical contraindication, the further ability to ambulate and to work." (Munro, 1952)

Munro described various splints and braces in detail including braces to cover the knees and the use of a pelvic band and discussed the importance of eliminating spasms in the muscles before getting patients to walk. An analysis was made of the type of gait that should be used depending on the patient's function. In cases of cauda equina he recommended just a cock-up splint for the ankle and he discussed the need for a swing through and swing to gait. The necessity for grading the exercises was stressed, i.e. patients were not supposed to start walking until they could balance.

"A period of intensive mat work and other callisthenics designed to strengthen the muscles of the pectoral girdle and arms to a point that will permit them to meet without fatigue the stress of weight bearing that is demanded for ambulation." (Munro, 1952)

15.2 Stoke Mandeville Hospital's debt to Deaver

In the United Kingdom Elvira Hobson (1956), Superintendent Physiotherapist at Stoke Mandeville Hospital in *Physiotherapy in Paraplegia* also acknowledged the debt owed to Deaver:

"A tabulated list of simple everyday movements (Activities of Daily Living or A.D.L.), the achievement of which is essential for self-care and independence, was first drawn up by Deaver and Brown (1945) and by the Veterans Administration (1946). An illustrated manual has been published by Buchwald (1952) and another by Rusk and Taylor (1953). These tables are used to provide an objective check of the progress of each patient and the full accomplishment of these activities is considered one of the most important goals in the rehabilitation programme." (Hobson, 1956)

15.3   Summary

The Americans were ahead with their bracing, walking, standing and sending patients home. They were better organised, produced better figures and were documenting their results, trying things out, publishing papers and reviewing their experiences to see how better results could be achieved.

16.   SURGICAL CONTRIBUTIONS

Surgeons in the United States made a significant contribution to the surgical treatment of acute spinal injuries.

Burrell recommended immediate surgery. He analysed the results of surgical treatment concluding that the critical factor was cord involvement and recommending that each case merited separate evaluation.

Under Cushing's direction the special field of neurosurgery became recognised as an independent specialty and he founded a school which had many followers. He was the first to develop the use of electric cautery in operations. However, the results of surgery were appalling in the First World War with a high mortality and few patients surviving to be repatriated.

Elsberg evaluated the importance of operative treatment and recommended incision into the cord to relieve pressure in certain cases.

Frazier, who trained Munro, had a thoroughly modern approach. He made a detailed statistical analysis of his own cases and over 700 from the world literature. He concluded that the recovery or improvement was better in the surgical than non-surgical cases and reported a reduced mortality following operative treatment than had been seen previously. He considered immediate reduction to be ideal and discussed the merits of open versus closed reduction.

Allen's experimental work in animals produced controlled trauma to the spinal cord and he then carried out a laminectomy in an attempt to evaluate different forms of treatment. Many of the questions he raised are still relevant today, in particular the problem of performing a laminectomy on a slightly injured patient immediately or waiting until the patient's condition becomes hopeless.

In contrast Munro insisted on non-operative treatment by gentle traction. Laminectomies were abandoned and a 30% reduction in the mortality of cervical cases followed.

The surgical emphasis in the United States has continued until the present day. Richard Schneider (1913-1986) saw 141 serious or fatal injuries among American football players, many of whom were tetraplegics. He delineated the mechanism of injury in cervical spine injuries and established a correlation between neurological damage and the nature of the injury. This formed the foundation of the modern management of cervical spine injury.

R. Cloward appreciated that injury to the spinal cord arose anteriorly (Cloward, 1961) either from a fracture or disc injury and pioneered the anterior surgical approach.

Bohlman (1979) carried out post mortem studies on patients with spinal injury, particularly cervical injuries, and delineated the importance of damage to the discs intruding on the spinal cord as part of the acute injury.

17. WHY DEVELOPMENTS DID NOT TAKE PLACE

By 1900 the United States was already a wealthy, well-developed country with high standards of medical care and well-trained physicians and important papers had been written on the management of spinal injuries, particularly by Frazier. One has to look at why developments did not take place. This can almost entirely be attributed to the fee-for-service payment of American doctors:

> "...the emphasis remained on the market not the state, and on the private consumers rather than organised labour or citizens...One of the consequences of the Flexner Report (1910) was the elimination of over half the existing medical schools; this reduced the quantity and improved the quality of medical graduates. Fewer doctors meant higher status and incomes. It became more common to visit a private doctor for a check-up, or for vaccines and routine ailments, rather as people were increasingly opting for elective and not just emergency surgery." (Porter, 1997)

The position of the American doctor in society was assured:

> "...the AMA resisted the Sheppard-Towner Act, which provided federal subsidies for states to establish maternal and child health programmes; it also opposed the establishing of veterans' hospitals in 1924. (Both were

seen as taking the bread out of the mouth of the private physician.) As group hospitalisation plans developed, the AMA at first expressed reservations and by 1930 was denouncing them as socialist...President Franklin Roosevelt's New Deal, designed to steer the nation out of the Depression, seemed to be leading America in the direction of a national health programme... The Depression and the popularity of President Roosevelt – himself a polio victim – forced the AMA to temper its views, although it constantly warned of the danger of the government encroaching upon the domain of medicine...charity hospitals began to introduce voluntary insurance schemes ...leading to the Blue Cross (hospital) and Blue Shield (medical and surgical) pre-paid programmes...Private health insurance became big and lucrative business. Hospitals in turn became the great power-base for the medical elite...Funds for flagship hospitals and research and teaching facilities were prised out of Washington, state governments and notably from philanthropic bodies such as the Rockefeller Foundation. Between the wars, the Foundation gave millions to university departments and hospitals in many countries to support the science-based medicine Flexner had envisaged..." (Porter, 1997)

While American medicine could provide superb care for discrete medical conditions, particularly surgical, and was in the forefront of research, this did not produce a comprehensive medical service.

Surgeons faced the twin demands of tempting fees and pressure from relatives to operate upon the spinal cord to see if anything more could be done. Patients would remain under the care of the initial doctor until all their insurance money was used up and while they may have had dramatic surgery, the rest of the body was managed in a fragmented manner, without any holistic approach. Patients were often covered with pressure sores. There was no integrated programme of rehabilitation and patients were just discharged into the wilderness when their insurance money was exhausted. The public resented this.

The Kennedy administration tried to introduce some form of comprehensive care. This, again, was opposed by the medical hierarchy and, eventually, under Lyndon Johnson, specialised centres for burns and spinal injuries were set up on the pretext that they would be for research. It was pointed out in the teeth of opposition from the American medical profession that you could not do research on spinal patients unless you had units to treat patients in. Eventually, in the 1970s, a chain of units was set up on an experimental basis. Each one had a different framework. Some were based in private hospitals, some in insurance hospitals, some in Veterans' Hospitals with the staff being provided by the university and others were university hospitals. As part of this development I was invited to take charge of a spinal unit based at the Veterans' Hospital at St. Louis with a university appointment at Duke University.

It was recognised that each of these provided better care than were available in the community at large. Despite this, today less than 20% of spinal injury patients are treated at these model centres (Go *et al.*, 1995). The rest are still being treated at random. There are still problems today. When the Clintons attempted to give the American people a National Health Service, this was supported by the American Association of Retired People (AARP) but they were immediately and strongly opposed by their own members who insisted that they must never be deprived of their right to choose their own physician. The proposal went down to defeat because it was opposed by elderly Americans, lawyers, physicians, pharmaceutical companies, insurance companies and other corporations.

Munro delineated the fundamentals of treatment, demonstrating how the work could be done, in particular, early transfer to a specialised centre. Bors followed these precepts but had difficulty in getting patients in early. He produced an integrated programme and, because these spinal patients were veterans, they could be cared for at home on a lifetime basis. Veterans' Hospitals served as a model of how spinal injuries could be treated

The United States was the first in the field, through Munro, to develop treatment but this was restricted to servicemen for political reasons and properly co-ordinated units for the treatment of all patients with spinal injuries had to be developed elsewhere.

Chapter 5

Canada

1.   INTRODUCTION

Munro, Watson-Jones and Ernest Alexander Nicoll (1902-1993), who visited the Lyndhurst Lodge Unit in the late 1940s, reported that Canada had outstanding clinical units and had made important contributions to the comprehensive care of the spinally injured. Military and civilian patients were admitted soon after injury and because the units were opened as early as 1944, the Canadians wrote some excellent clinical papers particularly on life expectancy. These are by Harry Botterell (1906-1997), Al Jousse (1910-1993) and Wynne-Jones.

Professor Mary Tremblay studied rehabilitation in Canada. She interviewed the founders and many early patients, and produced a comprehensive history and evaluation of the development of spinal injury management in Canada. I was fortunate to interview her and much of this section is derived from her papers.

2.   SOCIO-ECONOMIC BACKGROUND

Canada has a triple tradition. It has looked to Britain and France culturally. Because of its situation, dominated by its giant neighbour, America, Canada was regarded in North America as another state of the United States. Canada fulfilled a very important role in the treatment of spinal injuries. Innovative social aspects of rehabilitation were developed there which have not received the recognition they deserve.

135

3.   SPINAL CORD INJURY BEFORE THE SECOND WORLD WAR

Following the First World War, in common with the United Kingdom and the United States, Canada had a few surviving spinal injury patients. A dozen or so paraplegics lived in a chronic pensioners hospital, Euclid Hall, Toronto, Ontario (Morton and Wright, 1987). These patients lived in squalor and unhappiness. They were abandoned and ignored. No records have been found to show that veterans with spinal cord injuries were considered for the newly developed retraining programme offered to veterans with other disabilities such as amputations or blindness.

In contrast, there is an interesting group of civilian patients who sustained spinal injuries, were rehabilitated in their homes by their families, and survived. Professor Tremblay interviewed some of these patients and wrote several articles in Caliper:

> "Lorne (Cotsford) is one of the very few quadriplegics in Manitoba. He is believed to be also the only paralysed veteran in Canada whose father is also a paralysed veteran...Arthur Cotsford is a resident of the Veterans Home on Academy Road. He has a spinal cord lesion resulting from injuries sustained in World War I...Lorne lives with two other wheelchair veterans at their home on Atlantic Avenue." (Tremblay, 1995)

Irving Hoffman was a premedical student at the University of Toronto in 1927 when he became quadriplegic as a result of a diving accident. After physicians gave up on his care his mother took him home from hospital where together they developed methods to prevent respiratory and urinary infections. Hoffman graduated in commerce from the University of Toronto in 1935 and obtained a Master's Degree in Educational Psychology in the 1940s. He lived and worked from his home in Toronto for 60 years, and died in 1987 (Tremblay, 1995).

4.   KENNETH G. MCKENZIE (1892-1964)

Treatment of spinal injuries in Canada began with the appointment of McKenzie as the first neurosurgeon in Canada.

In *Fracture, Dislocation and Fracture-Dislocation of the Spine* presented to the Canadian Medical Association in 1935, he described the diagnosis and treatment of spinal fractures 'If the patient is paralysed, with retention of urine, immediate steps must be taken to prevent the development of bed sores and cystitis.'

He advised that the bladder should be regularly emptied and should not be allowed to distend and overflow (this had been advocated as a method of treatment in the First World War).

He described the treatment of the dislocated cervical spine and the management of upper thoracic fractures. He suggested that patients with incomplete lesions of the cord could be mobilised in a wheelchair but was opposed to open reduction of the fracture or dislocation.

McKenzie's views were conventional and the same as those of Lorenz Böhler (1885-1973) in Austria and Sir Geoffrey Jefferson (1886-1961) in the United Kingdom. He trained Harry Botterell.

5.   HARRY BOTTERELL (1906-1997)

In her article Tremblay says:

"Having graduated in medicine from the University of Manitoba, Harry Botterell completed his training as a neurosurgeon in 1937 at the Toronto General Hospital, where he was the chief resident of Kenneth McKenzie, the first Canadian neurosurgical specialist. Beginning in 1936 Botterell undertook the treatment of three men with incomplete lesions of the spinal cord who were admitted to the Toronto General Hospital and St Joseph's Hospital in the east end of Toronto..." (Tremblay, 1995)

Botterell did not accept that there was no effective treatment for spinal cord injuries. He undertook to coordinate every aspect of the patient's care. He assembled a group of nurses, orderlies, physical training specialists and physiotherapists to provide a coordinated programme of active nursing care and physical retraining. He also treated the bladder using Munro's tidal drainage apparatus to irrigate the bladder and prevent infections. His orthopaedic colleague Dr Robert Inkerman Harris (1885-1966) brought this apparatus back to Toronto.

All three patients survived and, because they had incomplete lesions of the spinal cord, were able to regain the ability to walk. They were all able to return to live and work in the community. This experience was filmed and presented to the Canadian Medical Association.

From this experience, Botterell developed his ideas about rehabilitation and the team approach. Even at that stage, before the Second World War, he far-sightedly urged the appointment of one physician to assume overall responsibility for the treatment of the individuals. The emphasis was on integrated care.

6.   THE SECOND WORLD WAR

The outbreak of the Second World War put a halt to progress in Canada. Botterell joined the Royal Canadian Army Medical Corps. With Dr William Cone (1897-1959), he helped establish the No.1 Canadian Neurosurgical Hospital in Basingstoke. In the early 1940s he was appointed chief neurosurgical officer, a post he held until 1945. He collaborated with Jefferson who was one of the few people to have an interest in the management of spinal injuries in Britain.

At Basingstoke, Botterell developed a specialised medical, surgical, nursing and physiotherapy team to provide care for soldiers with spinal cord injury. He developed his ideas and achieved a superb standard of rehabilitation and treatment in Basingstoke. Such a centre did not exist in Canada or in the United Kingdom until the unit at Stoke Mandeville was functioning.

No 1 Canadian Neurological Hospital was mobilized in December 1939, and went overseas in June 1940. In May 1943, it was re-designated Basingstoke Neurological and Plastic Surgery Hospital. This centre made an important contribution to neurosurgery since they developed specialised studies and techniques.

During its period of operation Basingstoke treated 3774 neurosurgical cases of which 221 were incomplete cord lesions and 154 complete cord lesions (Feasby, 1953). There was close collaborative work between all the departments and initially civilian patients were treated. They did not believe that gunshot wounds of the spine needed immobilisation since these fractures were stable. The value of treatment in a specialised centre with specialised equipment such as braces, wheelchairs, crutches and special toilets was practised. Their policy was to perform suprapubic catheterisation to control the bladder during transportation of the wounded; and management of the bowels by enemas on alternate days. Patients were turned every two to three hours day and night and wet beds were changed immediately to prevent the development of pressure sores. Interestingly they carried out plastic closure of sores before 1945 following the practice in the United States. Adequate nutrition was considered paramount and they prevented malnutrition by eradicating infection, controlling pain and depression and increasing protein intake. Sometimes transfusions of whole blood or plasma were necessary. They were conservative in their neurosurgical procedures on the cord for pain and believed that their treatment programme was a model, which other nations followed. Limited statistics are provided giving the classification of wounds and number of cases.

There is a personal account from Gustave Gingras (1918-1996) who arrived at Basingstoke in 1944 having just graduated from medical school.

He did not acknowledge the work of Botterell, but did discuss the high morale of the centre.

7. THE ROLE OF JOHN COUNSELL (1911-1977): THE SETTING UP OF THE CANADIAN PARAPLEGIC ASSOCIATION

At Basingstoke Botterell met Captain John Counsell, a patient who suffered a gunshot wound to the spine in August 1942. Botterell discussed with him the idea of establishing an organisation of veterans with spinal cord injury.

Following treatment at Basingstoke Counsell returned to Canada in 1943. On his return home he received care at the Montreal Neurological Centre. Later he and his wife returned to Toronto and lived with his sister and her husband. Counsell found that there were no rehabilitation programmes for veterans or civilians in Canada. He met Lewis Wood, a wealthy businessman, who also encouraged him to develop an association for veterans and civilians with spinal cord injury (Tremblay, 1995).

Counsell initially used a large wooden wheelchair to get himself from his bedroom to a sun-porch but an American veteran friend obtained an Everest and Jennings collapsible, self-propelled wheelchair for him (which had been developed in the 1930s in the United States). It is interesting that this chair existed but no one used it, even Roosevelt, who was crippled by poliomyelitis. Previously chairs were wooden or wicker, and in hospital the chairs were assigned to the ward not to the patient.

Counsell taught himself to transfer independently in and out of the wheelchair and into a car. He later learnt to drive a car with hand controls. In 1944 Wood and Counsell joined with Botterell to lobby the newly established Department of Veterans Affairs to turn Lyndhurst Lodge into the first Canadian rehabilitation centre for spinal cord injury.

Counsell and six other veterans with spinal cord injury founded the Canadian Paraplegic Association on 1st May 1945. It was the first organisation in the world founded and administered by individuals with spinal cord injury. Counsell was elected as the organisation's first President. The first constitution of the association had nine goals, which addressed the needs of all men and women who were disabled by paraplegia. Goals addressed three broad areas: medical treatment, training, and civil re-establishment.

The outstanding feature in Canada was that it was a cooperative effort between Botterell, Jousse and Counsell and the Canadian Paraplegic Association. Such cooperation was not universal as many doctors feared that their authority would be undermined by the development of patient support groups.

8.   HARRY BOTTERELL'S RETURN TO CANADA IN 1945

Botterell returned to Canada in January 1945. Impressed from wartime experience of the pitiable lot of the patient with spinal cord injury, he put his organisational skills, foresight and drive to work on their behalf. He accepted re-appointment in the Royal Canadian Medical Army Corps as director of the Neurosurgical Service of the Christie Street Military Hospital with responsibility for Lyndhurst Lodge.

Together with Jousse, he described his programme of treatment in Paraplegia (Botterell & Jousse, 1946). He acknowledged that he had looked to Munro, Deaver and Brown for his ideas (quite clearly the influence of Deaver, Physical Medicine Consultant, was seminal as Jousse went to spend a fortnight with him). Botterell made no reference to Guttmann's work but he had begun his work in 1940 whilst Guttmann did not start until 1944.

In this article Botterell described the superb programme of practical treatment, which was being carried out in Canada. From 3rd February 1945 until 1st June 1946 paraplegic patients from the armed forces were treated in Christie Street Hospital and Lyndhurst Lodge, Toronto. Pressure sores commonly developed during the period of evacuation. Suprapubic cystostomy was to be done on all patients with serious spinal cord injury. The abolition of sexual function made many men fearful of meeting their wives or fiancées. He described how this combination of circumstances made them despondent. Interestingly he said:

> "...One of our colleagues was reminded of the moving pictures of a German concentration camp – feverish, listless, undernourished, hopeless patients; spontaneous activities reduced to a minimum, the patients doing little or nothing for themselves, believing that they should not or could not." (Botterell & Jousse, 1946)

These are what Guttmann used to describe as 'the Buchenwald patients'.

8.1   Botterell's Credo

Botterell stressed the need for a team approach but emphasised that 'one doctor is required who appreciates the total problem and who will integrate all therapy.'

It was accepted that on the battlefield a suprapubic catheter should be used but under civilian conditions, tidal drainage was the treatment of choice. They also performed transurethral resections of the bladder neck. Twenty nine patients were studied who had 'on admission or have since developed calculi, 20 vesical, 15 renal and 6 with both renal and vesical calculi' (Botterell & Jousse, 1946). He demonstrated that if bladder function was satisfactory, patients did not get renal complications. He recommended that all patients should have an intravenous pyelogram every three months during the year following injury and at appropriate intervals thereafter. There were only 7 deaths in the 16 months between 3 Feb 1945 and 1 June 1946. He recommended that the bowels were managed by enemas every two days and showed that spasms could be managed by anterior rhizotomy. Pressure sores were closed by surgical treatment. Patients were given high protein diets with vitamins and blood transfusions.

Botterell's comments on rehabilitation illustrate why the Canadian experience was unique:

"Dressing and undressing, a bath and a multitude of other daily activities seldom considered in the life of a normal individual are tasks of some magnitude for the paraplegic; additionally there are the problems of the paralysed bladder and bowel as outlined above." (Botterell & Jousse, 1946)

Botterell paid tribute to Munro and acknowledged the Munro doctrine, which was the charter for all spinal injury patients. Botterell reaffirmed it as follows:

"To restore a paraplegic patient to a useful place in society, it is necessary that he learn to deal with his paralysed bladder and bowel, master wheelchair life, and if possible learn to stand and walk with braces and crutches. Unless self-care is mastered, the patient is dependent on others for his every need, and such dependency destroys initiative." (Botterell & Jousse, 1946)

He followed the Munro doctrine. The rehabilitation programme began immediately whilst the patient was in bed and continued until he was able to walk, live at home and work. The aim was a return to social and economic activities which would provide a happy and satisfying life. Patients were encouraged to attend hockey games, the races, concerts and restaurants. There was no barbers' shop at Lyndhurst Lodge as:

"...Patients are encouraged to use the stores of the neighbouring community. Diversional occupational therapy is reduced to a minimum and the patients are sent to vocational training and rehabilitation schools regularly used by non-disabled veterans. A motorcar transports the men to and fro and at school a wheelchair or brace walking is used." (Botterell & Jousse, 1946)

Interestingly Jousse was opposed to the Paraplegic sports movement. He thought that paraplegics should participate in sport with able-bodied people in such sports as bowling and moose shooting. The Canadians did not join the paraplegic sport movement until Jousse retired in 1968.

The idea that a patient with spinal cord injury should return home was advanced and visionary.

When Botterell arrived at Christie Street in January 1945 he found 100 paraplegics receiving basic nursing only. They were not being given any positive treatment, received excessive sedatives and their bladders were neglected.

Following unrest in the United States in 1944 when mothers and wives started to protest about the Pensions Hospitals, Roosevelt said no one was to be discharged from the services until they were fully rehabilitated and no further treatment could be carried out. Canada followed suit.

Munro visited Canada at Botterell's invitation. He supported Botterell's group and gave them the vision to succeed. Munro started to create havoc with the administrators (Munro, 1952). Lyndhurst Lodge opened in January 1945 and Jousse was appointed Medical Director in March 1945.

Spinal patients were initially treated at Toronto General Hospital under the care of Botterell but from the outset they were seen by Jousse and came under the umbrella of a comprehensive spinal injury service. When they were medically stabilised and ready to participate in rehabilitation they were transferred to Lyndhurst Lodge where they were encouraged to gain independence in all activities of daily living and return to participate as much as possible in their former civilian lives. Morale for the servicemen there was superb.

> "The atmosphere at Lyndhurst was: you are here to get going, to get back into the community. The nurses and orderlies, therapists, cleaners and helpers, maids, gardeners, everybody said that they knew what their purpose was." (Tremblay, 1995)

Lyndhurst Lodge emphasised physical retraining and education. It was the first institution of its kind in North America. The programmes provided individuals with the knowledge they needed to manage their own care when they returned to the community. By 1946 many veterans had purchased cars with newly designed hand controls. They used their wheelchairs to go to restaurants, barbershops and a local cinema.

In 1952 Botterell succeeded McKenzie. His career after 1952 was brilliant for the neurosurgical achievements it brought. He had boundless energy to carry plans to fruition, which endeared him to some but not to all. His greatest priority was training residents who subsequently moulded neurosurgery in many parts of the world but his intense relationship with his residents could be exhausting and frustrating.

9.   TREATMENT OF CIVILIANS

Treatment in Canada was more advanced than in the United States in that they began to treat civilian patients as early as 1946.   In August 1946 the Department for Veterans Affairs agreed to allow the admission of a limited number of paraplegics who were not veterans at a charge of six dollars a day. This was the first time rehabilitation had been available to civilian paraplegics.   Counsell and members of the association's divisions lobbied various local, provincial and federal governments to secure funding for civilians.   In 1950 the Association bought Lyndhurst Lodge from the Department of Veterans' Affairs for one dollar.

Securing funds for the costs of rehabilitation and retraining for civilians became a major focus of the association until the implementation of health insurance across Canada in the 1960s.   There was a concerted effort by administrators and servicemen to admit civilian patients so they could receive the same treatment as the veterans.   Well after the establishment of the Health Service there was a scandal that female patients could not be admitted to Sheffield for treatment as there were no female wards even though there was supposed to be a comprehensive health service in the United Kingdom.   Although the spinal unit at Stoke Mandeville took female service women, it did not take female civilians until 1948.

Canada also developed social policies enabling first veterans, then civilians, to recover the full cost of disability.   There was an advanced pension system, patients received attendance allowance and the cost of equipment was covered.   Veterans were welcomed for employment.   The Canadians rejected sheltered workshops.

10.   THE INFLUENCE OF THE CANADIAN UNITS

Canada achieved an excellent standard of treatment and rehabilitation from the outset, and both civilians and patients were being discharged home. Botterell, a very gifted doctor who devoted himself to his patients, understood the fundamentals of treatment. The Canadians achieved the best of both worlds, American technology and British comprehensive care.

Unfortunately the Canadians did not receive the acknowledgement that their work warranted, perhaps because they were not self-publicists and Jousse and Botterell stayed in Canada devoting themselves to their work. However, Munro, Watson-Jones and Nicoll who went to visit Canada, all acknowledged their work. The Americans did not recognise their work for cultural reasons, regarding the Canadians as backward while British units all looked to Guttmann.

In Europe in the 1950s German, French and Spanish doctors came to Stoke Mandeville to learn from Guttmann. A few Australian and New Zealand doctors visited the Canadian units.

Chapter 6

The German-Speaking World

1.   INTRODUCTION

Scientific medicine in the German-speaking world emerged early in the nineteenth century. Neurology developed as an independent discipline and Moritz Heinrich Romberg (1795-1873), Adolf von Strümpell (1853-1925), Wilhelm Heinrich Erb (1840-1921) and Hermann Oppenheim (1858-1919) wrote textbooks incorporating descriptions of spinal diseases. There were isolated descriptions of traumatic injuries of the spinal cord but no coherent pattern of treatment. It was at the end of the nineteenth century that Theodor Kocher (1841-1917) and Wilhelm Wagner (1848-1900) described a large number of cases with spinal injuries and showed how patients with traumatic spinal injuries could be successfully treated. Their work was recognised and served as a benchmark for doctors working in the field for the next thirty years.

It was not surprising that Kocher, trained by Virchow, an international figure, professor and Nobel Prize winner, and head of the Bern university department of surgery for 45 years, developed a scientific basis for treating these patients and dealing with the paralysis of the bladder. In contrast it is remarkable that Wagner, a self-taught general surgeon, working alone in a workers' compensation hospital, developed successful methods of treatment and published a textbook with Stolper (Wagner & Stolper, 1898) delineating all the problems, giving a prognosis and showing how patients could be kept alive.

The treatment and complications of spinal injuries in German combatants in the First World War were the same as those experienced by the other belligerents. At the end of this war, the management of these casualties was reviewed and there are well-documented accounts by Otto Marburg (1874-1948), Freih. v. Eiselberg, Oswald Schwartz and Otfrid Foerster on the treatment of spinal injuries.

After the rise of the Nazi party, and its concepts of eugenics whereby deformed and paralysed people were killed by starvation, toxic injections or other means, the idea of rehabilitating handicapped people was not welcome. The Nazis were opposed to specialisation in medicine of any sort, favouring general practice and herbal medicine, so that the progress of scientific medicine atrophied. The work of rehabilitating patients with spinal injuries had to start afresh after the Second World War when German doctors looked towards the United Kingdom and the work of Guttmann.

The role of Germany is critical. They were the leading country in the world in the development of the modern treatment of spinal injuries through the work of Kocher and Wagner. Their work during the First World War was in advance of the rest of Europe. Guttmann received his scientific training in Germany. Logically the comprehensive management of spinal injuries should have developed in Germany but it did not because of Nazi ideology and today German doctors deny all knowledge of this fine spinal tradition prior to the Nazi party, possibly because of the denial of everything that went before.

2.   THE PRE-EMINENCE OF SCIENTIFIC MEDICINE IN THE GERMAN PRINCIPALITIES

"The absence of clear-cut geographical boundaries and the movement of German-speaking people into Eastern and Central Europe over the centuries have made it difficult to define the frontiers of Germany with any precision." (Carr, 1979)

For centuries, Germany was split into many principalities with divergent cultures. Even when it was unified in 1871 these differences continued and one has to use the clumsy term of "German-speaking world" to embrace all the developments of science and medicine in such countries as Austria, Prussia, Bohemia (now the Czech Republic and Slovakia), German-speaking Switzerland and the German principalities.

Prussia, prior to the unification of Germany, led Europe from the 19th century to the mid 20th century, both in terms of industrial wealth and intellectual institutions. The sub-stratum was there. Prussia had the first social security system in Europe and there was a high standard of living and excellent academic standards in its many universities. The workforce was well educated. State training in technology put Germany at the forefront of industry and science. Technical precision and high standards were reflected in medicine. By now the centre of medical science had shifted from France to Germany. Microanatomy, physiology and organic chemistry flourished in university and independent institutes.

"In states like Prussia where princes promoted a service ideal, physicians tended to pride themselves on operating as civil servants. Top physicians and medical professors typically belonged to a Medical College (Collegium Medicum) attached to the royal court. Formal qualifications were valued. In Prussia, for example candidates for the MD were required to present a clinical case (Casus Medicopracticus) before the Collegium Medicum and Medicochirurgicum (state board of health). Similar requirements applied in the Habsburg Empire, where licenses were conferred by the universities of Vienna and Prague. In the German principalities, chains of command and responsibility descended from the Collegium Medicum through city councils to town and village physicians, whose local status was dignified by bureaucratic titles and sheaves of parchment diplomas. Official title conferred upon the licensed practitioner the exclusive right to local practice." (Porter, 1997)

The doctors were very proud of their titles. They achieved high ranking in the civil service and distinguished doctors, such as Virchow, entered parliament.

There were disadvantages to this hierarchical system, which stifled initiative. The doctors related only to their place in the firmament, if you were the director/head of department you were everything, the source of all knowledge, all wisdom, and all authority. Unless you were the head of the department you could not undertake independent research. All initiative, responsibility and authority stemmed from the director of the unit, making it possible for large numbers of patients to be assembled and undergo a comprehensive, unified system of treatment under the professor.

High standards of education were reflected in high standards of medicine. In all fields there were giants. In basic physiology these were Johannes Müller (1801-1858), Carl Ludwig (1816-1895), and Jacob Henle (1809-1885). In neurology these were Romberg, Erb and Oppenheim. In neurosurgery, Otfrid Foerster (1873-1941), Rudolf Ludwig Carl Virchow (1821-1902) and Kocher founded the neuropathological department linking clinical disease with neuropathology.

3.   THE DEVELOPMENT OF NEUROLOGY AND DESCRIPTION OF SPINAL INJURY THROUGHOUT THE 19TH CENTURY

3.1   Johann Peter Frank (1745-1821)

Frank was a pioneer in the study of diseases of the spinal cord and a founder of public health in Vienna. He published the first book on the systematic discussion of spinal cord disease and described the spinal cord as being made up of a chain of ganglia. He founded a school.

3.2   Johannes Müller (1801-1858)

Müller did not treat spinal patients but his studies form the basis of our understanding of nerve function. He worked on the reflex function of the spinal cord at the same time as Marshall Hall. Müller founded a school where Robert Remak (1815-1865) was one of his pupils and Virchow was one of his assistants.

3.3   Heinrich Romberg (1795-1873)

Romberg was the first physician to give particular attention to altered structure. Following twenty years research he published the first textbook of neurology, *Lehrbuch der Nervenkrankheiten des Menschen* (Romberg, translated 1853). This was the first systematic book to attempt to classify neurological diseases. The classification of diseases is curiously based on how particular nerves were affected so that diseases such as sarcoidosis or connective tissue disorders, which could affect different parts of the nervous system, would not be recognised. He did not describe disease entities and the conditions are not recognisable by modern standards. He talked of neuralgia and hyperaesthesia of the different nerves. He gave an excellent description of hysterical and pain behaviour:

> "A middle-aged man complained of an agonising pain in the whole back. The moment he entered the room he sat down upon the first chair within his reach, and pressed his spine in a peculiar manner against the back of the chair. He soon, however, rose again and walked up and down the room in great pain, stating that he only found relief by pressing his back against the wall or the chair, or by walking up and down. If anybody assisted him in undressing he would turn round suddenly in the greatest excitement, and request that his back be taken care of. It was evident that the removal of single parts of his dress caused great pain. He would stop

when he began, and then suddenly throw them off by a jerk. The pain extended over the entire back, passing equally to both sides. A gentle pressure of one finger upon the skin brought on a violent attack of pain, during which the patient twisted about and stamped with the foot. If firm pressure was applied he did not complain: on the contrary, he found relief from it, for which reason he took refuge to strong pressure and powerful friction. Four years previously, shortly before the attack of the pain, he had suffered from haemorrhage from piles, which ceased on their removal by excision. The back exhibited traces of the various remedies applied, on the supposition of the affection being of an inflammatory character; but the treatment had remained ineffectual, or rather the pain had increased in severity." (Romberg, 1853)

His descriptions of spinal lesions are cast in almost medieval language:

"A predisposition to vesical paralysis exists in old age, and especially in the male sex and after excess venery."

He quoted Paré:

"A young serving man was returning from the country with a respectable young lady, his mistress, riding behind him, and with suitable accompaniment; and while on horseback, he was seized with a desire to micturate; he did not venture to dismount and still less to make water in the saddle. Having reached this town, and wanting to discharge his urine, he could in no way do so, and was seized with great pains; he was covered with perspiration, and almost fainted away. I was then sent for and the people said it was a stone, which prevented him from making water. When I arrived and I put a sound into his bladder and pressed to the belly; and by this means he discharged about a pint of water, and I found no stone, nor has he experienced any inconvenience since." (Romberg, 1853)

He distinguished between cerebral and spinal paraplegia and drew attention to the importance of the acuteness of the onset of injury in producing symptoms. Thus, acute compression of the cord was more likely to give rise to a complete transection and after this, patients were likely to develop pressure sores. On the other hand, a gradual onset was less likely to give rise to complete paralysis. He attributed it to the loss of resisting power, which caused the parts most exposed to pressure to be attacked sooner than others.

He described gangrenous bladders (blisters) on the ankles and the dorsum of the feet. He investigated the function of the acidification of urine by the kidneys, by washing out the bladder and checking the acidity of the fresh urine entering the bladder. (If infected urine is allowed to stagnate, it rapidly becomes alkaline due to the action of ammonia splitting bacteria.) He drew attention to the development of stones within the bladder and kidneys, described paralysis at different levels of spinal cord transection, priapism, progressive deformity of the lower limbs and contractures. Spinal bifida is mentioned and treatment discussed. He concluded that any treatment of the spinal cord was useless but recommended water baths, vapour baths, friction, movement and walking exercises.

3.4   Nikolaus Friedreich (1825-1882)

Friedreich worked with Virchow and was appointed professor of pathology at Heidelberg in 1880. He correlated the pathology of the spinal cord to the clinical manifestations. Friedreich made extensive studies of spinal cord disease, delineating various conditions to which his name was attached (Friedreich's ataxia). He began to teach neurology systematically. Although a pathologist by training, his greatest skill was in clinical medicine and he wrote extensively on internal medicine but his main interest was in neurology. He was succeeded in his post by Erb.

3.5   Adolf Strümpell (1853-1925)

Strümpell followed Erb at Heidelberg. Based on personal experience he wrote a thousand page textbook of internal medicine of which 292 pages were devoted to neurological diseases (Strümpell, 1888.) Although the spinal cord was protected by the vertebral column, he showed that damage could occur when the spinal column was disrupted. Dislocation or fracture of the vertebra would impinge on the vertebral canal resulting in traumatic damage to of the cord. Attention was drawn to the total loss of function immediately following cord injury, with partial anaesthesia, and when the roots were involved, there would be shooting pain with abolition of tendon reflexes and fluctuations in temperature. In the worst cases death occurred immediately, otherwise the patient might recover but would die from the sequelae of cystitis and bedsores. In mild cases there would be complete recovery. He was in favour of referring the case to a surgeon to relieve the pressure on the cord by trephining it, otherwise, the patient should be confined to bed and nursed on a waterbed to try and prevent the development of pressure sores and cystitis. The application of ice to the spine was advocated and railway spine (the whiplash injury of the 19th century) was described. Like Romberg, he recognised the important prognostic significance of the difference between gradual compression, such as from tuberculosis of the vertebrae, to which the cord can adapt, and rapid compression, to which the cord cannot adapt. There is detailed discussion about the abolition of tendon reflexes and the impairment of bladder and bowel function. Strümpell postulated that trophic and vasomotor influences might play a part in the development of sores and recognised that they were caused by pressure and uncleanliness:

> "The more faulty the care of the patient is, the easier bedsores arise. With completely paralysed and anaesthetic patients, with incontinence of urine and faeces, of course they sometimes cannot be wholly and permanently avoided, even with the most careful management. The extent to which a bedsore may reach is sometimes absolutely frightful. A large part of the sacrum may be laid bare, after the overlying soft parts and the periosteum have become gangrenous and been thrown off." (Strümpell, 1888)

Drug treatment was not thought to be helpful but practical treatment was recommended such as the use of electrical stimulation, baths and cold water cures; and sending patients to spas. There was detailed discussion about how the bladder was to be managed, when catheterisation should be done, and the importance of cleanliness: the catheter had to be sterilised and disinfected otherwise cystitis would develop. Unless there was total incontinence an indwelling catheter to drain the bladder was not recommended. Strümpell had many years experience of these problems and gave practical advice as to how patients should be treated.

4. CLINICO-PATHOLOGICAL CORRELATION OF DISEASE

The great strength of the German school of medicine, of which neurology was an integral part, was in correlating disease, symptoms and clinical findings with the pathological processes in the brain and spinal cord. Virchow was one of its founders.

4.1 School of Berlin

Berlin was a new university and served as a stimulus for new ideas. Amongst the extraordinarily able group of doctors working there, Virchow, a professor of pathology, and Remak, initially a spinal physiologist and pathologist and later an electrotherapist and rehabilitation doctor, demand special attention.

Virchow, although he did not treat any spinal patients, influenced or trained Friedreich, Frazier, Kocher, Romberg, and Cushing, who incorporated his ideas into their practice. In contrast to Virchow, all these physicians and surgeons actively treated many patients with spinal injuries and set up systematic methods of care.

Remak carried out outstanding anatomical neurophysiological work in his early life and later applied his ideas to rehabilitation.

4.2   Rudolf Virchow (1821-1902) and his School

There could be little understanding of disease processes and the function of the spinal cord until pathology was linked to manifestations of disease.

Virchow dominated German medicine and was a founder of scientific medicine. Before' him, German medicine was obsessed with the humoral theory of disease. Virchow was the first to stress that disease was on a cellular basis. In an effort to dismiss romance from medicine he founded several scientific journals. He studied the relationship of paralysis to spinal cord disease and published some thirty-five papers on the subject. He was a pathologist and had no responsibility for treating patients at any stage of his career. When he attempted to treat a patient who was having an epileptic fit in the street, he was arrested because he had no licence to practice. Despite this, such was his erudition, intellect and force of personality that numerous practising clinicians sought his advice.

4.3   Robert Remak (1815-1865)

Remak was a Polish citizen who went to Berlin to study medicine and on graduation worked with Müller. There were only five microscopes in Berlin. Despite this he carried out basic work on the axons of the nerves and seminal work of the physiology of the spinal cord. As a Jew, he could not achieve a permanent university post and had to go into private practice in Johann L Schönleim's (1793-1864) clinic to support himself. His large private practice was extremely successful but nevertheless the prejudice that he had generated on the scientific side followed him and intensified because of his success. In later life he became devoted to the practice of electro-diagnosis and electrotherapy on which he became an authority. His work was comparable to that of Duchenne. He wrote a textbook advocating electric treatment for paralysed muscles, substituting galvanic for induced current, and introduced galvanic therapy for some diseases of nerves and muscles. He was the first to describe ascending neuritis.

He disagreed with Duchenne, whom he went to visit in Paris. They had an acrimonious dispute during which he accused Duchenne of murdering one of his patients. Invigorated by this he returned to Berlin where he advertised for patients. Such was the force of his personality and his reputation that the streets around his practice were filled with patients. He then decided he had too much work to do and went on holiday. This naturally endeared him further to his colleagues, being good at his work, a fundamental scientist, a practical physician and extremely successful financially. In the midst of this, he went off to deal with a cholera epidemic – he was an altruist as well. He made startling contributions in three fields, anatomy of the nervous system, embryology and electrotherapy.

Up to this point, attention had been directed to the underlying physiological and pathological concepts of spinal injury. The long-term provision of care had not been addressed.

5.   ORTHOPAEDICS

The practical aspect of caring grew out of a sense of social responsibility for disabled people. In 1838, George Friedrich Louis Stromeyer (1804-1876) advocated special institutes for the treatment of poor children with clubfeet. General hospitals were not considered suitable as the assistant doctors changed too frequently. Johann Friedrich Diefenbach (1792-1847) put the need for specialist care more strongly in 1841 when he said that special institutes 'for care of clubfeet and other curable contractures' were of no use 'without a doctor conversant with the treatment of the same'. If this was the small beginning of orthopaedic specialisation, public sympathy lagged behind. In 1876 the sight of deformed people was still considered to be a public nuisance and the superstition persisted that deformed babies were born to women who, during pregnancy, saw a deformed person (Le Vay, 1990).

6.   SPA MEDICINE AND PHYSICAL MEANS OF TREATMENT

At that stage in Europe there was great faith in spas where fashionable doctors worked, treating (rehabilitation was not an expression that was used then) patients who were crippled, mainly by arthritis but also by nervous diseases and neuraesthenia. The work of Frenkel, a spa doctor, was on a different plane. He carried out beautiful applied physiological studies on patients to delineate proprioception. Incredible studies were carried out by means of simultaneous photography on different planes to analyse gait by Braune and Fischer (Braune & Fischer, 1895-1904) so that very real academic progress was taking place in what today is called physiotherapy.

6.1   Summary

By the end of the nineteenth century, the understanding of the pathophysiology of spinal injuries in the German-speaking world was more advanced than the rest of Europe and the United States but there was no comprehensive method of management.

There were accurate clinical and pathological descriptions of diseases of the spinal cord. Experimental work, both in animals and humans, delineated the tracts of the cord and the manifestations and aspects of treatment. Methods of draining the bladder, the perennial controversies between intermittent and continuous drainage of the bladder were discussed and evaluated, as were the controversies of surgery and decompression of the spinal cord. The management and pathogenesis of pressure sores was understood. The rapidity of the onset of the paralysis, the importance of the extent of the lesion in the prognosis was appreciated but there was no systematic description of these lesions and how the level of paralysis affected patients who were still dying soon after injury.

This was all to change as a result of the work of Kocher and Wagner who wrote textbooks in which they described a systematic way of treating spinal injuries. These textbooks became the benchmark of spinal injury management for the next forty years.

Kocher's work on *Injuries of the Spine and a Contribution to the Understanding of the Physiology of the Human Cord,* published in 1896, was 243 pages long. Wagner's textbook written with his former pupil, Paul Stolper, on *Injuries of the Spine and Spinal Cord*, was 564 pages long and was published two years later.

These books describe in detail the anatomy, the pathology, the manifestations, and methods of treatment of spinal cord injuries.

7.   THE FOUNDATION OF SPINAL INJURY MANAGEMENT

7.1   Theodor Kocher (1841-1917)

Kocher came from a wealthy background. He was a native of Bern and studied in Berlin but could not obtain a university position with Virchow because he would not change his religion and take German nationality. He married a wealthy woman from Bern and was able to systematically pursue his studies for the rest of his life without financial burden. He returned to Bern in 1866 where he was made reader then professor in 1872 and he remained there for fifty five years. Holmes had a similar experience when he was working in Frankfurt as an assistant to Ludwig Edinger when he was told that he could not receive a university appointment unless he took up German nationality. Remak and Oppenheim could not obtain university appointments because they were Jewish.

As an undergraduate Kocher became interested in surgery, particularly the surgery of the many trauma patients. He speculated whether he could tackle surgical lesions at Virchow's cellular level hoping, by removing the damaged cells, to cure the patient. He was aware of the problems of surgery, wound infection, haemorrhages, poor outcome and high mortality.

He was acknowledged as the outstanding surgeon in Europe, if not the world, due to his work on thyroid function for which he received the Nobel Prize for medicine.

It is little appreciated or documented that he carried out extensive research on the function of the nervous system. Cushing carried out research in his department in 1905 and wrote a thesis on the circulation of the cerebrospinal fluid. It is his extensive but little known writing on the spinal cord, which is of particular interest to this study.

Working with Hugo Kronecker, Kocher began to study patients with spinal cord lesions. He wrote a thesis initially based on his work as a student and his subsequent research was based on a large number of patients diagnosed at operation or autopsy. All Kocher's students remembered how tedious it was working at night and at weekends, all around the clock, studying the reflexes of these unfortunate sufferers (Fulton, 1946). His exacting method of working was typical of Kocher and equally typical was the way he drew conclusions from the material. In 1896, having studied spinal lesions at every level, he was able to put this huge jigsaw puzzle together. Kocher's work is quoted in detail by Wagner and Stolper (Wagner and Stolper, 1898).

His researches on the innervation of muscles and skin could be utilised by surgeons and physicians alike. He, along with Head and Foerster, pioneered the concept of the dermatome in man. Kocher achieved this by correlating the clinical observations and post-mortem findings, both in his cranio-cerebral topography and his classification of fractures, by detailed record keeping over a period of more than twenty years. As first shown by Macewen and Horsley, it was necessary for a surgeon to determine the site of the abnormality in the spinal cord. At that time there was no X-ray, myelography, Magnetic Resonance Imaging (MRI) or Computed Tomography (CT) and localisation depended on clinical observation, which involved the disciplines of anatomy and physiology.

Head subsequently mapped out the dermatomes by determining the areas of referred pain and herpes from visceral ailments. Foerster experimentally divided the sensory nerves but Kocher relied on clinical investigation.

7.1.1 The emergence of publications devoted exclusively to the treatment of spinal injuries

Unfortunately many of Kocher's papers were published in an obscure local journal in Switzerland which made them difficult to access. Kocher

(1896) analysed 383 cases which were treated in a general surgical unit. Amongst these there were 80 12th dorsal, 78 1st lumbar, 37 11th dorsal, 32 10th dorsal and 23 2nd lumbar (Kocher, 1896).

7.1.2   Management of the fracture

Kocher recognised the dangers of a dislocation of the vertebra and described how reduction could be achieved. Spasm of the muscles could make this difficult. Attempts were made to try and relax the muscles in spasm and traction was used to disengage the dislocation. He warned against the dangers of forceful manipulations which could damage the cord and described the use of a Glisson sling with an assistant exerting even traction. One patient died during this manoeuvre. Once reduction had been achieved the vertebrae were maintained in correct alignment by means of immobilisation in a Glisson sling for 4-6 weeks throughout the 24 hours with heavy traction up to 5 Kg in weight with a firm roll placed under the site of the dislocation.

The clinical manifestations of traumatic injuries of the spinal cord were presented. He believed that an injury to the cord could not occur unless there was a bony injury, usually a fracture dislocation. The differential diagnosis between cord injury and a peripheral nerve injury was described. The dangers of producing a dislocation of the cervical spine by incorrect handling following an accident was presented and he graphically described how a doctor was examining a patient when he redislocated the spine and the patient developed severe symptoms, thus emphasising the importance of careful handling of the patient.   A male with a cervical dislocation at the 6th cervical vertebra had improved following traction but when this was discontinued, the vertebra redislocated and all his symptoms returned.

7.1.3   Level of injury

The different levels at which spinal fractures occurred with the damage to the cord and roots at different levels were analysed.

It was emphasised that in an injury of the spine there would be a kyphus with a gaping of the spinous processes but he advised strongly against eliciting crepitus in a spinal fracture.

7.1.4   Ill effects of unopposed action on the muscles

The importance of muscle balance was emphasised and he showed how contractures could be produced when a normally innervated muscle was not balanced by a paralysed muscle. There is a graphic illustration of a patient with a 4th upon 5th cervical dislocation who shows clawed hands and flexed elbows.

7.1.5   Compensation

He was aware of the deleterious effects that compensation could have on the patient's recovery and gave an example of a workman who fell, was unable to walk, could not work, who went to bed although he was able to move all four extremities. Kocher was of the opinion that if the patient did not have any insurance he would return to work.

He stressed that a fracture could cause increasing pain which could make the symptoms worsen and the doctor would be asked to adjudicate by the insurance company as to whether the patient was malingering or not.

7.1.6   Prognosis relative to the level of cord transection

He recognised that transection of the cord above the 4th cervical segment was incompatible with life.

Patients with incomplete lesions improved but warnings were given that patients must be carefully mobilised with correct positioning, traction and prolonged further management.   Incomplete lesions had mainly motor effects and had a more favourable prognosis. If there were only sensory changes then only the nerve roots were thought to be involved. A right sided dislocation of the 6th cervical vertebra gave rise to a left sided cord lesion. If part of the cord function was preserved the prognosis was good (a thoroughly modern approach).   The symptoms were much worse at the outset than later on because the force was dissipated and when the oedema of the cord resolved then function would improve.   Even though recovery of spinal cord function could occur the patient was at risk of developing pressure sores and bladder paralysis. It was acknowledged that very little could be done for patients with complete cervical cord transactions.

7.1.7   Pressure sores

He understood the pathophysiology of pressure sores.   The cause of pressure sores was not just the loss of sensation.   Motor paralysis makes it impossible for the patient to change his position and he recognised the danger of even a short period of immobilisation on the operating table, the patient having discolouration of the skin – congestion of blood in the dependent parts.

There is the first discussion of paralysis of the vasomotor nerves, which cause the blood to stagnate precipitating the development of pressure sores. He recommended the use of a water mattress.

7.1.8   Surgical treatment

It was thought that if the spinal fracture was treated carefully there would be improvement.   As a rule Kocher did not recommend surgical decompression, being of the opinion that haematomas would resolve spontaneously and surgery would only be indicated if the patient failed to improve.   He recommended the use of a general anaesthetic.

7.1.9   Sympathetic

The first discussion of sensory changes above the level of the lesion, (Sherrington Schiff phenomena) and ocular changes from involvement of the sympathetic nervous system in cervical cord transection were described. Kocher explained how the level of the injury could be determined by observing the alteration in sweating at the level of the cord transection.

7.1.10   Bladder

Kocher produced a large body of work, not all of which is readily accessible.   Wagner clearly regarded his work very highly and discusses the different methods of treatment that Kocher used.

Kocher recommended permanent drainage of the bladder, using a catheter, which was brought out under the surface of an aseptic fluid.   He would not practice intermittent catheterisation because he said it encouraged infection and he believed that permanent drainage of the bladder was best. (Wagner & Stolper, 1898)

7.1.11   Summary

There are accurate descriptions of the pathophysiology of spinal cord transection with detailed correlation of the symptomatology to the pathology.   There is discussion about the prognosis, in particular, how incomplete lesions may recover and that the damage was worst at the outset.

It is not surprising that Kocher, a Nobel Prize winner, who worked side by side with pathologists in a university department and with Kronecker, a notable physiologist, was acknowledged in his own lifetime as an outstanding surgeon who made contributions to so many fields.   He was so highly regarded that Cushing studied under him and wrote a thesis on the circulation of the cerebrospinal fluid.   Whilst immediately after his death his work on spinal injuries was quoted and recognised, today doctors never mention him and indeed some have never heard of him.   This is in contrast to Wagner.

7.2   Wilhelm Wagner (1848-1900)

Wagner was a self-taught industrious, versatile, courageous general surgeon. He worked alone in a small workers compensation hospital where he spent his whole career treating coal miners with spinal injuries (Ljunggren & Buchenfelder, 1989).   Wagner developed the practical treatment of spinal injuries. He showed how the patients could and should be treated.

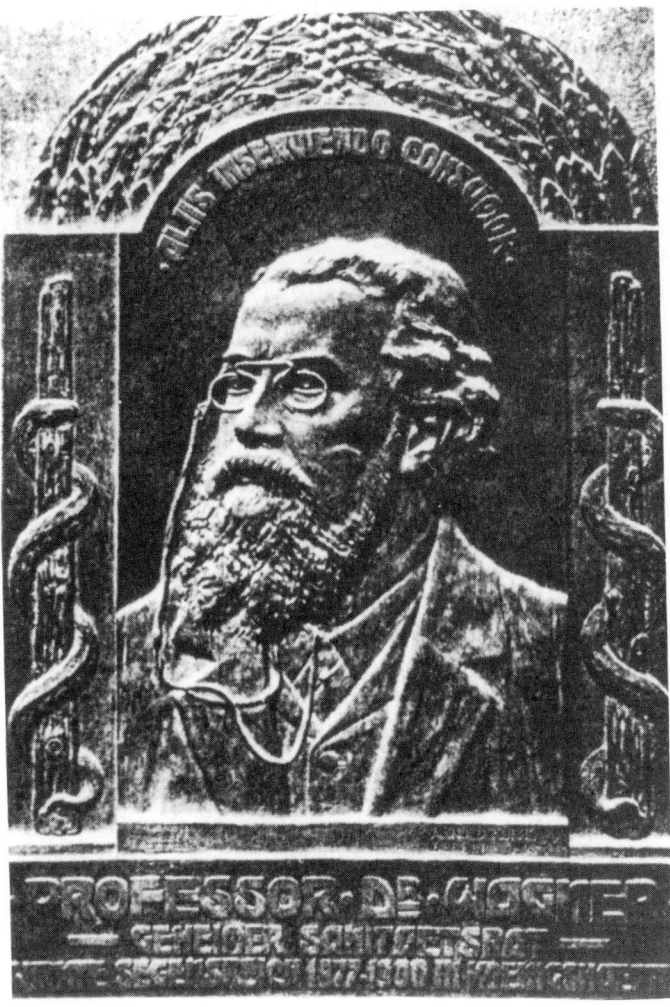

Figure 15. Wilhelm Wagner (1848-1900). This is the only illustration of Wagner from a commemorative plaque (Ljunggren & Buchenfelder, 1989).

After studying at Geissen and Marburg, qualifying in 1869, he worked as a physician in the Franco-Prussian war where he treated soldiers of both beligerents. He stayed on at Freiburg, writing many papers, until he obtained a position at a hospital in Königshütte, a small mining town in Upper Silesia with a population of 27 000. This is the town where the Guttmann family lived and its hospital was where Guttmann, prior to qualification as a doctor, worked as an orderly in 1918. (Goodman, 1986)

Wagner developed his interest in cranial and spinal injuries and rapidly achieved a local reputation, recognising the value of a plaster corset for the correction of kyphosis and scoliosis and for the treatment of spinal fractures. With his former pupil Paul Stolper (1865-1906), a paper on cervical spine luxations was presented in 1884 and in 1898 a textbook, *Injuries of the Spine and Spinal Cord*, was published. This book dealt with every aspect of the subject and was the most comprehensive text on spinal injury management until Guttmann's book in 1973. Anatomy, pathology, trauma, the symptomatology of the cord at different levels, practical treatment, the indications for surgery, relieving pressure, prevention of sores and deformity and physiotherapy were discussed and evaluated. It was seminal (Wagner & Stolper 1898).

Wagner identified six major problems; sepsis from pressure sores, treatment of cervical fractures, post-traumatic syringomyelia, infection of the chest, stones in the kidneys, sepsis of the renal tract and the necessity of immobilising patients in bed until the fracture healed.

7.2.1   Initial management

The chapter on treatment is superb and systematic. It had first to be decided how to transport the patient and even whether to keep them alive or not. The patient was bathed on a sheet to help prevent pressure sores and nursed on the sheet for inspection or palpation of the spine in order to avoid undue handling. The degree to which the deformity could be reduced could be estimated by exercising traction on the fracture and direct pressure upon the kyphus. Patients with spinal injury needed a long bed with all the facilities for traction and counter traction. A flat water-cushion, but not an inflatable ring, would be placed under the small of the back and under the buttocks. The whole of the sheet on which the patient was being nursed was covered with a layer of cotton. Particular attention was paid to the pressure points: heels, calves, buttocks and sacral area. Lint covered in boric acid was used. The legs were placed in slight abduction so as not to get pressure sores or gangrene on the medial sides of the knees. In this position it was easier to place the urine bottle between the abducted thighs. The buttocks had to be well cushioned with cotton wool under which a sheet of oilcloth was placed to keep the faeces away from the mattress. For doubly incontinent patients special beds were designed, such as those used for cholera patients, with a bucket underneath which could be removed. In the mining hospital these beds were found to be useful. for cleaning the patient without turning him over. This is the first description of specialised spinal beds and the recognition of the importance of turning the patient. From the illustrations it is clear that the patients did develop pressure sores. The practice of placing patients in a water-bath to prevent pressure sores was abandoned when it was discovered that sores could develop even when the patient was immersed. Fragments of the spinal fractures could not be immobilised in patients in a water-bath. Once the fracture had healed, the patient was mobilised and put into a bath, not only to clear up pressure sores but also to stimulate the locomotor apparatus. The concepts of the water-bath, low air-loss bed and air jets had to be rediscovered some eighty years later.

The treatment of spinal injuries had two main objectives:

1. To establish bony union of the vertebral fracture in the best alignment.
2. To bring about the best possible result by way of healing of the cord and nerves.

If the vertebral fragments were not too badly displaced then the spine had to be immobilised to avoid the risk of secondary displacement of the fragments. Another adverse factor was loading; the load had to be taken off the vertebrae. He recognised that patients should not be mobilised when they have a fractured spine. Mobilising a patient with a vertebral fracture and a cord lesion, even if the cord lesion is complete, can produce further damage to the spinal cord since, as a result of the fracture, the vertebra is compromised in its load-bearing capacity. Unless dynamic views are carried out, a standard x ray can fail to reveal the full danger to the spinal cord. In minor injuries this is of great importance since further damage can occur to the spinal cord.

Wagner was a practical psychologist who realised the psychological problem of keeping patients with an incomplete lesion immobilised. It was not sufficient to talk to them, as they were unaware of the severity of their injuries and the consequences of undue movement. It was necessary to tether the patients to their beds to keep them in a strictly supine position for 4 to 6 weeks, using light traction at the feet and head to keep them still. Traction was not used to achieve separation of the vertebral fragments but simply to keep the patient's spine in alignment. This may sound brutal, but when compared to the alternative, it was kindest form of treatment.

7.2.2   Management of the fracture: operative or conservative?

Wagner recommended treating the fracture or dislocation of the spine conservatively. Operative treatment was not considered beneficial. The patients were to be turned to prevent pressure sores and the bladder managed by intermittent catheterisation.

Luxation fractures, however, required correction. Avoiding secondary complications was the major goal. He was opposed to operative intervention and far-sightedly discussed the critical question of whether a completely severed cord could be regenerated or cured, and experimental work on salamanders and lizards, frogs and other animals quoted. While the stumps of a severed spinal cord could be accurately approximated they would only be healed by scar tissue and there would be no restoration of function and no conduction of nerve energies. A few sentences dealt with the prospective value that X-ray investigations might eventually attain in these kinds of injuries, a foresighted view at the time.

The management of cervical injuries with dislocation was prescient:

> "We may say nowadays that if a pure dislocation is diagnosed, then it must be reduced and even if the dislocation is complicated by a fracture, so it is a fracture dislocation. Proper reduction should not cause any major damage." (Wagner & Stolper, 1898)

Graphic descriptions are given as to how the fracture or dislocation should be managed. Reduction should be done swiftly without losing time. The method for reduction of a cervical vertebra depended upon the direction of the dislocation and on whether the facets were locked or not. The first thing to consider was how to unlock the dislocation of the articulate processes, and after that, reduction to a normal pattern was comparatively easy. Flexion without locking was described.

The method of traction was to place the patient supine on the operating table with the head and neck protruding beyond the edge of the table, held by the shoulders by an assistant who exerted distal traction. The surgeon held the patient's head or the upper part of the neck, pulling the other way. One or two fingers were placed on the spinous process to check neuro-relaxation. Once the facets were unlocked the whole complex could be reduced; a cracking noise was heard as the processes unlocked. Wagner recognised and showed that there was danger in reducing a dislocation of the spinal column. During this manoeuvre the cord could be further traumatised. The neck muscles would go into spasm as a result of the injury and were resistant to traction. He found that a dislocation produced by an extension injury was easier to treat.

Reduction should be carried out immediately; the complications of not carrying it out quickly were described. If a patient presented after many years, it was better to do nothing, as the spine would have fused in its dislocated position due to fibrosis. Anaesthesia could be dangerous to patients with severe cord injuries. If a patient was going to die anyway one would be wise not to anaesthetise him but every injury had to be considered on an individual basis.

The whole clinical approach cannot be bettered, even a century later. Today, with the advent of radiography, Computer Tomography (CT) scanning, myelography and Magnetic Resonance Imaging (MRI), the problem still persists today. Failure to follow Wagner's precepts has resulted in deaths, disaster, human suffering and numerous lawsuits.

The description of thoracic fracture is extraordinary because it applied the use of X-ray, which had only been discovered in 1898. The work was beautifully illustrated.

7.2.3   The bladder

There are eight pages of discussion on disorders of the bladder. Wagner favoured intermittent catheterisation, whereas Kocher favoured permanent drainage. Wagner, from practical experience, was aware that sores could develop within the urethra and give rise to abscess and fistula formation, which served as a sump of infection. This could be prevented, by washing out the urethra with a boric acid solution, which is still practised today. If the blood supply to the bladder wall had been compromised there could be meteorism and faecal retention. Patients died of cystitis and pyelonephritis. Well ahead of his time, Wagner described necrotising papillitis and stone formation in the kidneys.

7.2.4   Syringomyelia

Two cases of syringomyelia following spinal cord injury were described. It was postulated that when the vertebral column was kinked, it stretched the spinal cord and this, together with slight compression at the moment of trauma, caused an intramedullary cyst and fissuring of the spinal cord. This could happen without there being any haemorrhage. Clinical consequences could be so slight that people did not pay attention to it. However, there could be major bleeding into the cyst, which would rapidly produce the clinical picture of haematomyelia. These views on the aetiology of post-traumatic syringomyelia, advanced a hundred years ago, have not changed in the ensuing years. They are still rehearsed in journals without acknowledging Wagner's original description of the pathology (Silver, 2001).

7.2.5 Paralysis of the respiratory muscles

Chest complications were described, with patients dying of pneumonia. This was correlated with the level of the lesion. Patients with complete transactions of the cervical spine rarely survived the first month, and never the second month.

In a most interesting and far-sighted investigation, the level of the lesion was determined by the respiratory disturbance. In high transections, above the phrenic outflow, not much was known and the patients probably died. Interference with swallowing, tongue movement and movement of the palate in patients with high cervical cord transactions were described as was involvement of the hypoglossal nerves in the 2nd and 3rd cervical segments. If the 4th cervical segment was involved, there was paralysis of the diaphragm, which could only be seen in partial lesions but was absolutely unmistakable. The complete absence of respiration on the paralysed side was shown by failure of chest expansion. There were no normal respiratory sounds.

The higher the transection, the worse the prognosis. The lungs were affected because respiratory capacity was reduced when the thoracic muscles were paralysed and the vascular supply to the lungs was compromised. The lungs were over-distended with blood. Bronchial secretions could not be removed because of the paralysis of the respiratory muscles, that is the intercostals and the expiratory muscles. The stage was set for the development of hypostatic pneumonia.

Some of the patients were discharged as he described the benefits of spa treatment. One patient with an incomplete lesion survived for nine years after injury, was able to work, got married and fathered a child. Another partially paralysed patient survived for fourteen years.

7.2.6 Ancillary problems

Thoracic cord lesions complete and incomplete lumbo-sacral fractures, haemorrhage in and around the cord and spinal cord injury caused by lifting heavy loads were discussed. Diagnostic difficulties and lumbar puncture were described.

8. THE RECOGNITION OF WORK OF KOCHER AND WAGNER

The textbooks by Kocher (1896) and Wagner and Stolper (1898) became the standard reference work on spinal injuries and subsequent authors referred to them.

Head & Thompson (1906) refers to Kocher but not to Wagner. Holmes (1915) does not refer to either. Riddoch (1917) makes no mention of Wagner or Kocher. Frazier (1918) refers to Wagner and Kocher. Marburg and Ranzi (1918) refer to Wagner but not to Kocher. Thorburn (1922) does not mention Kocher or Wagner. Oppenheim (1911) gives full weight to their work. Jefferson (1927) refers to both Kocher and Wagner. There is no reference to Wagner or Kocher in Dick's thesis (1949). Benes (1968) does not refer to them.

The only person in modern practice who was aware of these textbooks was Guttmann. He did not refer to Kocher and Wagner in his 1959 monograph but does so in his textbook of 1973, although somewhat dismissively. It is fascinating that Guttmann had worked as an orderly at the Königshütte unit in 1918 some eighteen years after Wagner had died. However, by this time the hospital was no longer a spinal unit and Guttmann saw only one miner with a dislocated spine and he was told that the man would be dead in six weeks. He said that he only became aware of the existence of Wagner and Stolper's book many years later. (Goodman, 1986)

Until the work of Kocher, Wagner and Stolper, spinal injury treatment was the same throughout the Western world. There were good descriptions of isolated cases but most patients died soon after injury. There was no accepted method of management. After Wagner and Kocher's publications, most subsequent workers referred to them. There is a systematic description of the fractures, the pathophysiology, methods of treatment, the necessity for accurate diagnosis and immobilisation of the fracture, the dangers of moving an unstable fracture before union had occurred, the dangers of operative reduction and the complications which serve as a benchmark that could be read with profit today

9. THE EARLY 20TH CENTURY

Hermann Oppenheim (1858-1919) was the doyen of neurology in Germany but never achieved full professorship because he was a Jew. In the early part of the century he wrote a two volume textbook of neurology devoting 142 pages to spinal cord disease, of which twelve pages are devoted to fractures and dislocations of the spine (Oppenheim, 1911). This section is entirely based on Kocher, Wagner, and Stolper's methodology and researches, which were quoted extensively. Surgical matters were thought best to be left to surgical textbooks but the ill effects of early surgery were given. Methods of nursing the patient and managing the bladder were stressed.

Oppenheim recognised that the maximum injury to the spinal cord occurred at the moment of impact. He postulated various mechanisms whereby late changes to the cord could occur. There could be excessive callus formation at the fracture site causing secondary spinal stenosis which could ultimately impinge on the spinal cord. Incongruity between the site of the fracture and the site of the major neurological deficit, possibly due to injuries to the adjacent vertebrae, was recognised. X-rays were recommended. When the prognosis could not be determined, he advocated reduction of dislocation, conservative treatment and the use of water-beds. A poor outcome was noted.

It is a revelation as to how many of the ideas, predictions and mechanisms with regard to spinal cord pathophysiology, that Wagner, Kocher and Oppenheim were postulating, were a hundred years ahead of their time.

10.   THE FIRST WORLD WAR

10.1   Introduction

One and a half million soldiers of the Hapsburg Empire and two million Germans died. While there are accurate records of deaths, it is particularly difficult to elucidate the number of wounded but it could be anticipated that there were at least four million wounded Germans. It is striking that both Keegan (1998) and Gilbert (1995), whilst quoting the number of killed do not give the figure for the wounded. The surviving German 'grands mutilés' included 44 657 who lost a leg, 20 877 who lost an arm, 136 who lost both arms and 1264 who lost both legs. It is inevitable that there were a large number of spinal injured patients amongst the wounded but the majority of these would have died on the battlefield.

The large number of spinal injuries necessitated the setting up of spinal injury centres. Doctors from these centres met to discuss all aspects of treatment and at least two meetings were held in Germany.

The participants were Drs. Eiselberg (1916), M. Borchard, E. Payr, Steinthal, Fedor Krause, Kleist, Enderlen, Tilmann, Ludloff, Lobenhoffer, Krüger and Gaza.

The second reported in 1919 in the Medical Supplement (Borchard *et al*) was attended by the following:

August Borchard (1864-1940), Richard Cassirer (1868-1925), Wilhelm Keppler (1877-1919), Professor Fedor Krause (1856-1937), Herman Krükenberg (1863-date unknown), Otto Marburg (1874-1948), George Clement Perthes (1869-1927), Egon Ranzi (1875-1939) and Carl Schlatter (1864-1934). It is striking how many of these figures, sharing a common speciality during the war, developed international reputations subsequently with different eponymous diseases attached to their name.

The Medical Supplement article on gunshot injuries of the spinal cord, review of the foreign press (1919) provides an important summary of the papers produced by German surgeons during the war and also presents a discussion on gunshot wounds to the spinal cord, by these military surgeons in 1919 in Brussels. This gathered together accounts of injuries of the spinal cord, and their operative management. It is extraordinary that this summary of proceedings was translated and made available to English doctors in 1919 just after the First World War. (In the Second World War no such information passed between the belligerents.) These proceedings are informative in describing how spinal injuries were managed in Germany during the war (no such information exists for the Second World War in Germany).

10.2   Otto Marburg (1874-1948)

The most important paper presented at the meeting was by Marburg and Ranzi which was an abstract of their paper entitled *War Injuries of the Spinal Cord and Their Surgical Treatment* (1918).

Marburg was a very distinguished neurologist who worked in collaboration with Schwartz, a urologist, and Freih. v. Eiselberg, a physical medicine consultant, at a specialised unit set up by the army to treat patients with spinal injuries.

Marburg studied at the Vienna University Medical School, graduating in 1899. After a short postgraduate period there, he studied under Oppenheim in Berlin and received the degree of Privatdocent for neurology in 1905. He returned to Vienna, working as an assistant at the Neurological Institute. He was made a titular professor in 1912, becoming a professor in 1916.

This 210 page long monograph gives a very scholarly account (which is not surprising in view of the fact that Marburg was already a full professor at Vienna.) Only 4 pages out of the total of 210 are devoted to treatment.

There is a masterly review of the literature and he pointed out that Macewen was the first to perform a laminectomy in 1886 for the management of a spinal fracture. In contrast to the experience in the United States and the U.K. he saw no distinction between treatment in wartime and peacetime. Concerning wartime spinal injuries he reviewed literature from the Boer, Russian-Japanese and Balkan wars. The results of spinal injury treatment in the Balkans War had been disastrous reports only dealt with a small number of cases in contrast to the large number of cases cited in the literature of the First World War

Once the cord had been damaged there was no hope of recovery and suturing of the cord was rejected. There was no regeneration of the cord and transplantation of a rabbit's spinal cord had failed. Despite this some cases were amenable to surgery. It was impossible to distinguish between compression of the cord and damage occurring at the time of injury.

The army had set up one specialised unit to deal with spinal cord injuries at his hospital but it is not specified whether this was in Austria or Germany. Most cases came from the rear and were therefore late cases as acute cases were not transportable or perished soon after injury. Like other authors it was recognised that if a large number of acute cases were seen, there would be a high mortality because these patients were admitted dying from associated complications. Less seriously injured cases were admitted, the more seriously injured having died. As a result no statistical conclusions could be drawn.

The main emphasis was on gunshot wounds and there was discussion on:

- Retained bullets within the canal or the body
- Injuries caused by bullets that had penetrated – with or without demonstrable changes
- Blunt trauma

There were 142 laminectomies carried out at the centre: 27 cervical, 48 thoracic, 18 lumbar, 2 sacral, 6 conus and 41 cauda equina. Eighty four injuries were caused by rifle wounds, 33 to shrapnel, 16 to shells, 5 to rocks and 4 to falls. The pathology was meticulously followed up and scar and cyst formation were demonstrated. The clinical manifestations were discussed, not only of the 142 cases that were operated on, but also all the cases seen at the centre during the war years which totalled over 300.

10.2.1   The different levels of lesions

There was discussion about the differential diagnoses between spinal, radicular and plexus lesions, spastic lesions, improvement in the motor deficit, reflex changes, reflex patterns, sensory disturbances and sensory deficits.

10.2.2   Sensory changes

The sensory levels were mapped out with accurate illustrations. The authenticity of the work is demonstrated by the fact that several of the patients had pressure sores in the photographs.

10.2.3   Vasomotor and secretory changes

Vasomotor and secretory changes were documented including blistering, erythema and transient ulcers even on sites where there was no pressure.

Their practical application is shown by the fact that a large section was devoted to pressure sores contrary to the papers from France and the United Kingdom. They clearly understood their management and this is borne out by a paraplegic French prisoner, who was treated in Germany for two years when he was free of sores, but when he arrived back in France he rapidly developed them.

The suppression of sweating after spinal injury despite the injection of Pilocarpine, hyperhydrosis and anhydrosis was discussed. It was a major interest to Foerster since he produced many papers after the war on this subject in collaboration with his pupil, Guttmann.

10.2.4 Pre-operative investigations : determining the level of injury

The use of X-rays was well established and posterior and lateral views were used to gain a better understanding of the mechanics of the fracture.

Methods of determining the level of injury were discussed and attention was drawn to the fact that the site of the bullet and the clinical manifestations did not correspond and it was necessary to consider the trajectory of the bullet.

It was acknowledged that histories were frequently inadequate and the importance of obtaining a full history was emphasized. In the majority of patients paralysis came on immediately and remained unchanged. A smaller number of patients had a progressive paralysis until surgery was performed. The results of operation lead to an improvement in a small number of patients, particularly those with incomplete cervical lesions and cauda equina lesions.

10.2.5 Surgical treatment

No distinction was made between laminectomy in wartime or peacetime. Surgery was recommended under a general anaesthetic because they were afraid that under a local anaesthetic the violent manipulations and hammering of the spinal column would frighten the patient. The importance of identifying the correct level was stressed and that the vertebral level did not correspond with the level of cord damaged. The correct level was identified by counting the spinous processes and the vertebra marked prior to surgery by performing an x-ray. The stability of the spine was not necessarily affected even though five vertebral arches had been disturbed by surgery. Six patients were operated on under x-ray control. X-ray control was considered very useful in cases where the bullet was lodged in the soft tissue since any movement of the bullet during surgery would be immediately discernible.

A detailed analysis of the dangers of opening up the dura was made. It was recognised that the dura was the biggest protection to the spinal cord from infection. There is discussion on suturing of the roots of the cauda equina. Operation upon the cord produced problematic results.

10.2.6   Physiotherapy

Muscle wasting and stiffness were prevented by the use of massage. Swedish masseurs were trained to carry out exercises under medical supervision assisted by voluntary nurses. There was awareness of the dangers of contractures occurring. Attempts were made to alleviate spasticity by immediate massage. Splints were used to prevent contractures. If the paralysis improved, the patient with lower limb paralysis would be mobilised and attend a gait school. They would then be put in to a walker and finally canes would be used. Frequently the foot position would resemble a peroneal nerve palsy so orthopaedic footwear with elastic traction would be used.

Eiselberg (1916) concentrated on physical rehabilitation of these patients. The use of calipers is discussed and an illustration of a patient standing with calipers shows that the apparatus extended from the sole of the foot, right up to a waist band, shoulder band and with a harness over the shoulders.

In the upper limb, ulnar nerve palsy was the most refractory. Special splints were fitted to prevent finger contractures. Attempts were made to alleviate pain using serum therapy.

The post operative care of the patient by the nursing staff was stressed, particularly the need to position the limbs carefully. Treatment was not very successful as indicated by the many different methods of treatment that had been devised. The most far reaching suggestion had been by Wilms who suggested bilateral above knee amputation, a treatment that did receive advocates in the United Kingdom and I have seen patients who had this treatment carried out in the Second World War with distressing results. Apart from being unable to stand, the loss of the weight of the legs made it impossible for them to balance and had psychological consequences. Patients are unwilling to lose their limbs. It makes them feel unworthy and a bilateral amputation on top of being paralysed is an extra burden. This treatment was never carried out by Marburg and Ranzi. They gave paraplegic patients appliances to try and mobilise them again and referred to the work of Professor Eiselberg at Königsberger Hospital. The principles of the use of appliances were established. The lower limbs were splinted. The movement of the non paralysed trunk could then be transmitted through to the splinted paralysed lower limbs which had been rendered rigid. Improved versions of more primitive splints were used. The benefit of these appliances was that the partially paralysed patient would not develop pressure sores and there were aware of the psychological effect, that regaining some sort of motor performance would give patients optimism.

Appliances were used by all patients. In those who were slowly improving, parts of the appliance were discarded as improvement progressed. In totally paralysed patients, where there was no improvement the appliances might well be totally abandoned and discarded.

10.2.7 Pressure sores

For two years patients had been treated in a specialised 22 bedded ward in a general hospital devoted to the treatment of pressure sores, with all the latest equipment, headed by Professor Riehl. Patients from different departments of the hospital were also treated there. This was both revolutionary and visionary.

The prevention of pressure sores was considered to be one of the chief aims of post operative care. Frequently cases arrived at surgery with such extensive progressive putrid sores that the only course of action was to put the patient on to a water bed and wait until the sores had healed before surgery would be considered. With huge sores a bath was the only treatment and healthy granulation tissue was soon produced.

10.2.8 Bladder

The control of the paralysed badder was an insoluble problem and a separate monograph was produced by Schwartz, the Urologist to the Centre, entirely devoted to the subject and his published material was quoted (1916).

Schwarz approached the subject systematically and studied patients with other neurological disorders. A regular programme of catheterisation was set up monitored by manometry in an effort to establish automatic voiding.

There was no correlation between somatic spasticity of the body and spasticity in the bladder. Retention was more dangerous than incontinence. In their group of cases 46 had retention. A catheter was used to check the state of the bladder. Retention could persist for months. The significance of spasm of the external sphincter when they attempted to catheterise the patient was described. The typical presenting feature was retention. Descriptions were given of the different forms of bladder dysfunction, starting with the flaccid bladder with retention of urine. The bladder was emptied by expression, progressing to the autonomic bladder when the patients had no control of their bladders and the bladder emptied involuntarily. The significance of the residual urine was discussed together with the muscular tone of the bladder and the sphincter mechanism. Bladder washouts were carried out with benefit.

There was recognition that the bladder was innervated by the autonomic nervous system and had a different nerve supply to the rest of the body. This was in contrast to Head and Riddoch who believed that the bladder participated in a mass reflex of the striped muscles. It was only in the Second World War and subsequently that these problems were delineated and Schwartz's findings substantiated.

Combating ascending renal infection was considered of utmost importance. Bladder complications were the rule in cases of complete cord lesions. Many patients arrived at the centre with a severely infected bladder. Bladder irrigations were recommended several times a day and the internal administration of antiseptics but they warned against placing too much hope in these measures controlling infection. Even where bladder treatment was meticulous it was acknowledged that the temperature might suddenly rise with rigors, with flare up or progression of the urinary tract infection.

The insertion of an indwelling catheter for a few days was useful in some cases but they saw no benefit in performing suprapubic cystostomy prior to surgery as recommended by Schumm. Whether vaccination with Kolivakzin as recommended by Liepmann had any lasting effect could not be judged because of lack of experience. Nor could they comment on the use of Neosalvarsan which had only recently been introduced at the centre on any large scale. This is far-sighted and is the beginning of the introduction of the concept of antibiotics.

10.2.9   Social implications

The particular nature of spinal cord injuries and their complications (pressure sores and renal infections) meant that severe cases would need life long hospital care with medical and nursing staff skilled in the management of such cases. They had seen several patients perish because their complications could not be managed at home or in a hospital in their home country. In one case, a patient with severe contractures returned after being in hospital in his home country.

Specially designed facilities were set up for patients with spinal cord injuries where they could be cared for until their hospital treatment had finished and these facilities were attached to major departments of surgery so that the patients could be looked after by the surgeons and urologists working together.

This is the first discussion of a life after paralysis for paralysed servicemen and is in contrast to the situation in France and the UK. This is the first mention of social integration, and of segregation of patients in a pressure sore ward.

10.2.10   Results and prognosis

Marburg carried out a meticulous statistical analysis, attempting both a qualitative and a quantitative assessment of function. He analysed the results and found that of the 142 cases operated on, there were 42 deaths. Nine post operative deaths were related to sepsis of the spinal cord, 5 to pneumonia and 28 to renal sepsis and pressure sores. Urinary tract infection was almost universal.   Because of the poor condition of the patients, tuberculosis flared up. Two patients died of tuberculosis and it was a complication in a further 4.   Pressure sores leading to erysipelas was observed four times.   Some patients were in such a poor condition that surgery hastened their demise. An analysis was made of the timing of surgery to death.   Out of 142, 100 survived surgery.   A classification was made of how those who survived surgery improved.   No patient showed a complete recovery of function. Some patients with partial paralysis of their lower limbs who walked again with or without aids and patients who learnt to use their previously paralysed arms were considered to have improved.

A total of 71 cases showed some improvement.   Another group just improved a few segments sensory-wise or recovered some movement. (This is very similar to the classification used today.)

Discussion on selection of patients for surgery should include: which patients, when, where and which complications would be contraindications. He said not every case should be operated on. They saw over 300 cases but less than 50% were operated on which did not give a clear picture.   The surgical department received the worst cases, the mild cases stayed in the Neurology Department.   He thought a much larger number of cases should be operated on but was aware that milder cases may improve spontaneously.

The majority of cases were operated on within the first two months. Contraindications for surgery were: poor general condition (one patient died on the operating table) or infected wound surfaces close to the site of operation.   Intercurrent injuries such as pneumothorax were not considered a contraindication.   Indications for surgery included compression, retained bullets in the spine including intracord ones even if there were no neurological symptoms, fractured vertebrae with symptoms, indirect gunshot injuries with major nervous symptoms, patients with complete lesions and those with spasticity.

Where surgery was to be carried out depended on the circumstances. Marburg said surgery should be done where there is enough time and quiet for it to be done properly.   He advised against surgery at mobile surgical units advising that the patient should be taken to the rear or beyond.

It is striking that x rays were being routinely performed on spinal injury patients as early as 1917.

10.2.11   Marburg's later work

Marburg's superb practical work on the treatment of spinal injuries ceased at the end of the war when he returned to Vienna where he was appointed successor to H. Obersteiner as director of the Neurological Institute, which position he held until June 1938.   Despite the fact that Austria was under German influence, the Nazi laws did not apply. Jewish doctors could hold directorships of units and posts at the university and carry on independent work (Medvei, personal communication, 2000).

More than 200 papers on the anatomy, physiology and pathology of diseases of the nervous system were written by him. His interest in spinal injuries was retained but on a more theoretical basis. A textbook on trauma of the central nervous system was published and in addition he wrote a section in Foerster's textbook in 1936. The section on the management of spinal injuries is 53 pages long. This covered spinal cord contusion and concussion, haemorrhage, traumatic softening, disorders of the meninges and treatment of traumatic injuries and followed the conventional pattern of describing causes and levels of injury. Injuries were caused by puncture wounds, stab wounds and falls. Road traffic accidents came last on the list, in contrast to today.   Sports injuries were already occurring in skiing, tobogganing, discus throwing and hockey.

Marburg discussed the high mortality, nerve root irritation, progressive defect and post-traumatic oedema, but devoted little space to treatment. He made a distinction between those patients with a vertebral fracture without spinal cord involvement and those with spinal cord involvement. Marburg was the first to discuss the idea of accident prevention. He claimed that better traffic control, education and protection of workers would reduce accidents.   He also advocated prevention of sporting injuries. With regard to surgery, he recommended the removal of a foreign body in the spine and early operation after myelography. He discussed the prognostic significance of the completeness of the lesion and said that complete injuries could be incomplete – the important concept that when the cord is first injured there might still be preserved fibres, whose function could be impaired by oedema, which could later recover which has given rise to the great debate as to the completeness of spinal lesions. Discussion of treatment was perfunctory, covering pressure sore prevention by the use of a waterbed, the treatment of cystitis to prevent septicaemia and heat and massage to prevent muscular atrophy.

Marburg and Ranzi attempted a statistical analysis of the value of different forms of treatment. There was correlation between neurophysiological findings with the clinical presentation.

They developed the first effective spinal unit and outside experts were brought in.   The significance of the effect of renal sepsis and pressure sores on the general health of the patient was appreciated.   They were attempting to prevent infection by vaccination and were trying to use Neosalvarsan (the magic bullet of Ehrlich), the first antibiotic to combat infection. They were rehabilitating patients and getting them home.

Their work is full of practical ideas relevant to our treatment of spinal injuries today. Although Marburg ceased treating patients directly, he was the first to discuss the idea of accident prevention and advocated the prevention of sporting injuries.

10.3   Other work on the treatment of spinal injuries

During the First World War Marburg was meticulous in his treatment of patients with spinal injuries, achieving excellent results but he was not unique in this and discussions at the scientific meetings during the First World War by Kleist, Kruger, Keppler, Borchardt, Cassirer, Krause and Krukenberg delineate different schools of thought.

Kleist and Kruger (Eiselberg, 1916) were concerned that surgery had to be properly indicated and if the patient was too ill it could make their condition deteriorate.

Foerster did not participate in the meetings but his operation of dividing nerve roots to relieve pain was alluded to and was practised by other surgeons (Borchard *et al*, 1919).

Schwartz was not the only doctor to discuss the management of the bladder. Keppler (Borchard *et al*, 1919) described 54 cases, 38 of whom died within 74 days of injury. He drew attention to the dangers of failure to catheterise, giving rise to uraemia while the patient was being transported. The English doctors described similar problems and while the bladder management would be satisfactory in a base hospital or at the front, inevitably when the patients were held up on ambulance trains, disaster accrued. Keppler agreed that early surgery did not help.

Krause did not produce a statistical analysis (Borchard *et al*, 1919) but there was a description of 71 cases in military hospitals, drawing attention to paralytic ileus, distending the abdomen and causing heart failure. He also drew attention to the less serious prognosis when compression of the cord was from accumulation of cerebrospinal fluid or blood. He too was not in favour of immediate operation. He discussed the problem of regeneration of the cord, and the complication of excruciating pain. One of his patients was alive and well two years after injury. 300 cases of spinal injury were gathered together at Eiselberg hospital. Delaying surgery was considered undesirable. He drew attention to respiratory problems and described double amputation of the legs to prevent pressure sores developing on the useless limbs. The participants at the meeting did not agree with this. In particular, Krukenberg opposed it.

Krukenberg advocated grafting the ulnar onto the crural nerve and said he had performed this operation on two patients and had observed one long enough to observe slight abduction of the hip (Borchard *et al*, 1919).

German and Allied Military Surgeons experienced the same problems. There were a large number of paraplegic patients, and difficulty with transporting them. Management of the bladder was problematic and many patients died of uraemia while being transported. There was limited consensus about the indications and contraindications for surgery. There was no mention of the work of Kocher or Wagner.

10.3.1   Summary

As a result of the First World War, doctors in Germany, like other belligerents, were confronted with the problem of a large number of paraplegic patients and they made significant progress since the fundamental papers of Kocher and Wagner in that:

1. They recognised that severe spinal cases would need life long care and a specialised unit had been set up in Germany to treat soldiers with spinal injuries
2. Other consultants such as a urologist, a specialist in rehabilitation and a specialist in pressure sore management were attached to the unit where Marburg worked.
3. The difference between the diagnoses of cord plexus and peripheral nerve lesions had been discussed
4. Vasomotor changes had been elicited. There was discussion about the spinal control of sweating which had not been discussed previously.
5. The indications and contraindications for surgery on the spinal cord had been analysed
6. The use of physiotherapy (which was not discussed by Wagner or Kocher) including splinting, prevention of contractures and mobilising the patient had been discussed.
7. The concept of using antibiotics in the form of Neosalvarsan was being attempted to combat infection.
8. They were endeavouring to return the patients to their homes.
9. They had a greater understanding of the treatment and prevention of pressure sores than anyone else and had a specialised ward for patients with pressure sores.

After the First World War, just as in the U.K. and France, the spinal units closed down and doctors returned to their practice. Marburg went to Vienna to be director of the unit and Foerster carried on with his general neurological unit where patients with spinal cord lesions from different causes were treated.

11.   BETWEEN THE WARS

11.1   Frenkel and Foerster

Until the beginning of the twentieth century patients with spinal disorders were treated by neurologists and orthopaedic surgeons. Doctors in other disciplines treated patients with chronic neurological disease and the methods they developed were of practical importance to patients with spinal paralysis. They have passed the test of time and are now an integral part of present day management. Frenkel and Foerster were key figures in the development of these ideas.

11.1.1   Heinrich Frenkel (1860-1931)

Frenkel was a doctor in the spa town of Heiden in Switzerland. At that time the commonest neurological disease then was tabes dorsalis, which resulted in loss of the appreciation of painful sensations and loss of proprioception (position sense). The patients had preservation of motor power but developed ataxia (loss of co-ordination) as they were unaware of the position of their limbs in space and were consequently unable to walk and fell to the ground. In addition, as a secondary consequence of the loss of appreciation of pain they developed painless deformed joints (Charcot's joints). Until Frenkel, treatment consisted of strengthening the muscles but this was useless as the patients did not know where their limbs were in space and sat, terrified and immobile. He fortuitously discovered that by teaching the patients to compensate for the loss of position sense, using their eyes, they could learn to walk up and down stairs, backwards and forwards. He was not just an exercise or spa doctor but was carrying out practical neuro-physiological experiments upon the patients and made the discovery that ataxia was due to the loss of position sense and not due to weakness. Frenkel's exercises are still used today for the treatment of patients with spinal cord disorders. He considered that the bladder could also lose proprioception so he instituted a system of bladder training and stimulation by the use of boric washouts, a treatment still practised today (Frenkel, 1902).

In Germany there was a long and strong tradition of exercise and they extolled the benefits of exercise as a philosophy and a religion in its own right. It became incorporated in the Nazi philosophy of "Health through Strength". There were camps where youngsters went on marches and mass exercises in the mountains and forests. In 1936 Lord Horder recommended to the House of Lords that a programme of exercise similar to Germany should be introduced in Britain. After the First World War the Germans were the first to introduce sport for the disabled and amputees, even arranging competitive games.

11.1.2   Otfrid Foerster (1873-1941)

Foerster was born in 1873 in Breslau. A brilliant student, he worked with Carl Wernicke (1848-1904) and Emil Kraepelin (1856-1926), Joseph Dejerine (1849-1917) in Paris and met Marie and Joseph Babinski (1857-1932). During the summers, he observed Frenkel's neurological patients in Switzerland and published papers with him on ataxia (Foerster & Frenkel, 1899, 1900).   Foerster was interested in practical therapy. In those days there was no curative therapy for syphilis (penicillin therapy had not yet been introduced) and the underlying cause, just like spinal injuries today, could not be treated: only the secondary effects. Foerster tried to work out a scientific basis of practical therapy and never lost interest in the theme of physical therapy and physiotherapy. He had been impressed by the methods of Duchenne and Dejerine and by the English school of physiology, Hughlings Jackson and Sir Charles Scott Sherrington (1857-1952), whose work he referred to as his bible.

As he had no laboratories or research institute, his research was carried out in the basement of the Wenzel-Hanke Hospital in Breslau, probably financed from his private practice until the Rockefeller Foundation built him a Neurological Research Institute in 1932. This was too late to significantly improve his research output. He was offered a Chair at the University of Heidelberg and a post in Berlin but chose to stay where he was. (McHenry, 1969)

Foerster was a medical scientist. He correlated structure and function and his interest in the practical therapeutic efforts was a major part of his work. He studied co-ordination, which was the subject of his professional thesis in 1902. Following his work with Frenkel he demonstrated that hemiplegia of cerebral origin was spastic, whereas in tabetic paraplegia it was flaccid. He understood the significance of the spinal reflex arc and undertook the operation of posterior root section to eliminate spasticity in cerebral palsy. This became known as Foerster's operation. This operation also eliminated the root pain in tabes. He proceeded to delineate the sensory dermatomes, by operating on the posterior nerve roots. He then moved proximally and carried out anterolateral transection of the spinal cord for intractable pain. These procedures, root section and cordotomy, have been adapted today to treat pain in spinal patients by total destruction with alcohol block. (Haymaker & Schiller, 1970)

His major work was on peripheral nerve injuries. He set up a peripheral nerve injury unit and operated on patients with spinal injuries.

He was criticised that so many of his staff were Jewish but he said he did not choose his staff on the basis of their religion but on the basis of their intelligence. This may have been because his wife was half-Jewish. When the Nazis came to power his children were expelled from school as they were of Jewish descent.

This is a sanitised account of a man who was, by all accounts a singularly unpleasant person with whom no one wanted to work. He was an enthusiastic therapist. His chief, Wernicke, once said of him:

> "I now have an assistant who makes lame walk and blind see."
> (Haymaker & Schiller, 1970)

When Guttmann in 1923 unsuccessfully applied for a job in paediatrics at Wenzel Hancke Hospital, he was told to go downstairs where he was given a job, without interview, working for Foerster. He worked in the neurosurgical department intermittently for ten years, initially unpaid, eventually becoming Foerster's assistant. When people remonstrated with Guttmann in later life about his unreasonable and autocratic behaviour, he replied, "You think I am bad. You should have seen what Foerster was like".

Guttmann fled to the United Kingdom in 1939 and was co-author of a chapter entitled Rehabilitation After Injuries to the Central Nervous System in *Rehabilitation of the War Injured* (Doherty & Runes publication date unknown) in which he acknowledged Foerster's patterns of treatment of peripheral nerve injuries:

> "General Organisation – The installation in this country of several centres for the treatment of peripheral nerve injuries is a great step forward. The congregation of cases is a single department under the same specialised staff, with continuous treatment under the same supervision, is certainly the best guarantee for the systematic study of the whole question, for better results. The success of a centralized treatment and the care of peripheral nerve injuries in other countries was shown by the 'Peripheral Nerve Centres' in the USA during the last war and particularly by Foerster's work in Germany during and after the last war. His material included about 4,000 cases. Although he worked under conditions by no means ideal compared with those of a modern centre in this country, his results were remarkably good and better than those of many other authors of that time. Foerster has emphasized again and again the secret of his better results. It was only in some respects a specialized surgical technique; the main reason was a better and systematic after-treatment and after-care, in other words, a good understanding of rehabilitation.

> The installation of centres for peripheral nerve injuries, however, does not cover the whole problem of organisation in the rehabilitation work.

In practice it is not possible to bring all cases into these centres, particularly in the early days after injury. Therefore precautions should be taken in all General and Military hospitals, particularly in military base-hospitals, that the injured can be seen immediately by a Nerve Specialist versed in the after-treatment of peripheral nerve lesions. Neglect of this vital principle of rehabilitation in the first period, even in the first days after injury, accounts for much of the prolonged disability of the injured person, with all its economic consequences. The importance of this point can hardly be exaggerated. An integral part of the organisation of which might be called 'Primary rehabilitation service' is a thorough record of all treatment given in the first period after nerve injury. Undoubtedly such a service would greatly facilitate the work of the centres for peripheral nerve injuries and would play a big part in improving the end-results.

Of the same importance as the primary supervision immediately after injury is the late supervision of these cases after their discharge from hospital, from the centres and from the Army. This late supervision also includes the post-war supervision of peripheral nerve injuries. Experiences in all countries after the last war have clearly shown that any successful late supervision of these cases can only be achieved by a loyal co-operation of the medical authorities with the public health services and – as Cairns and Young pointed out (1940) – with the Ministry of Pensions, and last but not least, with the employers. Such an organised co-operation of the various authorities concerned with the rehabilitation work is of particular importance in the reconditioning period of the injured. One of the main tasks of the 'after-care service' is (1) to provide the injured man with light and graduated work in the former occupation until he is fit for heavy work, (2) to supervise this light and graduated work. In my own experience the best results in supervising the injured persons during the reconditioning period were obtained with the help of industrial medical officers and general practitioners. Experiences in all countries have shown that many patients, left alone in their reconditioning period, will never make sufficient effort to reach their full working capacity.

In discussing some methods of particular importance for a speedy and, if possible, complete rehabilitation only a few points can be considered. Cases with peripheral nerve lesions can be grouped into those in which restoration of nerve conduction is possible and those in which there is no chance of nerve regeneration. In regard to treatment, however, this distinction is not an absolutely strict one, as similar principles have to be considered in both cases up to a certain point."

All these methods were directly applicable to spinal cord injury. In fact the actual words have been used subsequently to describe spinal injury management. Guttmann's chapter discussed the positioning of paralysed limbs, strengthening of the synergists, electrotherapy, remedial exercise and occupational therapy but it is remarkable that in this discussion there was no mention of spinal cord injury.

In retrospect Foerster's major role in the history of the treatment of spinal injuries was that Guttmann spent 10 years working for him and learned from him how to be a fine neurologist and how to rehabilitate peripheral nerve injury patients. Later Guttmann adapted these methods for the treatment of spinal injuries. Guttmann also learnt about destructive procedures, that is, posterior nerve root section and cordotomy and popularised alcohol blocks, which he used to treat spinal patients with intractable spasm. Foerster was particularly interested in thermo-regulation and Guttmann took this further by studying sweating by means of spreading powder impregnated with starch which changed colour when it became wet. Guttmann's interest was maintained in this field in the United Kingdom while he worked at Oxford and subsequently at Stoke Mandeville where we collaborated together and produced further papers.

Foerster wrote a seventeen-volume textbook of neurology (Foerster, 1927-1936).

12.   WORK IN AUSTRIA AND CZECHOSLOVAKIA

Unfortunately, the fine foundation in the understanding and treatment of spinal injuries by Wagner, Kocher, Foerster and Frenkel was not developed in Germany. The position of spinal injury management can be derived from Böhler's standard textbook, *The Treatment of Fractures*, (1935). This book served as the bible of orthopaedics between the wars.

Lorenz Böhler (1885-1973) started as a country doctor and was in charge of a military hospital in the First World War. In 1925, he was invited to Vienna to take charge of an accident hospital founded and funded by the Austrian social security authority. This was a unique hospital, which pioneered the treatment, which led the world in the treatment of all forms of fractures. His textbook described fractures of the spine in a dogmatic but conventional manner. He divided them conventionally into fractures, which involved injury to the spinal cord and those that did not. He recommended reduction of dislocation of the cervical spine by means of a Glisson's sling; a strap placed beneath the chin of a subject; a method of treatment, which is painful and useless in reducing dislocations and can produce pressure sores under the chin. He used local anaesthesia in the reduction of dislocations, instead of general anaesthesia, which is also useless in view of the local spasms at the fracture site. According to Wagner this can be both useless and dangerous. With regard to major fractures of the thoraco-lumbar spine, he advocated splinting and immobilisation in a plaster of Paris jacket, which could only produce pressure sores. With major fractures, he used a plaster bed and said that the patient should be mobilised within two days: a prescription for disaster. He thought that the bladder should be managed by regular washouts and asserted that he had prevented pressure sores by splinting the paralysed patient by their legs and driving traction through their knees. He claimed that the patients could lift themselves up by their arms after two days. His son, an orthopaedic surgeon, retrieved a film of his treatment of spinal patients which shows that he was treating spinal cord injuries by an active programme of exercise. He was a pioneer in the management of spinal fractures and established the importance of rehabilitation.

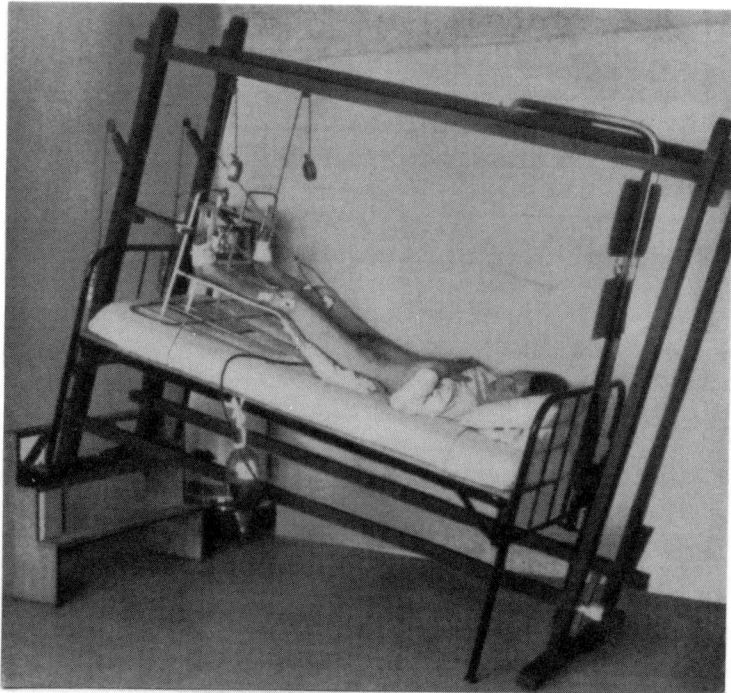

Figure 16. Böhler's method of treating spinal injuries. The immobilised patient could not possibly be turned and would inevitably get pressure sores on the dependent areas such as the buttocks (Böhler, 1935).

There was already a divergence. Although Austria was under the domination of Germany with economic union and a common foreign policy, Austrian universities and medical training were different and Austria pursued an independent medical policy until the Anschluss. Jews, as shown by Marburg, could hold full university appointments and professorships. Bohler was doing advanced work there rehabilitating spinal patients in advance of Germany.

Vladimir Benes, Deputy Head of the Neurosurgical clinic in Prague, reviewed the work in Czechoslovakia in the interwar period (Benes, 1968) and quotes A. Jirásek in 1929 being in favour of an open surgical approach. There were no spinal units. He states that the first comprehensive work was the rehabilitation lecture by Z. Kunc published in 1950.

13. THE DECLINE OF GERMAN MEDICINE IN THE INTER-WAR PERIOD

During the First World War spinal management in Germany was more advanced than in France and the U.K and even until the advent of the Second World War, management of spinal injury in Austria was at least comparable with the best treatment in the United States of America. Why didn't spinal injury development take place in Germany after the First World War?

The sad decline in the management of spinal injuries is only a reflection of the decline of German medicine in the inter-war period. It is facile to attribute this to the rise of Hitler to power. It is not as simple as this. There were several reasons:

- **Volk** politics and racial myths
- The science of **eugenics.** Arising from this was the philosophy that mentally and physically damaged people should not be a burden on the state and should be destroyed as not being worthy of life and that all resources should be directed to the physically fit.
- **Racism**.
- **The role of Nazi science**. The emphasis was on positive health. They abhorred deformity and practised selective euthanasia. There was opposition to specialisation. General practitioners and lay healers were favoured. Individual training was shortened.

13.1   Pre-Nazi ideas

13.1.1   The Volk

At the end of the 19th century and until the rise of the Nazis, extremely nationalistic right wing views were current in Germany. These involved the concept of the Volk, a series of myths, which were compromises between pagan memories, dynastic ambitions and the teachings of the Church. The blood of the Volk (the Germans), even if they lived outside Germany, was everything and entitled them to a superior place in the world. Thus Germans living in Sudatenland and in the Volga in Russia were considered part of the Volk.

13.1.2   Eugenics

Galton, an uncle of Darwin, founded the science of eugenics in the United Kingdom. It was believed that various characteristics such as genius could be inherited and this led to the concept that by selective breeding, the race could be enhanced. Conversely desirable factors could be bred out of the race and lost by interbreeding with "inferior" people and this led to the science of racial hygiene.

These ideas were reinforced and given spurious scientific backing by a study published in 1913 by the anthropologist, Eugen Fischer, on German settlers in East Africa who had interbred with the local Hottentots. He concluded that their offspring were invariably of an inferior type (Weale, 2001). He made no comment on social stigmatisation but his study resulted in the mixing of races being regarded as leading to spiritual and cultural degeneration and dilution of race.

Such ideas were not restricted to Nazi Germany but were being practised in the United States and France, leading to legislation whereby mentally defective people were institutionalised and sterilised (Weale, 2001). Attempts, in the United Kingdom to legalise sterilisation and euthanasia did not succeed but in Sweden 63,000 people, mostly women, were sterilised between 1934 and as recently as 1975 when the policy was halted.

In fact the United States was more advanced in these policies than Nazi Germany and the Germans looked to the United States where half the States were practising compulsory sterilisation. By 1929 nearly 15 000 people had been involuntarily sterilised in the United States during the previous 20 years mainly prisoners and those in homes for the mentally ill (Caplan, 1992).

In Germany whilst this policy was favoured, it was open to discussion and legislation had not been implemented.

This was compounded by racism.

13.1.3   Racism

Today racism is regarded as being an extreme example of prejudice, which culminated in the horrors of the extermination camps, and it is rejected out of hand but it is necessary to understand what it meant at the end of the 19th century and in the early 20th century before Germany was taken over by the Nazi party under Hitler's leadership.

It was a pseudoscience given some semblance of respectability by referring to eugenics and had been given a philosophical basis by J. Gobineau and H.S. Chamberlain (Weindling, 1993). Essentially it consisted of studying the different types of people based on anthropological measurements of bodily structure combined with an enquiry into the psychological composition properly belonging to each race.

A race shows itself in a human group which is marked off from every other human group through its own proper combination of bodily and mental characteristics, and in turn produces only its like (Günther, 1927).

It was postulated that different races could be categorised as superior, the Aryan, fair and intelligent and warlike and meant to rule and lead; and various inferior categories, the lowest being the Negro. As this was on a hereditary basis, the only way the inferior races could improve was by being exterminated, conquered and colonised by the superior Aryan races that would transform their role in society. Initially Jews were to be classed along with the Nordics as one of the superior, cultured races of the world. Races were delineated by blood and any dilution of the blood was said to lead to a deterioration in the race. These prejudices could give seeming legitimacy to the subjugation, colonisation and ill treatment of the indigenous population of Africa, South America and anyone who was not of the Aryan creed, and were unquestionably accepted as the way the world was ordered. In Europe black people were regarded as being inferior breeds who were discriminated against in employment, education and social conditions.

Today we regard these as aberrations but at that time they were mainstream science and by 1932 more than 20 institutes for racial science and racial hygiene had been established at German universities and at least 10 journals were being published on racial hygiene (Caplan, 1992). They gave a theoretical basis for Nazi policies and reading literature prior to 1933 sets the scene for Hitler's policies:

"The influence of the Jewish spirit, and influence won through economic predominance, brings with it the very greatest danger for the life of the European peoples and of the North American people alike. 'For what is here at stake is the unhindered development of the bearers of the highest culture of mankind, who, if the process of amalgamation with these emissaries of the East goes further, run the risk in mind and body of wandering off those paths which their own genius has marked out for them." (Günther, 1927)

The Germanic tribes were in possession of certain traditional eugenic customs, and of a traditional but more unconscious, aversion to mixture with the blood of the dark European races.   The Germanic father recognized a newborn child, which was laid before him on the ground in solemn form, as fit for bringing up by lifting it.   Deformed and sickly children were set out.   The Germans looked on the criminal as a degenerate, from whom his clan cleansed itself through the death penalty. 'By the public death penalty the society wished as energetically as possible to rid itself of something which had been untrue to its kind. The public death penalty, therefore, was born of the effort to keep the race pure.' The penalty for deliberate injury to the sexual powers was death; abortion was punished with slavery."

This was linked to politics. They were against equality as shown by the Enlightenment.

The biologically untenable theories of the French Revolution (that is, of the Ages of Enlightenment and of Rousseau) as to the 'equality of all men' ended, as in France, by tearing down all over Europe the last barriers against race mixture.

The differential birth rates could lead to the "nation being utterly impoverished in its capable, gifted, and strong-willed elements."

They were in favour of eliminating the weak and the infirm "That which falls must be pushed as well."

Lenz said:

"It is all the more needful for the European States and their representatives to give heed to the demand made by eugenics, in that the Great War has brought incalculable losses on them through the contra-selection of the most capable. The pick of these stood for four years in the fight, and suffered heavy losses."

"it is the Nordic section in the warring nations that has suffered the heaviest losses"

"The question is not so much whether we men now living are more or less Nordic; but the question put to us is whether we have courage enough to make ready for future generations a world cleansing itself racially and eugenically."

Whilst in prison in 1924, Hitler read a textbook entitled *Outline of Human Genetics and Racial Hygiene* by Fischer and Lenz. He incorporated these ideas into *Mein Kampf* thus his racial policies were ready made for him (Caplan, 1992). People at the time, who read Hitler's writings, dismissed them as the rantings of an ignorant man. Max Planck went to see him when he came to power to reason with him but said:

> "He has lost all contact with reality. What others say to him is at best an annoying interruption, which he immediately drowns by incessant repetitions of the same old phrases about the decay of healthy intellectual life during the past fourteen years, about the need to stop the rot even at this late hour, and so on. All the time, one has the fatal impression that he believes all the nonsense he pours forth, and that he indulges his own delusions by ignoring all outside influences. He is so possessed by his so-called ideas that he is no longer open to argument. A man like that can only lead Germany into disaster." (Medawar & Pyke, 2000)

Unfortunately Hitler meant literally every word he said in *Mein Kampf* which serves as the template for his future work and when he came to power these rantings were turned into the frightful horror of the extermination camps where 10 million Jews, gypsies and other unfortunate people were systematically exterminated.

13.2   Practical implication and implementation

During the First World War, owing to the Allied blockade, there was a shortage of food in Germany. People survived with difficulty, on rations and by buying food on the black market. This did not pertain in mental hospitals where the inmates could not obtain food by such means.

> "During the First World War, 140 234 people died in German psychiatric asylums. Assuming an average peacetime mortality rate of 5.5% per annum, this means that 71 789 people died as a result of hunger, disease or neglect, about 30% of the entire pre-war asylum population. Psychiatrists watched and recorded mortality rates, weight loss and the progress of epidemic diseases, impotent in the face of governmentally decreed wartime rationing." (Burleigh, 1994)

These people died in squalor. The debate on the right to die and negative human worth began in the late nineteenth century. A law sanctioning voluntary euthanasia was drafted in 1913. Ernst Heinrich Philipp August Haeckel (1834-1919), a Darwinist and Monist wrote:

> "...fused the notion of killing as an act of mercy with the crudely materialistic argument that this would save a great deal of public and private money." (Burleigh, 1994)

Instead of being just a theoretical problem, euthanasia became a practical post-war policy but it was not implemented because of objections by the courts and socialists. Germany was impoverished and was paying heavy reparations. It was thought that the State could not afford to bear the burden of mental asylum provision:

"In future an impoverished state will be unable to bear the type of mental asylum provision which developed extensively in most of the regions of Germany before the war."

The number of patients in mental institutions increased dramatically:

"Between 1924 and 1929 the number of psychiatric patients rose dramatically, from 185 397 to more than 300 000. There was no commensurate increase in bed capacity."

It became recognised that:

"...caring for chronic or geriatric patients was a 'luxury that Germany could not afford'. A financially constrained nation was in the process of 'caring itself to death'."

The state psychiatrists recognised that on economic grounds they could not keep large numbers of mentally defective patients in the asylums and they started to practice a very active programme of rehabilitation. Instead of just providing custodial care they were carrying out electric shock and insulin shock therapy and discharging patients into the community (Pross, 1992). German psychiatrists were very systematic and when they followed patients up in the community they recognised that the families of these psychiatric patients showed a higher incidence of mental illness (Burleigh, 2000) and the idea of selectively eliminating these whole families or at least stopping the mentally subnormal from breeding became accepted policy. Whereas before the Nazis it was up to discussion and debate, when the Nazis came to power the machinery was in place to implement this and it became compulsory.

13.3   The Nazis

When the Nazis came to power in 1933 Germany was virtually bankrupt and they said that they could not afford to keep mentally subnormal patients in hospitals ("life unworthy of life"), choosing to spend the money on healthy people instead. When they talked of "life unworthy of life" they meant that the life was unworthy because it did not contribute to the health of that mysterious racial entity, the Volk (Macklin, 1992).

The Nazi euthanasia programme was never intended to benefit the individual but to further the objectives and goals of the "volk", a term that in the abstract means "nation" or "people" but, as the Nazis used it, meant the German Aryan people whom they regarded as inherently superior (Cranford, 1992).

There was therefore a double attack: on people who would contaminate the pure blond Aryan race and there was the idea that mentally subnormal people, schizophrenics etc. would reproduce at a greater rate and this would destroy the race whereas intelligent people who practised birth control had smaller families. Women were encouraged to have large families. In 1938 the Nazis instituted Mothers' Crosses in bronze, silver and gold for women 'rich in children' (Burleigh, 2000).

The Nazis believed that it would be possible to solve social and political problems by biological means. They introduced eugenic legislation: the Law for the Prevention of Genetically Diseased Offspring, which was passed on July 14 1933. This permitted sterilisation of anyone suffering from "genetically determined" illnesses, including feeblemindedness, deafness, blindness, severe alcoholism, Huntingdon's Disease, schizophrenia, severe malformations and insanity. The Nazis' views fell on fertile ground since prior to 1933 psychiatrists had advocated sterilisation but this was on a voluntary basis and the Orthopaedic Surgeon, A. Lorenz, who was the doyen of European orthopaedics recommended that patients suffering from hereditary defects should not be treated (Weindling, 1993). After July 1933 sterilisation was compulsory.

By 1934, 181 Genetic Health Courts and Appellate Genetic Health Courts had been established to administer the Law for the Prevention of Genetically Diseased Offspring. Doctors were required to register all genetic defectives and to undergo training in genetic pathology. In the first year in which the sterilisation law was in operation, nearly 400 000 people were denounced to the Hereditary Health Courts, 75% by their doctors. Only 80 000 cases came before the courts, of which some 62 000 were made the subject of a sterilisation order, of these a little under half were sterilised (Caplan, 1992).

Doctors benefited financially by this and moved from being concerned about sick individuals to being concerned about the health of the nation.

In September-November 1935 the Nuremberg Laws were passed that excluded Jews from citizenship and prohibited marriage or sexual intercourse between Jews and citizens of German or related blood. All prospective marriage partners had to be examined by a physician to prevent 'racial pollution' (Caplan, 1992).

Hitler regarded it as right that the worthless lives of seriously ill mental patients should be eradicated but euthanasia was not legalised until war was declared.

In 1939 Hitler's physician, Theo Morrell, wrote a memorandum framing a possible law: "…for the destruction of life unworthy of life".

On 18 August 1939, the Reich Committee introduced the compulsory registering of all 'malformed' newborn children, echoing both the language and the methods of Morrell's memorandum. In return for a payment of 2RMS (Reich Marks) per case, doctors and midwives were obliged to report instances of idiocy and Down's syndrome, microcephaly, hydrocephaly, and physical deformities such as the absence of a limb or late development of the head or spinal column and forms of spastic paralysis. On 1st September 1939 the Second World War began.

In October 1939 Hitler issued an order allowing German doctors to perform involuntary mercy killings of patients. In the case of children, the Reich Commission examined them for the Registration of Severe Diseases of Childhood. This was intended initially to examine the cases of infants up to the age of three but was extended until the upper age limit was sixteen. Once the selection for euthanasia had been made, the children were transported to a group of specially selected clinics – usually on the pretext of receiving better treatment. Some were killed by having serious respiratory diseases induced, some with drug overdoses, and some were experimented on. Their parents were usually told that they had succumbed to pneumonia.

Pfannmuller, who was the director of an institution, describes how he killed children: "we do not kill …with poison, injections, etc;…No, our method is much simpler and more natural, as you see…" Sudden withdrawal of food was not employed, rather gradual decrease in rations. A lady questioned whether a quicker death with injections would be more merciful (Macklin, 1992).

After the declaration of war when the Germans occupied Poland, Polish patients in mental institutes were gassed at Posen by the German army.

Also in 1939 the euthanasia programme for mentally ill adults started (the orders were backdated to coincide with the start of the war). German psychiatrists regarded these patients who could not be discharged, cured or put to work as liabilities. The money that was being devoted to treating them could be used for the healthy. Specially designated physicians examined questionnaires returned by mental hospitals on each patient. Gassing was done in rooms built to resemble showers. The purpose of elimination was not only to continue the struggle against genetic disease but also to release hospital beds for the war

The euthanasia programme was suspended in August 1941 because of public disquiet and protests by the church, particularly the Bishop of Limburg and Archbishop Galen who preached sermons attacking this policy. The RAF printed Galen's sermons and dropped them as propaganda pamphlets. The original plan had been to eliminate 70 000 patients.

Instead, a second phase started of so-called 'wild euthanasia' so the killing continued in hospitals. It was carried out by special nurses by injections supervised by doctors.

In September 1944 German patients in mental hospitals were killed in Bavaria to make beds available for war casualties. Responsibility for selecting and killing patients was left at this stage to individual doctors in the mental hospitals (Caplan, 1992).

13.4   Gradual extension

The extermination started with the newborn then extended to the age of 3 then to 16. The climate in Nazi Germany was that of selective killing of the mentally or physically abnormal adults, sterilisation to prevent hereditary medical and antisocial diseases, and killing defective children.

It was not just Jews and the physically and mentally deformed that were killed. Killing became a method of treatment for anyone who did not measure up to the norms.

Patients committed to mental hospitals were killed to make room for soldiers. This included people who became distraught in Germany's burning cities who were committed to mental hospitals as "disturbed air-raid victims". (Pross, 1992)

In a 9 February 1942 order "on treatment of soldiers with hysterical and psychogenic reactions" the head of the military medical service, Siegfried Handloser, decreed "War hysterics who cannot be cured of their symptoms through treatment are to be committed to the hospital sections of mental institutions." (Aly *et al*, 1994) 15 000 German soldiers on the Eastern Front, who were suffering from shellshock and deserted, were executed by court martial   (Burleigh, 2000) whereas the Air Force crews were treated in psychiatric units.   Severely injured German soldiers were not treated and subjected to euthanasia (Lifton, 1986).

By the time the war ended only 15% of patients in mental hospitals had survived (Caplan, 1992).

14.   THE DESTRUCTION OF GERMAN MEDICINE BY THE NAZIS

Nazi ideology destroyed German medicine but this was not directed uniquely against medicine – it was part of a much larger Nazi philosophy. The Nazis were hostile to conservative or reactionary bodies like the church and armed forces.   In many ways they were innovative and progressive. Nazi thinking permeated all branches of life and thought.

They introduced the concept of Nazi physics and were opposed to the theoretical physics of Fermi and Einstein who were Jewish so their progressive ideas were not thought worthy of consideration (Heinemann-Grüder, 1994).

Nazi art favoured realistic images of muscular soldiers and supermen whereas the German impressionist/expressionist movement, especially work by Weiss and Gross, showed people to be deformed. This deformity was loathed by the Nazis. Jewish art was thought to be decadent.

Wagner's music was popular. Apart from being a master musician, Wagner was the father-in-law of Chamberlain and a rabid anti-semite. Jewish composers such as Mahler and Mendelssohn were banned and there was opposition to Negro music on racial grounds.

Mendelssohn's statue, which had stood in the front of the Leipzig Gewandhaus, was removed. But that was far from the end of it: Händel's Old Testament oratorios lost their original titles and were Aryanized so that *Judas Maccabeus* turned into *The Field Marshall: A War Drama* or, alternatively, into *Freedom Oratorio: William of Nassau*, the first version rendered by Hermann Stephani the second by Johannes Klöcking. Three of the greatest Mozart operas, *Don Giovanni, Le Nozze di Figaro,* and *Cosi fan tutte*, created a special problem: Their librettist, Lorenzo Da Ponte, was of Jewish origin; the first solution was to abandon the original Italian version, but that did not help: The standard German performing version was the work of the Jewish conductor Hermann Levi. There was a last way out: A new translation into purer, nonpolluted German had to be hastily prepared. The new German translations of Da Ponte's libretti to *Figaro* and *Cosi* were by Siegfried Anheisser, a producer at the theatre in Cologne, and by 1938 they had been adopted by seventy-six German opera houses......the new masters of Austria were astonished to discover that there were Jews in "Waltz King" Johann Strauss's extended family, and his birth certificate disappeared from the Vienna archives. (Friedländer, 1997).

The Nazis were anti-intellectual. They were hostile to Jewish authors and there was a mass burning of Jewish books in 1933.

Nazi architecture was brutal, extolling the Fuhrer principle and intimidating people.

The Nazis introduced their own calendar (Burleigh, 2000).

Jewish scientists could not have their work quoted and Jewish musicians could not have their music played. Their work was considered a threat to traditional German values. Initially discounted by W. Heisenberg and others as crackpot ravings, Nazi racism gradually forced its way into German universities and rapidly took over.

14.1   The role of doctors in the Nazi party

By January 1933 when Hitler came to power 2800 (6% of the total) doctors in the Weimar Republic had joined the Nazi Physicians' League, their trade union. The medical profession became the staunchest supporters of the Nazi regime and 45% were members of the Nazi party. Doctors prospered under the Nazis. They had a higher status and their wages increased because they received fees for the sterilisation. They received jobs in the insurance scheme, university posts vacated by Jews (Proctor, 1992) and when the Jewish General Practitioners had to give up their practices, these were taken over by German doctors.

Doctors were the driving force in much of the Nazi legislation: running courses on racial hygiene, drafting the racial legislation, giving evidence in court (which was so time consuming there was no time for other work) and becoming the bureaucrats and administrators of the medical aspects of the regime.

By the time the war ended more than 38 000 physicians, almost half of all doctors in Germany, had jointed the Nazi party. More than 7% of all physicians were members of the SS compared with less than 0.5% of the general population (Caplan, 1992). It is comfortable and a conventional fallacy to believe that the doctors who did these tasks were isolated and mad and had nothing to do with mainstream life in Germany. This was not the case.

There were also well-trained, reputable and competent physicians and scientists who were ardent Nazis (Caplan, 1992). Those physicians and public health officials, who staffed the camps, murdered the demented and advanced theories of racial hygiene were according to this myth, simply lunatics, charlatans and quacks (Caplan, 1992). They volunteered to work in the camps because of the opportunities for experimentation. Serving in the camps advanced their academic careers, enabling them to carry out research and experiments and to write theses. They were well paid and fed. They made the selections on the ramps at the death camps as to who was to work and who was to be exterminated.

14.2   How the Nazi party influenced treatment

The doctor was to be a Führer of the Volk to better personal and racial health. He was to be a servant of the state and his greatest responsibility was to the health of the state not to the health of the individual patient

In 1935 new regulations were imposed on doctors by a small number of Nazi colleagues. A 'doctor Fuhrer' controlled all doctors and had to report everything back centrally. A two tier system of staggered penalties was introduced. Lower courts issued warnings, assigned demerit points, fines or suspensions. Higher courts ordered striking off. Contracts had to be approved and if a doctor received higher qualifications, these too had to receive approval.

Cases of alcoholism, incurable hereditary or congenital diseases, and contagious diseases such as venereal disease had to be recorded (this information could then be used in the sterilisation programme). To be upgraded doctors had to attend special courses run by Nazi fanatics.

The Nazis exploited the traditional physician-patient relationship. Confidentiality between patient and doctor was eroded by an ordinance in 1935, which stated that a medical secret could be laid bare if the common sense of the people demanded it. As a result doctors became legally obliged to inform on their eugenically infirm patients to the Nazi health authorities. Anyone who dared to oppose Nazi "scientific' racism risk losing their jobs, freedom and even their lives. In March 1942 the Reich Health Leader publicly repeated the regime's desire to establish a 'health file' on every German from the cradle to the grave which again violated the principle of confidentiality.

When the Germans conquered the Netherlands doctors were asked to report on patients and breach confidentiality but the Dutch doctors, to their eternal credit, refused and several hundred were transported to the extermination camps. There was the change in the professional role.

It was planned to nationalise all the doctors and pay them a salary. In August 1944 Himmler said that doctors should be put on fixed salaries and made financially accountable for every day their patients were sick.

The actual treatments were Nazified. They were not based on what was good for the patient but what the state wanted. For example, abortions and sterilisation were banned for normal people but were to be carried out on Jewish people for moderating the race but if you were a healthy German you were not to have an abortion. Similarly with fertility treatment, if you were a Jew you were to be sterilised, but if you were an Aryan and could not have a child, you would be offered fertility treatment. If you were an air force pilot and were needed by the state you got psychiatric help but if you were a German deserter you were shot. So the high-grade people got the best treatment.

In the SS this was taken to a higher degree. All prospective marriage partners had to be examined by a physician to prevent "racial pollution."

The Nazis believed that it was healthy to experience pain.

There was aversion to the concept of institutionalised care so existing clinical facilities were not enlarged. There was a decline in hospital building from the beginning of the Nazi regime so there was increasing pressure on beds. As a consequence, there was a rise in industrial injuries, scarlet fever, typhoid and diphtheria.

14.3   How the Nazis took over

Universities were no longer regarded as ivory towers but became organs of the state. The doctors' trade union movement became an organ of the Nazis and the Neurological/Psychiatric Association was dissolved.

Doctors lost their independence and their responsibility shifted from the individual patient to the state. They had a dual role as executors of a criminal regime (executors on German submarines, selections in the camps) and healers concerned with professional corporate progress, technicians of people's health, charged with preserving civilian and military manpower resources. Medicine served as a disguise for executing people (Proctor, 1992).

As a result of the Editors' Law, passed on October 4 1933, German-Jewish medical scholars were forbidden to publish the results of their research in German books or journals (Kater, 1989). German doctors could not quote work by Jewish authors.

14.4   Natural healers

Promising natural lay healers were channelled into the regular medical student body thereby safeguarding the ideals of New German Healing in a formal academic setting. Quack doctors were allowed to practice and the Nazis decreed that regular doctors should assist registered natural healers at their request. In Britain it was an offence to work with or cover a Quack. Hitler and other members of the hierarchy pursued bizarre forms of natural healing and drug taking under Morrell. This was not unique since it seems to be a trait amongst leaders of countries to fall into the hands of charlatans.

14.5   The attack on the universities

M. Heidegger said: 'The much praised academic freedom will be rooted out of the German university.'

The Nazi movement's calls to restore traditional values to education appealed to the conservative academic establishment, which trained Germany's civil servants. Nazism was enormously popular among students, who eagerly responded to appeals to join the common cause of rebuilding Germany's greatness.

Jews were driven out even before Nazi legislation was introduced.

Hitler said:

'Nowadays the task of the universities is not to cultivate objective science but soldier-like military science, and their foremost task is to form the will and character of their students.'

His idea of a good education was: One that produced a sound physique and a 'good firm character'; scholarship and research produced pacifist weaklings. (Medawar & Pyke, 2000).

In Germany university appointments were state appointments controlled by the civil administration. Prospects for achieving a teaching job in the universities were almost guaranteed by a candidate's membership of the SS and anyone with affiliations to political or religious organisations not aligned to National Socialism were passed by or even dismissed. In Leipzig assistants and medical students agreed to use the Nazi salute. It is estimated that Germany may have lost as many as 40% of its medical faculty to racist fanaticism. Jews and socialists were removed from university posts. It was necessary to be a Nazi to be appointed so second or even tenth rate people were appointed if they were Nazis. Vacancies were filled by enthusiastic Party members (Medawar & Pyke, 2000). Consequently the universities became downgraded.

14.6   Academic standards

There was a specific attack on academic aspects of the universities. There was an emphasis on practical work and natural subjects. Entrance was restricted. Members of the SS were given preference. Jews were not allowed in so the standards of entry were debauched. Time was taken up at the universities for special courses on marching and politics so instead of attending lectures, students were being marched around the countryside getting themselves fitter and so violent were the activities that they broke limbs and consequently lost further time from their studies. The professors were attacked and not allowed to lecture by their students at the outset, if they were Jewish professors, they were booed and shouted down and thrown out. The higher examination, the habilitation examination, was abandoned in some instances and a lower standard was accepted. There was a lack of foreign travel. German doctors and scientists could not attend meetings. There was restriction of interchange of ideas with other countries throughout the Nazi doctrine. Heisenberg wrote:

"The immediate pre-war years or rather what part of them I spent in Germany struck me as a period of unspeakable loneliness." (Medawar & Pyke, 2000).

German scientists could not accept the Nobel Prize because one had been awarded to a Jew. The Austrian physiologist, Otto Loewi, was forced to transfer his Nobel Prize money from Sweden into a Nazi-owned German bank.

German medical students had to show commitment to the National Socialist concepts of health and medicine and their loyalty to the party was regularly monitored. The role of the "Fachschaften" in medical schools was to organise lectures to indoctrinate students with Nazi ideology. Students became accustomed to brutalisation in the classrooms and carried this on when they graduated.

From 1935 both general practitioners and specialists were required to attend training courses every five years run by fanatical Nazi instructors.

14.7 The change in the training of doctors

Jews were excluded from universities. The curriculum was made more practical and new subjects such as racial hygiene were introduced. Students lost time from their studies because they were required to participate in exercise programmes and attend courses on political indoctrination.

14.8 New subjects

The Nazis modified the medical curriculum adding Rassenkunde (race hygiene) and more conventional subjects were gradually squeezed out. They tried to biologize a broad range of social problems including crime, homosexuality, the falling birth rate, the collapse of German imperial strength and the Jewish and gypsy "problems." Endurance of pain was regarded as a mark of character. The Jew was believed to be less able to tolerate pain than the "Aryan".

14.9 Changing the curriculum from academic to practical

Nazi doctors rejected modern "mechanistic" medicine favouring a holistic approach. They were opposed to both institutionalised patient care and specialisation, preferring general practice. The völkisch physicians strove for a return to a preindustrial state, where the forces of nature, rather than synthetic pharmacological products and the technology of a laboratory or operating room, were enlisted to aid the human body in maintaining or recovering its balance. It was their conviction that healing was a craft to be executed on the basis of intuition rather than reason. Applied medicine based on hunches and experience was rated far more highly than theoretical medical science practiced at the universities.

14.10 Shortening the curriculum

Apart from the loss of the curriculum by the introduction of new valueless subjects, when war broke out in 1939 the medical curriculum was shortened by two years. This left little time for the perfunctory dissertation; it had to be done in the second, clinical half or right after the final state examination (Kater, 1989). Disastrous understaffing led to senior medical students being conscripted to the medical corps after provisional final examinations or none at all. These specifically Nazi-trained young doctors entering medical practice in the late 1930s had standards that left much to be desired. Because medical teachers continued to be drafted, professors were kept on well beyond retirement age.

14.11   The responsibility of the individual

It was the citizen's duty to the state to be as fit and healthy as possible. The Nazis put the concept of obligation for health into practice (Pross, 1992). Smoking, drinking, homosexuality and illegitimacy were discouraged but this was practically impossible to implement, as it was too widespread particularly in the Nazi party.

Early research showed that cancer of the bronchus was linked to smoking. The citizen had to exercise, march in the woods and eat a healthy diet. Women were not allowed to wear make-up (Proctor, 1992).

Nazi physicians recognised the importance of a diet high in fruit and fibre. Every German bakery had to produce whole grain bread. Restrictions were introduced on the use of DDT (Proctor, 1992).

15.   EXPERIMENTATION IN THE CAMPS

It was the advent of the inhuman experiments in the camps and the resultant Nuremberg trials that drew the world's attention to the practice of experimentation on human subjects but there is a long history of patients and soldiers being used as subjects for experiments in the late 19th century that would not be accepted today.

Doctors were criticized for treating the poor in hospitals as no better than laboratory guinea pigs. Other vulnerable groups were children and the mentally ill. Doctors in the colonies became notorious for experimenting on native peoples, especially in the concentration camps where sufferers from sleeping sickness epidemics were herded. Scientific medicine became stigmatised as inhumane. The attack on medical science was spearheaded during the 1890s by socialist newspapers, anti-vivisectionists and nature therapists, many of whom combed the medical press for evidence of scientific atrocities. Besides bacteriology, experiments in other surgical and physiological areas were condemned. Examples were the transplantation of cancerous tissue, the deliberate implanting of worms in children, and the injecting of gonococci for the study of the resulting inflammation. The state was criticised for lack of controls on experiments and for the failure to invoke legislation against assault resulting from medical malpractice.

A classic example of protests against human experiments was the scandal over the research by the dermatologist A. Neisser who in 1879 had identified the gonococcus as the cause of gonorrhoea. In 1895, inspired by Behring's successes with anti-diphtheria sera, he injected young prostitutes (the youngest aged 10) with a cell-free syphilis serum in the hope that this would provide immunity.   Instead, the effect was to infect some with syphilis.   In 1898 a scandal erupted over these experiments.   Medical colleagues such as the dermatologist A. Blaschko and the medical historian Julius Pagel rallied to Neisser's aid, as did state officials such as Althoff to whom Neisser owed his appointment.   As had been the case with animal experiments, professors were confident that the state would approve of their work.   Althoff and his medical advisers were a significant lobby in support of the extension of clinical research.   In the event, Neisser received only a formal censure from the state.   Henceforth, he used Java apes for experiments on a state-funded expedition.   In 1905 he was one of the first to observe the syphilis spirochete, and with August von Wassermann he developed a diagnostic test for syphilis based on analysis of blood serum.   Neisser's prestigious supporters in the medical profession and public health administration argued that a certain amount of sacrifice was justified to maintain the forward march of science. (Weindling, 1993).

It is a horrifying omen and paradox that Neisser was himself a Jew.

When the Second World War began human experimentation was rationalised on the grounds that animal experimentation had taken the researcher only so far and better results would accrue only after transfer to humans.

Experimentation in the camps was not just an aberrant performance by demented SS doctors.   The medical profession took the lead and instigated certain aspects of this work.   The doctors were well-qualified, working in collaboration and under the direction of prestigious scientific institutes in Germany, such as the Kaiser-Willhelm Institute who encouraged, formulated and supervised it.   They used material from it and they monitored it.   It was presented at scientific meetings and is still being used.

The pattern of the research followed an aberrant but diabolical logic.   The root causes of the concentration camp experiments were (Katz, 1992):

Obedience to the Fuhrer

The ideology of race

The ideology of science

The ethos of professionalism

The impact of war on soldiers and civilians

15.1   Eugenic work

Much of the eugenic and hereditary work was based on twin studies.   The aim was to populate the world with Aryan stock so there was interest in how to produce multiple births.   This was part of the twin study work carried out by Mengele.   In 1935 Mengele was awarded a PhD entitled "Racial

Morphological Research on the Lower Jaw Section of Four Racial Groups."
He was trained in eugenics and was interested to learn from his twin studies
how the population could be increased.   Much of Mengele's work when he
was infecting children and then executing them seems wild and ill-conceived
but he was trying to see if the infection could modify the twin.   He sent
material back to the Kaiser Wilhelm Institute, which was internationally
renowned for this type of surgery work with many Nobel Prize winners.
F. Sauerbruch was on the Research Review Committee that approved grants
for Mengele's work (Pross, 1992).

Abderhalden showed that the hereditary basis was transferred through
proteins (Weindling, 1993).   He believed that if you could isolate these
proteins then you could work out the basis of hereditary.

Conversely experiments were being carried out to sterilise people by the
use of x-rays and injections.

15.2   Applied work

15.2.1   Survival at sea

Specific work was ordered by the Air Force on survival in the sea, which
was carried out by the camp doctors.   The German Air Force was concerned
that many of their pilots were being shot down in the channel and lost by
hypothermia so experiments were carried out to determine where people
should be reheated quickly or slowly.   Prisoners (not volunteers) were
plunged into freezing cold water and reheated by different means, the one
attracting the most attention was by using women to reheat them.

It was necessary to determine over a longer period the effect of drinking
seawater.

15.2.2   High altitude compression experiments

In order to intercept allied bomber planes, the Germans had to produce
fighter planes capable of flying at high altitudes and experiments were
carried out to enable pilots to be able to withstand such high altitudes.
These were completed by Sigmund Rascher, a scientist, who was under
supervision of the university and the Luftwaffe, at Dachau in May 1942.

15.2.3   Wound experiments

The army was concerned about treating wounds on the Eastern Front so
they were producing fractures and infecting them and then treating them
with different means but there was no control.

A separate series of experiments were carried out after Himmler's deputy, SS Obergruppenfuhrer Reinhard Heydrich, was mortally wounded and there was dispute as to whether he should have received sulphonamide so they produced some gangrenous wounds in camp inmates and carried out experiments on different forms of treatment.

15.2.4   Cholera experiments

There was an epidemic of cholera on the Eastern Front. People were deliberately infected with cholera to assess different forms of treatment.

15.2.5   Surgery

Doctors and medical students came to the camps and carried out operations on healthy (if that term can be used under those circumstances) prisoners, such as gall bladder operations, to learn the techniques. Among the prisoners were doctors who were enlisted to show the visiting Germans how to operate.

15.2.6   Brain and tissue research

Brains of different ethnic types were obtained for research purposes Victims were killed and their brains were sent off to form a museum. Unfortunately these brains are still being used for teaching purposes.

Injections were carried out on individual cells to investigate their structure. It would seem as though the inmates were being injected and then killed so that staining of the different tissues could be seen.

15.3   Presentation of the work

This work was known about and was presented at different scientific meetings. Data on hypothermia studies was presented to 95 physicians in October 1942 at the annual meeting of the Luftwaffe medical service in Nuremberg in December 1942, at a conference of Wehrmacht physicians in Berlin and to a select group of physicians at a meeting in Berlin including Sauerbruch in May 1943. Results of the Ravensbruck experiments were reported at a Congress of Reich Physicians in May 1943 (Caplan, 1992).

There has been much debate, not just about the ethics of this experimentation, but as to whether this work should be used as the data now exists. It is considered that much of it was so badly controlled that it is valueless but some of the high altitude and hypothermia work formed the foundation of our current knowledge.

Doctors believed they were being 'good doctors' because although they were perhaps producing brief suffering of their patients, in the long term, they would create a healthy race. Not one of the doctors or public health officials at Nuremberg pleaded for mercy on the grounds of insanity (Caplan, 1992).

16.   ANTI-SEMITISM

There has been reference to anti-semitism and how different aspects affected Nazi medicine but at this point it is convenient to gather the threads together to show how it was implemented and its effects.

In the eighteenth and nineteenth centuries, there was structured anti-semitism in Austria and the German principalities so that to obtain a university appointment you had to be a German citizen of the Christian faith. Consequently, Jewish doctors could not obtain official appointments. Nevertheless Germany was regarded as having less anti-semitism than Poland, Russia and Hungary and Jews went there, particularly to Berlin, because they could study and experience less anti-semitism. The well-publicised case of Freud, who initially trained in neurology but was unable to secure a position and instead founded psychiatry, is not the only example. Henle, a Jewish convert and Romberg, a Jew, both obtained official appointments. By contrast Remak could not obtain a post and worked in private practice. Oppenheim, the outstanding German neurologist, was not appointed to a university post but received an honorary title. Despite the stipulations of the Weimar constitution:

> "...the stipulation of the Weimar constitution in respect of equality of treatment for *all* German citizens in *all* spheres were unacceptable to great and important segments of the population...on the eve of the Nazi take-over there were still only two Jewish professors in all Bavarian universities." (Vital, 1999)

Jewish doctors had the greatest difficulty in obtaining university appointments and as neurology/psychiatry was not looked upon as prestigious, they gravitated to these fields. As soon as the Nazis assumed power the situation reached its climax with the Enabling Laws. Possession of even a single Jewish grandparent disqualified academics from teaching the German Master Race (Medawar and Pyke, 2000). At Tübingen the number of Jewish faculty members dismissed was distinctly low – for a simple reason: No Jew had ever been appointed to a full professorship at this institution, and there were very few Jews among the lower-ranking appointees (Friedländer, 1997).

Jewish doctors were forbidden, by law, to hold state appointments, university appointments or treat German patients but had to have a degraded title as 'attendants to the sick' and could only treat Jewish patients. Guttmann had to cease his post as first assistant to Foerster at the Wenzel Hanke Hospital. He worked as Director of a Jewish Hospital and at the outbreak of the Second World War fled to the United Kingdom. Bors, who had worked in Czechoslovakia, went to the United States of America. Marburg, who remained the outstanding contributor to spinal injuries in the inter-war years, fled Austria in 1939 and also went to the United States. Schwartz, the urologist to the centre, was also Jewish. Thus Nazism's gift was to expel all these pioneers from the Third Reich, bringing their outstanding training in spinal injury treatment to the Free World, where they were responsible for the development of spinal injury management. These points are amplified in Silver, 2003.

Jews constituted a considerable proportion of the German medical profession. In certain specialities such as neurology and psychiatry there was preponderance. Jews were not allowed to practice as GPs and were driven out of the universities. Civil servants filled all the teaching hospital posts so they were driven out of these.

Jews lost their jobs with the universities. Many of them were brilliant and were Nobel Prize winners such as Paul Ehrlich, Fritz Haber and Otto Warburg. Ehrlich died before the Nazis came to power. Haber was thrown out of his post and died of a broken heart. The case of Warburg is extraordinary since, while under constraints, he carried on working at the Kaiser Willhelm Institute throughout the Nazi period.

Jews could not get fees from insurance companies. They were not allowed to treat German patients. Their property was confiscated. Germans could not treat them. They were not allowed to call themselves doctors. They could not get their work published. They were not allowed to refer to Jewish doctors nor could they treat German patients.

National Socialist student leaders strove to remove both Jewish university professors and Jewish students, who were renown for their examination success and were strong competitors for their jobs in an overcrowded profession. At the University of Frankfurt in 1933 even before any laws had been promulgated German medical students drove out their Jewish fellows, confiscating their student identity cards and chasing them off campus. Many university departments with Jewish staff were closed down. Embarrassingly for the Nazi regime, a large number of civil servants and members of party organisations still consulted Jewish doctors despite being forbidden. They valued the confidentiality of Jewish doctors, fearing that if they visited Nazi doctors they would be denounced to Reich Hereditary Courts. So, in 1934, the Nazi Physicians' League issued a directive admonishing all non-Jewish patients to see only "Aryan" doctors. German physicians persecuted their own Jewish colleagues, for example, by getting their mortgages foreclosed to cause them financial ruin.

Finally in July 1938 Hitler decreed that all Jewish doctors were to be decertified save a few exceptions in areas of dense populations of Jews. Those who were retained were no longer to be regarded as members of the German medical community, lost the designation of "physician" and all memberships of professional organisations. They were known as "Krankenbehandler" (sick-treaters). As the Jews fled the Jewish Hospitals in Leipzig, Mannheim and Breslau were closed by the authorities.

17.   WHY THE GERMANS DID NOT TREAT SPINAL PATIENTS

Initially German neurology was leading Europe and they were doing excellent work in the First World War comparable, if not ahead, of France and the U.K. After the First World War extremely fine rehabilitation work was proceeding in Foerster's Unit and during the war V. von Weisacker set up a Head Injury Unit. Amputees were well rehabilitated and sport was developed as a method of rehabilitation in Germany. Bohler's work demonstrated that results could be achieved.

Despite the high profiles of the Kaiser, who had a withered arm from a birth palsy, and Goebbels, who had a club foot from polio, rehabilitation did not achieve priority in Germany.

Rehabilitation of spinal injury patients demands resources, energy and belief but this thankless task can be achieved. This was contrary to the Nazi philosophy of positive health. They did not believe in scientific medicine and anyone who was deformed or diseased was considered 'unworthy of life'. Selected killing of deformed mental patients and latterly their own soldiers could not lead to meaningful rehabilitation of the spinally injured in Germany.

Economically there is no profit to be made in rehabilitating sick people. In 1962 when Enoch Powell was Minister of Health he gave an address to the Royal Society of Medicine in which he made the following statement:

"It is not the health services which produce wealth, but wealth which makes possible expenditure upon the health services, like all those other expenditures of which neither the purpose nor the outcome is economic benefit but which are the specific mark of a human society and in their elaboration and refinement distinguish a civilised nation from an uncivilised, and advanced culture from a backward one." (Powell, 1962).

Chapter 7

France

1.   INTRODUCTION

The first description of traumatic spinal injury in the French literature was by Ambroise Paré (1510-1598). Nearly a century and a half was to elapse until Jean Louis Petit (1674-1750) and Guillaume Dupuytren (1777-1835), made a clinico-pathological study of traumatic spinal injuries. This was followed, in the first half of the nineteenth century, by the work of Jean-Martin Charcot (1825-1893), Guillaume Benjamin Amand Duchenne de Boulogne (1806-1875) and Charles Edouard Brown-Séquard (1817-1894) when as part of their general neurological studies, they described injuries of the spinal cord, delineated the pathological changes and correlated them with symptoms and signs. They also applied their patho-physiological findings to the treatment of patients with spinal injuries, particularly in investigating the development of pressure sores.

Pierre Marie (1853-1940), a pupil of Charcot who succeeded him at the Salpêtrière continued his work. During the First World War, there were many French casualties with spinal injuries and several spinal units were established to treat them. George Guillain (1876-1961), Jean Camus (1872-1924), J.A. Barré (1880-1967), Jean Lhermitte (1877-1959), Gustave Roussy (1874-1948) Professor Dejerine (1849-1917) and Mme Auguste Dejerine-Klumpke (1859-1927), and Pierre Marie were attendant physicians.

They contributed to the development of treatment and described the early causes of death, the development of heterotopic calcification, pressure sores and the psychological aspects.   They emphasised the importance of meticulous nursing care and of mobilising the patient. The mortality was high. When the war ended, this work ceased. No scientific papers or any record can be found on the treatment of patients with traumatic injuries of the spinal cord in the neurological or orthopaedic literature between the wars and why this should be is a matter for comment.

The occupation of France by Germany in the Second World War led to an end of all medical advances and it is not surprising that there was no recorded work on injuries to the spinal cord. Furthermore, the speed of the German blitzkrieg in May-June 1940 meant that there would have been few military spinal injuries compared with the 1914-1918 trench warfare. It was only in the 1950s when a series of French doctors came to the United Kingdom and learned Guttmann's methods that spinal units were re-established in France.

The work in France was at its most innovative, original and fundamental at the time of Charcot, Duchenne and Brown-Séquard and declined later. By contrast in Britain and the United States progress was gradual and their experience in and after the First World War led to further scientific advances and the development of modern treatment.

2.   THE TREATMENT OF SPINAL INJURIES FROM THE 16TH TO 19 CENTURY

2.1   Ambroise Paré (1510-1590, general surgeon

Paré, a barber surgeon, dominated surgery in France in the sixteenth century, gave the first description of traumatic paraplegia. He worked at the Hotel Dieu, an old charitable foundation, one of the main hospitals in Paris. Paré was an army surgeon under Henri IV and subsequently treated a succession of French kings. His work on war wounds and developing prostheses was revolutionary and was acknowledged by other surgeons. In 1564, he published his Magnum Opus textbook on surgery, *The Works of Ambroise Paré*. It is over a thousand pages long and published not in Latin, but unusually, in French. The English translation (1649) is used for all citations. He made many contributions, in particular on amputations where he used a tourniquet. He discontinued the use of boiling oil to cauterise wounds and used maggots to clean up dirty wounds.

Paré recognised cord compression could occur in vertebral fractures, and lead to paralysis of the bladder so that "the urines and excrements came from them without their will or knowledge" (Paré, 1649). He recommended laminectomy for a patient with a spinal injury, removing the splinters of broken bones, and he used a fearsome Hippocratic apparatus to reduce the dislocation by direct compression with a board.

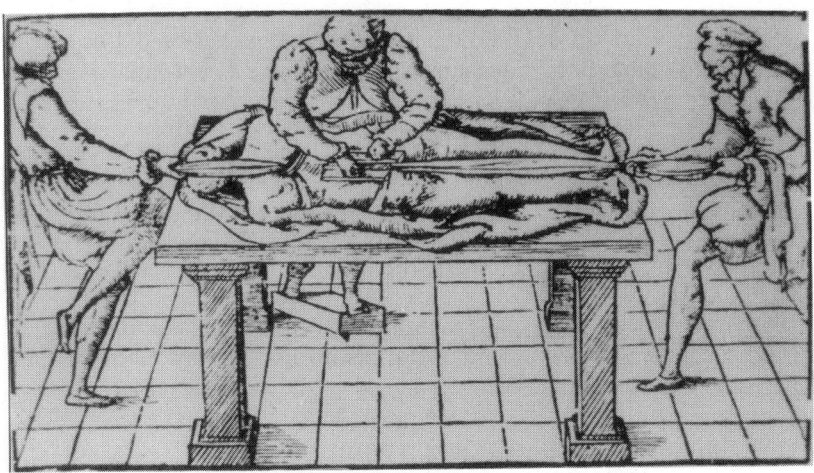

Figure 17. Paré's method of reducing a dislocation by traction. Note the direct pressure with a board (Paré, 1649).

He distinguished between a cord lesion with a bad prognosis and a cauda equina lesion, which could be caused by a fracture of the 'rump' when someone fell heavily on their buttocks which had a better prognosis. This lesion caused weakness of the hamstrings so that the patient could barely flex their knees and as a result of the total flaccidity of the ankle joints the feet could be forcibly flexed towards the buttocks. Paré also described how this fracture of the coccyx could be reduced, by inserting a finger in the fundament (anus). The patient should be kept constipated for twenty days. Clearly patients with low lesions did survive.

Paré made a distinction between the problem of a single vertebra being prolapsed (where the prognosis was poor as the acute gibbus impinged on the cord) and when multiple vertebrae were prolapsed (where the cord would not be so acutely traumatised and where the protrusion was gentler so if the compression was slow, the cord could adapt to the compromised canal). He thought that all spinal curvatures (idiopathic scoliosis) were due to dislocations and he attributed the scoliosis of young girls to habitual malposture. He used a corset or sheet of iron to correct it, and recommended changing the corset every two months. Thus his observations in the 16th century were valuable and far-sighted.

2.2   Dalechamps of Lyons (1513-1588)

Dalechamps did not describe traumatic paraplegia but he did described paraplegia resulting from tuberculosis of the spine two centuries before Percival Pott (1714-1788):

> "These patients are subject to abscesses, which are difficult to cure and point in the loins and the groins. When the back or the neck is displaced, all the parts below loose sensation and movement. If they are displaced in a rounded form, not sharply angulated, the sensation is little or not affected." (Le Vay, 1990).

Nicholas Andry (1658-1747) although credited with the founding of orthopaedics did not mention traumatic paraplegia, but described postural scoliosis and its treatment.

2.3   Jean Louis Petit (1674-1750)

Petit was the greatest French surgeon after Paré. He wrote a book on general surgery (1705), translated into English in 1726. He described traumatic paraplegia as:

> "Giving rise to impossibility in walking, a numbness of the parts that are beneath a dislocation from whence follows instantly or sometimes afterwards a palsy in the lower extremities. The belly becomes bound. The urine is stopped in the first days and afterwards runs involuntary. Then comes mortification and death is not far distant." (Petit, 1726)

He attributed the inability to walk to the bending of the spine and his description of the paralysis prior to Bell gives a very interesting insight to the neuro-physiological concepts of the time.

> "What causes a difficulty of walking is that the compression of the marrow interrupts the course of the animal spirits in the muscles. Of progression, which are sometimes not only weakened, but entirely lose their elasticity in the 21 hours or sooner according to the degree of compression."

He recognised the relationship of incontinence to the paralysis and to pressure sores and described how the weight of the patient lying on his back compressed other parts of the body.

> "Gangrene comes at the spiny epiphyses of the spine's patient...because the patient is always lying upon his back and these parts are compressed by the weight of the body between the bones and the bed whence the blood vessels are depressed there and the humour is stopped. More

because the parts are paralysed and have lost their elastic force and suffer themselves to sink down and cannot stand the compression."

He made the distinction between a complete and incomplete spinal cord transection and described how a dislocation should be reduced 'although incomplete lesion luxations be the most difficult to reduce yet it is less dangerous than the complete one because the marrow is less compressed in one than in the other'. He did not advocate extension and counter traction. He recommended hyperflexion to disengage the locked facets of the vertebral column. Whilst this manoeuvre would relieve the vertebral problem, it would only damage the spinal cord still further. He recommended a full debridement of the pressure sores. He understood the psychological implications to patients and doctors alike and stressed that treatment should still continue despite the bleak prognosis:

> "It remains to this subject that I exhort the surgeons who have such melancholy cases under their cure to have abundance of temper to keep their patients in as proper a position as they can, to lift them often, to visit them often in order to prevent all their wants, to hear their complaints for I dare venture to say there are none greater objects of pity. Besides, they must have their beds provided with a half sheet and an oil cloth both one and the other to keep the bed dry and the skirt in particular so as to turn the patient and place him upon his belly for more convenient dressing of him."

He described a series of cases at all levels: 10 cases of dislocations, 12 fractures of the spine, many of them accompanied by spinal cord injury with post mortem findings. He gave an account of ascending lesion causing death as a result of paralysis of the diaphragm when the phrenic nerves were involved. Much of the description concentrated on the mechanics of injury. In the absence of X-rays he considered that fractures were less prevalent than dislocations. He was aware of the work of Bell and François Magendie (1783-1855). He gave a very interesting account of using a gum elastic catheter to drain the bladder, and a massive abscess in the scrotum, which had tracked to the abdomen. This was no doubt due to a traumatic fistula.

2.4   Joseph-Clement Tissot (1750-1826)

The use of exercises to mobilise the patient was first described by Tissot, who in 1780, published *Medical and Surgical Gymnastics*, a book advocating moving the paralysed parts of the body to 'awaken the weakened parts of the brain'. He, like Paré, recognised that moving the patient regularly could alleviate the risks of pressure sores and renal calculi. He gave a very modern description of pressure sores:

"The weight of the body pressing on the side on which the patient lies results in changes in those parts which are prominent, especially on the coccyx. The pressure, which these parts suffer, soon results in inflammation and gangrene unless care is exercised. These changes come from poorly arranged bed linen, from moisture of putrid discharges, which irritate and erode the skin. The remedy from these conditions we have borrowed from Dr Stephen Hales. It is to change the position of the patient often to avoid the formation of kidney stones, to minimize compression of the parts, to change the linen often and to avoid the bad effects of perspiration and putrid discharge... All those methods will not suffice to restore strength to the wounded. It is also necessary to get them off their beds." (Licht, 1965)

As in other European countries, there was little progress in spinal management in France, until the time of the French Revolution. There were a few institutes for scoliosis where mostly young girls were treated as private patients (Le Vay, 1990). Although traumatic paraplegia was recognised, there was no mention at all of pressure sores or bladder management and presumably, the patients died before such complications could develop.

2.5   Antoine Louis (1764-1792)

Louis was an illustrious surgeon who was one of the three perpetual secretaries of the Royal Academy of Surgeons. The secretaries recorded surgical observations and carried out a synthesis of accepted surgical practice (Brockliss & Jones, 1997). Louis's observations, made in 1774 were published again in 1836. He commented that failure to administer first aid could greatly reduce survival of the injured. He believed that help of the surgeon is always useful and beneficial but he acknowledged that they could not save the patient as it was 'beyond the useful means of our Art' (Louis, 1836).

2.6   Baron Guillaume Dupuytren (1777-1835)

Dupuytren trained in medicine in Paris. In order to become the second surgeon to the Hotel Dieu hospital, he took a competitive examination, writing a thesis on lithotomy. He rapidly became the principal surgeon in Paris. Very hard working, he would carry out a ward round surrounded by students first thing in the morning, he would then teach and in the evening carry out another ward round. Wealthy, very unpleasant and with a disdainful manner, he criticised his colleagues and his rivals.

He did not write a formal textbook of surgery. He gave a series of lectures translated and edited into a book by Professor Le Gros Clark

(Dupuytren, 1846). Thirty pages are devoted to traumatic spinal injury with clinico-pathological studies. Dupuytren first described the anatomy of the vertebrae and their articulation and the importance of the angulation obliquity of the facetal joints in preventing dislocation. The vertebrae become progressively larger from the cervical to the lumbar region. He recognised and made the distinction between fractures of the articular processes, which had a good prognosis (as the cord was not involved) and fractures of the body involving the spinal cord (which were invariably fatal). Dislocation of the atlas upon the axis is discussed as is its mechanism. He stated that a laceration of the cord by the odontoid is not compatible with life.

He pointed out the risks (that others had noticed) of attempting to reduce a dislocation of the cervical spine, because the process of reduction would cause additional compression and stretching of the spinal cord. He recommended accepting the situation as it was.

"It must be admitted that the number and strength of the ligaments which unite the vertebrae together, the almost vertical or slightly oblique facing of their articular processes, and the mode in which they lock into each other, together with the extended surface by which their bodies are connected, and the small amount of motion admitted of between any two, I say it must be admitted that these points combined necessarily render dislocation very difficult. The relative arrangement of the articular processes no doubt constitutes the chief obstacle to dislocation of the vertebrae" (Dupuytren, 1846).

2.6.1   Dislocations of the vertebrae

Dupuytren described five cases of dislocation of the vertebrae, recognising that undue movement of the fractured or dislocated spine caused the lesion to ascend and this was directly the cause of death. When the spinal cord is injured the major trauma occurs at the moment of injury. When the vertebrae are immobilised, the lesion tends to improve. However, if the fracture is allowed to move, particularly in the first few days after injury the cord will be further traumatised and the damaged area will expand laterally and vertically thus leading to a deterioration in the patient's condition..

He attributed the fatality of patients with high traumatic injuries of the spinal cord to the upward extension of the traumatised segment of disorganised spinal cord, so that the origin of the phrenic nerves is ultimately involved and respiratory death follows. His was probably the first account of the dangers of moving a patient with an acute injury of the spine.

There was a thoroughly modern discussion on the propriety of attempting to reduce dislocations where only the articular process in the cervical spine was dislocated.

"Even could such reduction be effected without further injury to the cord, it is reasonable to believe that there would be little or no relief to the symptoms, as illustrated in the operations for fractured spine, which have been uniformly unsuccessful. It is the lesion of the cord at the time of the accident, which appears to be irremediable by surgical interference: perfect rest is the only chance of the patient."

The question was addressed scientifically by remarking that: "the force requisite to effect the desired object would necessarily involve the spinal cord in the tension and would thus complete the mischief which compression had already begun. A late reduction was invariably mortal." The timing and the propriety of carrying out this manoeuvre is still a matter of debate.

Medico-legal implications were discussed as early as 1830.

"Thus the violent extension of the neck of a child or of a feeble or intoxicated person may occasion death. Indeed, instances are recorded in which the first vertebra has been dislocated from the second, in consequence of lifting young children by the head."

He recorded the experimental work of M. Richond who had recourse to a series of experiments on dogs and cats. From these researches he inferred that the lesion of the cord between the first and second vertebrae would cause instant death. When a corpse was found with a dislocation of the cervical spine, the question arose: Was the dislocation found on the dead body effected-during life or after death? Was it done accidentally or intentionally? The mechanism of forced flexion was described and ante-mortem and post-mortem studies carried out. There was no aversion to furthering knowledge by practical experiments on patients.

The famous Paris hangman assured Louis, the illustrious secretary of the Royal Academy of Surgery, that he could cause very speedy death by twisting the body round when the head was fixed, and that life was extinct when a remarkable flaccidity succeeded the general rigidity. The distinction was thus made between strangulation which can cause a slow death lasting over half an hour and is the basis of people being hung, cut down, recovering and subsequently living a normal life, as opposed to a hanging by large drop through a trap door when the neck is broken causing a fracture of the atlas and a high cord section leading to instantaneous death. The vertebral column is so firmly knitted together, that great violence alone can separate it. He concluded that a dislocation could only have occurred during life if there was discoloration of the face, dullness of the eyes, general paralysis (muscular relaxation), congestion of the internal organs, especially of the heart and lungs.

2.6.2   Fractures of the vertebrae

Dupuytren described three patients with incomplete lesions of the spinal cord who survived the initial accident.   After bloodletting, two recovered; one died 45 days later, and a cyst of the cord was found at post mortem. All the patients had gangrenous pressure sores over the sacrum.

Dupuytren advanced our understanding of spinal injuries in many ways. By seeing the patients twice daily, he categorized their clinical conditions, made clinico-pathological correlations of the relation between the anatomy of the spinal column and the pathological changes within the spinal cord, described the causation of pressure sores, and carried out experimental work on spinal column trauma. However, he did not discuss management of the bladder nor how to prevent pressure sores.

His management of the fracture and of the spinal cord damage was centuries ahead of other practitioners.   Many of the fundamental principles of treatment were recognised by him, in particular personal supervision of the patient twice a day.   He was responsible for the patient's care and described the dangers of moving recent fractures.   He was against operative intervention and realised the dangers of trying to treat a unifacetal dislocation, relating the dangers of manipulation to traction on the cord. Such knowledge in the absence of a radiograph let alone Computerised Tomography scanning or Magnetic Resonance Imaging is remarkable.

3.   THE FOUNDERS OF MODERN NEUROLOGY

Whilst the rest of Europe were still discussing sterile ideas (Sigerist, 1943, Porter, 1997), French doctors were teaching at the bedside and making clinico-pathological correlations from autopsies and experiments on animals and humans (Haymaker and Schiller, 1970).

Charcot and Brown-Séquard made fundamental contributions.   They described spinal cord diseases, particularly traumatic injuries of the spinal cord, and delineated treatment.   In contrast, Duchenne did not have any hospital beds but his examination and experimentation on the patients was the basis of the present clinical examination of the nervous system.   Just as Foerster and Head delineated the dermatomes which we use every day in clinical examination, Duchenne's description of the nervous system and its role in controlling motor function and the activities of the individual muscles set out the principles on which neurological examinations are based today. The men who established the modern practice of neurology, Charcot,

Brown-Séquard and Duchenne, were not aristocrats, most were self-made men who had to fight their way to the top. Charcot was the son of a carriage maker, Brown-Séquard and Dupuytren were poor orphans and Duchenne was from a sea faring family (Haymaker & Schiller, 1970).

The school of French neurology made a quantum leap forward. Magendie founded experimental medicine and vivisection was taking place. 'Why think when you can experiment' Claude Bernard (1813-1878), (Haymaker & Schiller, 1970). They all stressed how vital it was to look at patients and experiment.

3.1   La Salpêtrière

The birth and development of French neurology are inseparable from the name of the Salpêtrière as it was the centre for Charcot's scientific interests.

Charcot opened a new chapter in the medical history of the Salpêtrière when he became chief of the medical service in 1862. His work greatly contributed to the Salpêtrière's international renown to this day (Guillain, 1959).

3.2   Jean Martin Charcot (1825 -1893)

Charcot became chef de clinique in the faculty of medicine from 1853 to 1855 and medecin des hopitaux de Paris in 1856. Initially, he was a general physician and his first papers were on diseases of the elderly and on gout. Charcot was appointed Medecin de l'Hospice de la Salpêtrière in 1862, a great asylum holding a population of 5000 people. At that time, neurology did not exist as a separate discipline and there were no research facilities but Charcot immediately remedied this by establishing a research laboratory (Guillain, 1959).

In 1881, Charcot became the first professor of neurology in the world. He instituted new teaching methods and appointed pathologists and psychiatrists to the service. Over a period of eight years, he described many diseases of the nervous system and founded modern neurology. He made a great contribution to the treatment of spinal injury.

He saw the necessity of obtaining autopsies to correlate clinical science with pathological anatomy (Owen, 1971). His lectures and clinical demonstrations are legendary.

3.2.1 Charcot's specific contribution to our understanding of spinal injury management

3.2.1.1 Pressure sores

Charcot made the first scientific analysis of pressure sores by full description of the pathogenesis of sores in diseases of the spinal cord and of the nervous system (Charcot, 1877). His work was seminal, and as it has either been ignored or misquoted it is important to study his concepts in detail. He stressed that the causation of the sore in cerebral and spinal cases was the same, that anaesthesia of the paralysed part was not the sole cause, that the patients with incomplete lesions also acquired sores, that rapid atrophy of the tissues contributed, as did immobility. He also recognised the role of pressure but considered it secondary. He tried to alleviate pressure by turning the patients regularly, the first recognition of its value. Sores could appear in two days and carried an ominous prognosis, and indeed they were called 'ominous' sores.

"When acute bed-sore appears under the influence of a lesion of the spinal cord, it shows itself in the very great majority of cases in the sacral region and consequently above and internal to the chosen seat of eschars of cerebral origin. Here it occupies the median line and extends symmetrically on either side, towards the adjacent parts. It may, indeed happen that only one side will be affected, in the case, for instance, where a lateral half of the cord is alone engaged then the cutaneous lesion frequently shows itself on the opposite side of the body from the spinal lesion."

"The influence of attitudes here plays an important part. Thus it is customary when the patients are so placed as to repose on the side, during part of the day to find, besides the sacral eschar, vast necrosive ulcerations developing on the trochanteric regions. It is also common enough to see, contrary to what happens in cerebral cases, that the different parts of the paralysed limbs which are exposed to even slight and brief pressure, as the ankles, heels and inner surface of the knees, present lesions characteristic of an acute bed-sore. Eschars may also show themselves, but indeed very rarely, on a level with the apex of the scapula, or over the olecranon process. Speaking generally, we may say that the spinal lesions, which produce acute bedsores, are also those which give rise to rapid muscular atrophy and to other disorders of the same class. The almost simultaneous development of these different consecutive affections makes it seem probable, already, that they have a common origin." (Charcot, 1877)

These pressure sores became infected and dangerous, and commonly gave rise to fever in the acute stage and relapsing fever in the chronic stage. Infection could spread and disseminate septic emboli. Thus he acknowledged that sores are always infected. He made minute descriptions of the superficial vesicular eruption and of the underlying tumorification and cellulitis of the tissue. He was aware of the dangers of maceration of the skin caused by continuous seepage of urine, which he tried to avoid by means of intermittent catheterisation. He noted that paralysis of the sympathetic nervous system could give rise to hyperaemia and a raised peripheral temperature of the tissues, but he did not believe that this retarded healing provided the animal or patient was fit; He also demonstrated the role of infection.

> "...there are circumstances in which, contrary to the usual rule, local nutrition may receive a serious blow from the mere fact that a part has been withdrawn from vasomotor innervation. This happens as experiments attest when the whole organism has been subjected to potent debilitating causes. Thus a vigorous animal has long had the greater sympathetic nerve divided on the side of the neck: nevertheless, no injury has been experienced in the parts corresponding to the distribution of the divided nerve. But let the animal fall sick or be deprived of food then the scene changes immediately and we see, says M. Claude Bernard, an inflammatory phenomenon ensue in that side of the face which corresponds with the experimental section. On that side, even without the intervention of any external agent whatever, the conjunctiva and pituitary membrane rapidly begin to suppurate. In man, the same concurrence of circumstances ought necessarily to determine effects analogous to those observed in animals. And we may indeed question whether some of our trophic derangements are not really produced in this manner. Such is, perhaps, the case as regards the acute bedsore of apoplectic patients. Here, in fact, the general condition is most unfavourable and the gluteal eschar occupies precisely that side of the body, which on account of the motor paralysis presents a relative elevation of temperature evidently connected to the vasomotor hyperaemia." (Charcot, 1877)

It is the role of trophic nerves that is most widely misquoted and misunderstood, and Charcot interpreted it in the following words:

> "...before adopting a theory which cannot subsist without calling out a whole system of nerves whose existence is as yet problematical, it is necessary to make sure, by every means, that it is really impossible to explain the phenomena, the interpretation of which is required, by appealing to the properties of the different nerves already known. We

must take care not to infringe the axiom of Logic, *'Haud multiplicanda entia absque necessitate'* ('One must take care not to multiply more entities than necessity dictates.') Now, the vasomotor theory being eliminated, there yet undoubtedly remains much to be done from this point of view." (Charcot, 1877)

3.2.1.2   The Relationship of symptomatology with the vertebral lesion

Paré had described the different prognosis of acute angulation of a single vertebral fracture but Charcot took this study further by studying the relationship between the spinal cord symptoms and vertebral fractures. Paralysis in Pott's disease is not related to the severity of the angulation because paraplegia from Pott's disease could occur without any trace of deformity. By contrast, the spine could present the most extraordinary deformities yet the cord remained intact.

Charcot considered in detail slow compression of the cord and posed the question as to whether the subsequent paralysis was due to direct pressure from the vertebra or was secondary to impairment of the blood supply, a long-standing question that is still pertinent. Paraplegia could be painful when the peripheral nerves were involved (Charcot, 1889).

3.2.1.3   Bladder function

Charcot distinguished between different types of paralysis of the bladder. In an upper motor neurone lesion, the reflexes were preserved and detrusor contractions occurred, whereas in a lower motor neurone the bladder was atonic. This is an original and thoroughly modern observation (Charcot, 1881).

The nerves that cause the bladder to contract originate in the crura cerebri. The function of the bladder governs the morbidity and mortality of the patient hence the importance of understanding the anatomy and physiology of bladder control. Charcot first described the anatomy of bladder control by making the important distinction that if the lesion was above the 3rd, 4th and 5th sacral nerve, reflex contraction may occur. If the lesion was lower, there was no reflex arc, the sphincter was paralysed and urine then incessantly dribbled out, drop by drop, because the bladder muscles no longer met any obstacle (Charcot, 1877).

3.2.1.4   Haematomyelia and Irritation of the spinal cord

Charcot worked closely with Duchenne and they pointed out that following spinal cord irritation there was a diminution of electrical contractility in the muscles of the paralysed part of the body (Charcot, 1877).

3.3   Guillaume Benjamin Amand Duchenne de Boulogne (1806-1875)

Whilst a general practitioner in Boulogne, Duchenne became interested in electro-physiology, a concept first developed by Magendie. He stimulated the orbital branches of the 5th cranial nerve with fine platinum needles. While testing one of his patients, Duchenne found it was unnecessary to pierce the skin to stimulate muscles as this could be achieved by two cutaneous electrodes after suitably preparing the skin. He built an electric shock apparatus and armed with this equipment arrived in Paris. Charcot acknowleged Duchenne as his master though they learned from each other. They were close personal friends and Charcot gave him facilities at La Salpêtrière. With Charcot's support, he pursued his studies on the action of the muscles of the human body by studying other doctors' patients, following them from clinic to clinic and to their homes (Poore, 1858; Haymaker & Schiller, 1970).

He studied patients with nervous diseases, experimented on recently amputated limbs and animals, and carried out animal dissections. He observed not only the superficial easily palpable muscles of the extremities but also those of the trunk and diaphragm. His work on the diaphragm was a most beautiful example of simple experimentation linked with careful observation.   There had long been controversy as to the action of this muscle.   Clinically, it was obvious that the chest expanded during inspiration, and yet when an animal was eviscerated and the diaphragm examined directly, the chest was sucked in by the diaphragm (Silver, 1971).

Duchenne resolved this problem by showing that the diaphragm was indeed an inspiratory muscle but that it expanded the chest only when it was in normal relationship with the abdominal contents. His work was published under the title *The Physiology of Movement* (1855). He showed how each muscle of the body could be examined clinically, how injuries to different nerves led to paralysis, and how muscles could contract synergistically and reciprocally.

Duchenne's work was the foundation of the examination of the individual muscles without which any orthopaedic or neurological examination would be impossible.

He discovered that extension and flexion of a joint could only be achieved by the combined action of muscles. He noticed that splints stop the joints from moving and used elastic cords and springs to emulate the action of the muscles in paralysed limbs.

He used muscular prostheses to:

- Supply the individual voluntary action of the palsied or wasted muscle
- Restore or facilitate natural movement

- Prevent or overcome deformities of joints by balancing the tonic forces, which control the normal relations of the articular surfaces.

He realised that the use of springs and elastic cords was not appropriate in the case of contractures and that rigid equipment should be used to prevent deformities. He used elastics or springs to extend the fingers of tetraplegic patients and also made apparatus to use on the lower limbs and correct saddleback and spinal curvatures. He noticed that women from Boulogne had a tendency to have potbellies after pregnancy. This is due to the development of the belly during pregnancy, and the looseness and weakness of its walls after delivery; so that in women with slight lumbosacral curve, the abdominal wall by its force offers more resistance to the development of pregnancy, and it recovers and remains firm and tense even after many pregnancies. Duchenne's approach in designing appliances was to observe and reproduce nature as closely as possible and he was a forerunner in this respect (Duchenne, 1855).

Despite the importance of this work nothing comparable has been written since. He received scant recognition at the time in France. In Germany, he was honoured and his book translated by Wernicke in 1895. His work was not translated into English until 1949 (Silver, 1971)!

Duchenne was influenced by Sir Charles Bell. It would seem that physicians and research workers of the time lived in a more leisured age, had more time for the philosophical side of their natures to develop and just as Bell wrote a book of *Essays on the Anatomy of Expression in Painting* (1806), Duchenne also attempted the difficult task of analysing the movement of the face. Duchenne had difficulty in obtaining satisfactory autopsies on the patients whom he studied because he had no hospital appointment. He showed that the lesion in Tabes dorsalis was in the posterior and lateral columns of the spinal cord and that weakness was due to sensory ataxia and not paralysis of the muscles. He correctly located the lesion in the spinal cord and not in the cerebellum. In poliomyelitis he demonstrated that the lesion was in the anterior horn cells and not in the muscles, as believed at that time. He pioneered and performed the technique of muscle biopsy. He wrote a short section on electrotherapy and paralysis from a purely neurophysiological aspect. However, there is a description in an obituary notice that to everyone's amazement he was able to make paraplegics stand. The circumstances are obscure and it is not specified if he used electro stimulation (if so, it would be the first description of practical application of functional electrical stimulation) or by physiotherapy alone or using an apparatus. Whichever method he used, it was extraordinarily pioneering.

His work on electrical stimulation of the muscles of paralysed patients was the trigger (Duchenne, 1872), determining the points of election where stimulation could produce contraction of the muscle enabling a paraplegic to stand some 150 years ago. This public demonstration excited crowds and were the first experiments leading to today's practice of functional electrical stimulation (Duchenne Obituary, 1875).

As a result of his industry, excellent clinical observation and original research work, Duchenne gradually gained international recognition and success in private practice, although he was never given an official appointment to a hospital in Paris (Haymaker and Schiller, 1970). It has been said that he founded no school but this is not true. He wielded a great influence and numerous doctors, including Foerster, the outstanding European neurologist between the wars, were profoundly influenced by his observations. Samson Wright (1899-1956), the influential teacher of physiology at the Middlesex hospital before and after World War II stressed that the only neurology textbooks needed were Sherrington's *Integrative Action of the Nervous System* (1906) and Duchenne's *Physiology of Movement* (1855) (personal communication, 1950).

His down to earth methods brought a breath of fresh air into clinical practice. With no patients of his own, he nevertheless saw spinal cases and described the loss in function electrically, and how the muscles could be examined. His methodology is still used today by all neurologists. Just as Head and Foerster delineated the dermatomes and segments on the sensory side, so Duchenne delineated the motor segments. He and Charcot founded the methodology of clinical neurological examination, the essential initial evaluation of a patient after spinal injury.

3.4   Charles Edouard Brown-Séquard (1817-1894)

, As a contemporary of Charcot and Duchenne, it is appropriate to consider him amongst the French neurologists. He worked in dire poverty for his MD thesis, with no facilities of his own, working in the laboratory of Dr Martin-Magron, an extraordinary achievement.

In 1859, he was one of the first consultants at the National Hospital, Queen Square, London and remained there for three and a half years. He left to become Professor of physiology and pathology of the nervous system at Harvard College. He resigned in 1867 and became Chargé de Cours in experimental and comparative pathology at the Faculty of Medicine in Paris. Not being a French citizen, he did not achieve the chair. He relinquished his position in 1872 and drifted between France and the United States of America. Eventually, in 1878 with the death of Claude Bernard, he returned to Paris, became a French citizen and was appointed Professor of Medicine at the Collège de France, a position he held until his death (Haymaker & Schiller, 1970; McHenry, 1969).

3.4.1 Brown-Séquard's specific contribution to our understanding of spinal injury management

In 1840, while still a medical student in Paris, he described the effects of sectioning the spinal cord. The first part of his doctoral thesis (Brown-Séquard, 1846) involved the study of reflex movements in frogs and provided an unequivocal account of spinal shock at about the same time (if not before) Marshall Hall (1790-1857) gave the phenomenon its designation (Aminoff, 1993). The second part was concerned with the functions of the columns in the spinal cord, and described the effects of selective lesions in different part of the cord in different animal species. At that time, it was believed by Bell and Magendie that all sensation travelled up the posterior columns (Aminoff, 1993). However, Brown-Séquard found that the posterior columns were not the main pathways taken by sensory fibres. He showed that transverse section of the posterior columns did not produce sensory loss but increased sensation to cutaneous stimulation distal to the lesion. Other experiments indicated that the sensory fibres traversed and decussated in the cord's central grey matter. Lateral hemisections caused hyperaesthesia on the same side with sensory loss on the opposite side. When he cut the cord at two different levels on opposite sides, the second lesion caused sensation to be lost on the side that was originally hyperaesthetic. He then carried out longitudinal sections on the cord at different levels. Brown-Séquard furthered his investigations by carrying out clinical observations of patients. In patients with unilateral cord lesions, he observed contralateral loss of sensation but preservation of power below the level of the lesion. This has all been confirmed by subsequent clinical observations and the lesion is known eponymously as Brown-Séquard lesion. Brown-Séquard also emphasised that different fibres mediate different sensory modalities, touch, pain, temperature and sense of muscle contraction (Aminoff, 1993).

3.4.2 Criticism

Brown-Séquards' work was criticised and his conclusions concerning the sensory pathways in the cord met much resistance. He requested an investigative committee, which was formed by the Société de Biologie in Paris, with Paul Broca as chairman and Claude Bernard and E. Vulpian, among the members. Broca was an admirer of Brown-Séquard and the committee reviewed his work, repeated certain experiments and came out in strong support of him:

"The doctrine (that sensory fibres travel in the posterior half of the cord, and the motor fibres in the anterior half), so seductive and widely accepted, is only one more deception...whose debris is scattered on the grounds of history. The beautiful experiments of Mr Brown-Séquard have just brought down forever this well-cemented edifice, the foundation of which was laid by Charles Bell and the last stone by M. Longet. It is indeed true that appearances are often misleading.... For a long time, as you know, our colleague has studied without a break the functions of the cord and six years ago, he communicated to you his first work on the subject. But minds were so biased in favour of the doctrine of Charles Bell and the first work of M. Brown-Séquard was received with a certain disbelief and received only passing attention..." (Aminoff, 1993)

3.4.3   Vasomotor function

Brown-Séquard complemented Claude Bernard's discovery of the vasomotor nerves. He was the first to show that stimulation of the cervical sympathetic in the rabbit caused blanching of the ear. As a result of these studies, he developed an interest in the influence of these nerves upon nutrition (Haymaker & Schiller, 1970). These experiments were also carried out in desperate circumstances in his apartment where his animals were housed. He worked all hours of the night and day and finally fell seriously ill from an infected wound sustained in the dissecting room.

3.4.4   Role of pressure in the development of pressure sores

Like Charcot he studied the aetiology of pressure sores. In 1853, he showed that in experimental animals with paraplegia, préssure sores could heal and be prevented, if the skin was not subjected to periods of sustained pressure, thus establishing that pressure sores were not directly related to the neurological damage.

Brown-Séquard was an innovative, elegant experimenter and it is extraordinary how he managed to do the technical feats of operating upon animals and keeping them alive for many months afterwards. In the early days, he worked virtually single handed in great poverty. His experiments upon pressure sores are unique, and a most beautiful example of his work. He devised a control trial (an achievement in itself). Both sets of animals were paralysed but only those subjected to pressure developed pressure sores.

"The frequent occurrence of certain pathological changes after section of the sciatic nerve in Mammals has been cited as a proof of the dependence of the nutritive operations upon nervous agency. I think the following experiments give evidence against that doctrine. I have divided the sciatic nerve in a number of rabbits and guinea pigs, and placed some of them at liberty in a room with a paved floor, whilst I confined the others in a box, the bottom of which was thickly covered with bran, hay and old clothes. In a fortnight, the former set exhibited an obviously disordered action in the paralysed limbs; claws were entirely lost; the extremities of the feet were swollen; and the exposed tissues were red, engorged, and covered with fleshy granulations. At the end of a month, these alterations were more decided, and necrosis had supervened in the denuded bones. On the other hand, in the animals confined in the boxes, no such injuries had accrued. And although some of them, have been kept living for four, five and even six months after the division of the sciatic nerve, no alteration whatever has appeared in the palsied limbs except atrophy. In these cases a portion of the nerve had been cut off, so that reunion was nearly impossible and did not take place. Experiments made on pigeons have given the same results. It is obvious from these experiments that the pathological changes which occur after the section of the sciatic nerve do not proceed directly from the absence of nervous action, but that they are consequent upon the friction and continual compression to which the paralysed limbs are subject, against a hard soil, owing to the inability of the animal to feel or avoid it. In similar experiments made on frogs, I found that no alteration took place, except when water penetrated through the wound, under the skin, and between the muscles." (Brown-Séquard, 1852)

He showed that it was not the loss of sensation that caused sores because burns, wounds and ulcers existing in paralysed parts after the section of their cerebro-spinal nerves, were cured as quickly and as well as those in sound parts. He reaffirmed this by further experiments:

"After the complete transverse section of the spinal cord in mammals or birds, I have found that the ulcerations, which take place around the genital organs, do not result directly from the absence of nervous action. One of the causes of these ulcerations is continued pressure, and another cause is the continual presence of urine and faeces." (Brown-Séquard, 1852)

He then looked at the deleterious effects of urine on the formerly unprotected skin showing that it was the urine alone which caused pressure sores, because urine was dried and then washed off in a further control experiment, no sores developed.

"My opinion is well proved by the following experiments: -

1st. I have put, three or four times a day and for many days, a certain quantity of urine on the posterior part of the neck, in the neighborhood of the scapulae, upon guinea pigs. Before a week elapsed, the skin at the place acted on by the urine had lost its hair and epidermis. After a week more there was an ulceration in the skin, and ten or twelve days later the skin was destroyed, and there was an ulcer with a very bad aspect. This fact proves how powerful is the action of urine on the skin.

2d. On guinea pigs, upon which the spinal cord was cut in the dorsal region, and on pigeons, upon which the spinal cord was destroyed from the fifth costal vertebra to its termination, I have found that no ulceration appeared when I took care to prevent any part of their bodies from being in a continued state of compression, and of washing them many times a day to remove the urine and faeces.

3d. In cases where an ulceration had been produced, I have succeeded in curing it by washing and preventing compression.

4th. I have found that in animals having the spinal cord cut across, every kind of wounds or burns were cured as quickly as in healthy animals." (Brown-Séquard, 1852)

3.4.5   Management of the spinal cord following injury

Brown-Séquard devoted a whole section to the implication of his researches for the management of spinal injuries. The controversy between the views of Astley Cooper who favoured operation and Bell who was opposed to it was and is still today a very live issue. Brown-Séquard discussed this in physiological terms and recommended carrying out the decompression by trephining of the spine. It had been suggested that laying bare the spinal cord was a dangerous procedure but by his meticulous experiments on animals as a medical student, he showed that exposure of the spinal cord to air was not dangerous so that operations on patients was feasible. Trephining might help because it was believed that death after a fracture was due to pressure causing irritation or excitation of the cord. Trephining could thus allow reunion of the spinal cord, which would allow function to return and the removal of some parts of the vertebrae would be followed by production of new bone.

Of particular interest is his review of operations at that time. He describes a remarkable operation done in 1832 by an Italian surgeon, A. Mercogliana, who removed the body of the third cervical vertebra through the throat leaving the spinal cord exposed. The patient had an ulcerated throat. He had no trouble whatever in the function of his nervous centres and recovered (Brown-Séquard, 1860).

Brown-Séquard gives the cause of death after a fracture of the spine. 'When the spine is fractured high up, if the spinal cord is crushed death occurs instantaneously after a very short time in account of a cessation of respiration and of a peculiar influence on the heart by the vagus.' (Brown-Séquard, 1860)

Like Charcot he was aware that in paraplegics, who had lesions of the sympathetic, the unopposed action of the vagus caused slowing of the pulse. He postulated that the cord could regenerate. Unfortunately, his farsighted observations have not been substantiated in this instance. He had appreciated the danger of immobilising people in bed, saying that the muscles would become weakened and he recommended establishing an electrical and massage room when he was a physician at Queen Square. He describes at considerable length acute myelitis. He recommended various forms of drugs to improve the blood supply to the cord and for the treatment of pressure sores 'to prevent the formation of sloughs, or to cure them when formed, and to prevent other alterations of nutrition in the paralysed parts'. He was already formulating the doctrine 'prevention is better than cure'. He suggested direct application of ice to the sores by putting ground up ice in a bladder and applying this directly to the sore (Brown-Séquard, 1861).

His clinical observations foresaw the work of Frenkel in that he recognised that when the posterior columns were damaged, it would give rise to a paralysis due to the patient's inability to recognise his limbs although motor power was preserved. So long as the patient could see his limbs, he could use them.

He gave the first fascinating description of phantom limbs seen in paraplegic patients. This has been denied for many years in the case of amputees.

"Sensations of cold or of heat, of touch (formication, tickling, pressure, tightness) of pain (pins and needles) and also sensations arising from muscles, and giving the idea that the limbs are in a different position from that in which they really are – in fact, all the sensations that pressure or some other cause of irritation may produce when applied to the ulnar or the sciatic nerves." (Brown-Séquard, 1861)

Charcot, Duchenne and Brown-Séquard's contribution was to delineate the function and structure of the spinal cord. They developed these ideas and applied them to the aetiology of pressure sores and were the first to show how pressure sores could be related to the different components: sympathetic innervation, somatic innervation, lack of movement and pressure. They described how pressure sores could be prevented and the bladder managed but there is little detailed description of how the patients should be treated.

Apart from two cases described by Dupuytren, there is no account of patients being discharged home. There is no mention in Dupuytren, Charcot or Brown-Séquard's work of turning the patient or of supervision or training of the nursing staff. The only successful and systematic spinal injury management appears to have been by Wagner in Germany.

3.5   Pierre Marie (1853-1940)

Marie worked with Charcot after being his pupil at the Salpêtrière and eventually succeeded him. He provides a link between the classic neurology of Charcot and the modern day because he died as recently as 1940. In his 511 pages long textbook on spinal cord disease (Marie, 1895), there is no description of traumatic spinal injuries. With the advent of the First World War, he contributed to many aspects of spinal injury management and virtually all the people who wrote on the subject paid tribute to Pierre Marie. Cushing upon meeting him at a scientific meeting in France during the First World War described him as 'A dear old man'. It is relevant to discuss Marie's contribution to spinal injury management in the First World War.

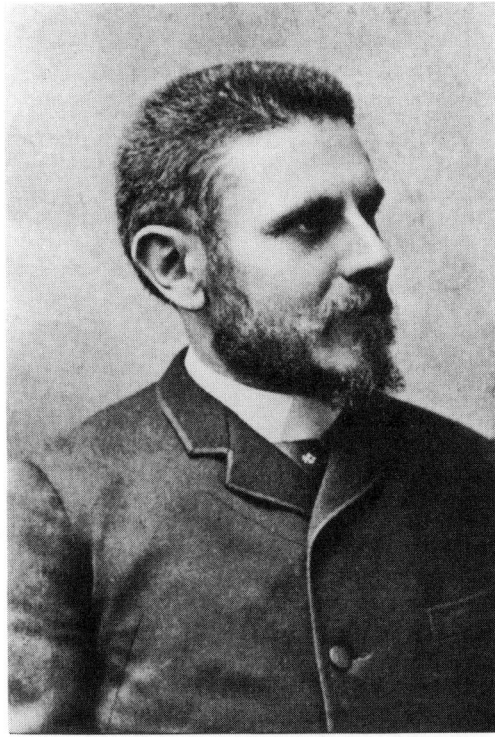

Figure 18. Pierre Marie (1853-1940) (McHenry, 1969).

4.   THE FIRST WORLD WAR (1914-1918)

4.1   Introduction

Just as with other belligerents, there were many French soldiers with spinal injuries during the First World War. A spinal injury seldom occurs in isolation and in war time where wounds are caused by missiles such as shrapnel, bone debris, bullets, and shell splinters, or mine explosions and land slides, the soldiers inevitably had intercurrent injuries, of the chest, abdomen, and skull and many died before they could arrive at treatment stations. French doctors recognised the prime importance of early transfer of the patients to spinal centres, the danger of sepsis from pressure sores and acute ascending infection from the bladder. It is not surprising that there was a high morbidity and mortality from these complications because even 25 years after setting up his superb unit, Ludwig Guttmann reaffirmed:

"Infection of the urinary tract resulting in chronic pyelonephritis resulting in renal failure was still the main killer of sufferers from spinal cord injury or disease." (Tribe & Silver, 1969)

4.2   Literature

There is a rich French literature on spinal injury in the First World War, in particular, a book by Roussy and Lhermitte devoted to wounds of the spine and cauda equina (1918). It is authoritative, cites more than 100 papers including some from Germany also written during the war and comparable to the British Medical Research Council publication.

Ten papers have been analysed in detail (Table 6).

The two papers by Bellot, and Dejerine and Jumentié do not refer to overall treatment but describe specific conditions associated with spinal injury. A meta-analysis of these ten papers provides an overall picture of French spinal injury management, comparable to British papers. The striking contrast is that French papers detail day-to-day management but make no statistical analysis whilst the British papers produced statistical analysis with few details of the clinical management.

The French with their great tradition of bedside neurology recorded striking clinical descriptions. They were more concerned with pressure sores, early transfer to specialised units and the general well being of the patients. The British, placed great emphasis on bladder management, performed fundamental physiological research, suggested alternative treatments, and were also concerned with operative management of the injured spinal column and cord.

Treatment is listed in Table 6 in decreasing order of importance and will be discussed in that order.

Table 6. Review of the French literature

Principles of treatment	Pierre Marie	Mme Dejerine & Ceillier (2 papers)	Camus, Couvreur, Hugonet (3 papers)	Calot	Lhermitte/ Claude/ Roussy (2 papers)	Guillain et Barre	No of recom- mendations
Prevention of pressure sores	+	+/+	+/+/+	+	+/+	+	10/10
Careful catheterisation	+	+/+	+/+/+	+	+/+	+	10/10
Specialised nursing staff, physiotherapists and doctors	+	+/+	+/+/+			+	7/10
Early transfer to spinal unit		+/+	+/+/+		/+		6/10
Frequent staff supervision	+	+/+	+//		/+	+	6/10
One doctor responsible for all aspects of care	+	+/	/+/+		/+		5/10
Specialist rehabilitation facilities		+/+	+/+/+				5/10
Vocational training and re- integration		+/+	+/+/+				5/10
Physiotherapy Maintenance of nutrition		+/+	+//				3/10
Opposition to early laminectomy					+/+		2/10
Postdural reduction of the fracture				+			1/10
Research, fundamental and applied		+					1/10
Statistics, living/ dying						+	1/10

4.2.1   Pressure sores

Everyone recorded pressure sores. Claude Bernard and Charcot had delineated their pathogenesis but did not discuss treatment. Marie realised the importance of pressure sores and devoted the whole of this paper to this topic. He misunderstood and misquoted both Charcot and Brown-Séquard when he stated that they believed pressure sores were caused by the injury to the trophic nerves. In reality, Brown-Séquard showed that the pressure was the cause of the damage (see section 3.4.4). Marie also said that Charcot and Brown-Séquard did not understand sepsis and the role of the aetiology of pressure sores whereas in fact, Charcot had shown very elegantly that damage to the sympathetic did not produce a pressure sore alone, it was only when the animal was malnourished or infected that sores supervened (see section 3.2.1). Although pressure sores had previously been accurately described by Petit in the eighteenth century, Marie's views on the treatment and causation of pressure sores were a step forward.

- He did not believe that pressure sores were invariably fatal but he gave no figures.
- He recognised that occlusion of the circulation was fundamental in the causation of sores and that these became infected, encouraged by maceration of the skin.

As today, he attributed sores to loss of sensation 'the patient can no longer feel that he has a sore. Whilst a normal subject would experience pain and move about, unconsciously even while asleep, the patient because of his paralysis and loss of feeling cannot move' (Marie, 1915). This is the fundamental pathogenesis of pressure sores.

First there is redness then bruising of the skin which eventually would turn into parchment then blisters formed full of blood stained fluid. In a patient with a complete lesion, although a dry pressure sore is thought to be benign, infection supervenes. Maceration occurred through the injudicious use of wet dressings and above all, by contact with faeces or urine. Urine would provide favourable conditions for anaerobic and aerobic growth, micro-organisms would penetrate to the tissue where the skin had disappeared and form huge foci of necrosis down to the sacrum and possibly fatal.

Guillain and Barré observed pressure sores on any areas exposed to pressure, even if the limbs were wrapped in cotton wool, the pressure was transmitted through the dressings. (Inappropriate dressing concentrates the pressure, thereby making a sore much worse). The trochanters were particularly affected, despite the care of the staff.

Roussy and Lhermitte agreed that the prognosis was not necessarily fatal, but gave no figures. They thought that the sores were due to the mass body weight being transmitted to the pressure points, without pain as experienced by normal people. Patients did not complain, the nursing staff were not informed, and they were not turned. They, like Marie knew that if a pressure sore was left to macerate, it enlarged. All their patients had bedsores and one prisoner of war who had no bedsores whist in Germany, developed them after a train journey to France, while he was being repatriated.

4.2.1.1   Treatment

Marie believed in the doctrine that pressure sores could and must be prevented by avoiding maceration of the skin by wet dressings or urine (Marie, 1915).

He dogmatically and incorrectly stated that if patients were continent, they didn't get sores, and if they were incontinent they always got sores. Marie recognised that following spinal injury there was retention of urine so the patient should be catheterised to prevent sores. The patient must be transferred to a specialised unit. The skin should be protected by using quinine powder. Patients should be put onto air cushions, which should be kept clean. They must be turned hourly during the day and two hourly at night. The medical staff should supervise the specialised nursing staff and personally inspect two or three times a day the heels and gluteal region of the patients to ensure that their instructions were being carried out. Thus, for the first time, the doctor was made responsible for the total care of the patient.

Once a pressure sore had developed, there was no mention of taking the pressure off the sore. Marie recommended that deep necrotic sores should be sprayed with phenol solutions. Lhermitte and Roussy suggested other solutions.

Camus recognised the beneficial effect of sunlight on pressure sores, the need for asepsis and changing the linen regularly because so many patients were incontinent.

Guillain and Barré also realised that sores could be prevented by proper care. They recommended protecting the areas liable to develop pressure sores by wrapping them in cotton wool. They did not mention turning the patients.

The ill effects of equipment were recognised by Jean-François Calot (1861-1944), who believed that sores could be caused by the mal application of a plaster cast and by Lhermitte and Roussy who opposed rubber rings or suspended beds (type Dupont) because the straps could cause complications.

Lhermitte and Roussy agreed on the dangers of urinary maceration of the sore, the need to turn the patient every hour by day and many times during the night and that doctors should inspect the pressure sites at risk. They were the only doctors to suggest that sores should be operated on; they used the expression "la moucheture", making a cut in the bruise and letting the tissues drain. They did not describe débridement, cutting the sore open or closing the sore by plastic surgery. They did not describe radiography of the sores to look for underlying osteomyelitis or sinograms. While they accepted the importance of sore prevention, they did not recognise that when a sore developed pressure on the sore must be stopped. They described overwhelming spreading sepsis, toxic complications and erysipelas.

Despite understanding the pathogenesis and need to prevent pressure sores, each paper recorded extensive sores. Thus both their theories and management plans were correct, but these were not implemented.

4.2.2 Bladder management

None of the papers were primarily devoted to bladder management. Apart from preventing incontinence to reduce the risk of pressure sores, there seems to have been little interest in the management of the bladder. When it was discussed it was only in relation to the management of pressure sores. By contrast some British papers were devoted entirely to the neuro-physiology of the bladder, with extensive discussions and experiments upon the different forms of bladder management.

The French doctors did not describe radiography of the bladder, cystograms or cystometrograms. Clinically, they warned against both urine macerating the skin and traumatising the urethra with a rigid catheter. They used both intermittent and permanent catheterisation and stressed the need for asepsis in the management of the bladder.

Marie suggested that the bladder could be emptied from time to time by a nursing orderly or by the patient himself. This prevented both intractable pain when the patient suffered from an over distended bladder during the rail journey while being transferred to the rear, and early occurrence of retention and overflow. This statement is particularly interesting because it implies that the bladder is normally innervated and is painful while the bladder outlet is paralysed. This phenomenon is only observed in very low lesions such as the cauda equina. This would suggest that more serious spinal injuries with higher cord transactions who had anaesthetic bladders probably died at the front line.

Guillain and Barré described uraemia in the early stage with haematuria preceding established urine infection and pyuria often leading to death. Haematuria was attributed to vaso-dilatation and bleeding of the bladder mucosa, to such a degree as to cause anaemia. Bladder management was paramount. Patients should be catheterised four times a day with their own personal equipment and soft catheters, straight or bent (coudée) with asepsis. If haematuria developed, a permanent catheter should be installed. The bladder was washed with warm boiled water. When the urine was purulent, irrigation should be done with a special 'goménolée' oil. Urotropine, a smooth muscle relaxant, was given to damp down the spasms of the bladder.

Roussy and Lhermitte accepted that every patient had a urinary tract infection. With purulent urethritis and overwhelming bladder sepsis they recommended intermittent catheterisation of the bladder, and were the only doctors to use supra pubic catheterisation. They too recommended bladder washouts, and prescribed diuretics.

The doctors did not appear to be intimately involved in the bladder management, which was probably carried out by nurses or orderlies.

4.2.3   Specialised staff and facilities

Although one or two patients may have been kept alive by Dupuytren and Charcot in peacetime, this was not possible in wartime, when many casualties would arrive at hospitals after offensives. At the front line and the receiving hospitals, doctors would sort the patients into those likely to survive who would be treated, and those who would probably die and would receive no treatment.   Many of the patients were in the latter category and even if they were not too badly injured, they would develop pressure sores and urinary infections because the fundamentals of management were being ignored. The only way that adequate care for spinal injury patients could be provided was in specialised centres with adequate staff.

4.2.3.1   The doctors

Camus, Roussy and Lhermitte recognised that there should be designated staff working full time.   This was the case at the Invalides hospital where one doctor was in charge of the organisation of the unit, another was in charge of the bladder management and pressure sores management and Mme Dejerine of neurological treatment.   The grouping of patients in specialised units allowed the Dejerines to do some extraordinary studies on heterotopic calcification.

4.2.3.2   The nursing staff

Camus, Roussy, Lhermitte, Guillain and Barré all pointed out the need for highly specialised, trained, conscientious and dedicated staff. For a hundred to 150 patients, Camus recommended that there should be, apart from the chief medical officer, a surgeon, an urologist, a neurologist, two 'masseuses' (physiotherapists) and two nurse assistants.   He would have preferred male staff, but because of the war effort, women had to provide the necessary care, even if they might have difficulty moving patients. Because the work was very tiring, there were no more than 4 patients per nurse, so that in a ward with 25 beds, the staffing should be one nurse, one strong nurse and two assistant nurses. Porters should be available all year to take the patients outside.   At night, it was also essential to have experienced and trained staff.

4.2.4   Early transfer and careful transportation

Lhermitte, Roussy and Marie believed that to avoid early death, early transfer to a specialised unit was essential, and this was one of the recommendations emanating from the Conférence Interalliée of 1917 (Camus, 1917). They identified the 'immediate phase', straight after the accident, when the patient is in a state of 'shock'. The 'later' phase showed signs of muscular vitality in the lower limbs, or improvements in the incomplete lesions.

Roussy and Lhermitte recommended that during transportation, the patient should have extra protection because of the incontinence, and to avoid diarrhoea, they should be given an opiate to make them constipated. They gave two examples of patients recently wounded. The first was wounded on 27th September and admitted and quickly transported by ambulance to a neurological army centre on 1st October. The other patient was wounded on 13th January and transported to the neurological unit on 19th January. Most patients were admitted urgently to specialised centres, but attendants at the front did not always have time to evaluate the patients properly and send them as early as possible, in a cast to the correct unit. If they were sent to the wrong unit, they might not be fit for later transport to the neurological unit. Kennedy and Cushing gave graphic descriptions of the long lines of casualties lying on stretchers by the side of the railway lines for hours on end, awaiting transfer (Cushing, 1936). Roussy and Lhermitte described a patient who was operated on in the ambulance where they took out the bone and shrapnel fragments. Roussy and Lhermitte do not appear to suggest that the patients should be catheterised during the journey. However, Marie understood the importance of dealing with the bladder at the front line hospital. Patients were to receive specialist treatment with many nurses to give extra care during transportation to the rear. The patient was catheterised with a soft catheter, allowing the bladder to be emptied by the nurse or the patient himself, especially during the long train journey. Patients with sphincter incontinence were placed on a hollow leather cushion. Nevertheless, all the patients arrived at specialised units with bladder infections and pressure sores.

4.2.5   Frequent staff supervision

The accounts are quite specific and recognise the strength of French clinical medicine, including bedside treatment and interactions between nurses, doctors and patients. Doctors were expected to give clear instructions to the nursing staff so that the patients were turned regularly and not left lying in the same position. All the authors emphasised regular frequent staff supervision by the doctors to check that their orders were being carried out.

Unfortunately, there is no evidence that these exhortations led to adequate performance.

4.2.6   Specialist rehabilitation facilities and equipment

There were spinal units. Patients were treated at the Hopital des Grands Infirmes du Système Nerveux at the Invalides, at the Centre Neurologique de Bourges, at the Salpêtrière and then at the new Institut National des Invalides and at the Army neurological ward of M. Fresson. Not all the hospitals were listed, possibly for reasons of military security. From the descriptions, some would be centres of secondary referral, and others without active surgical or diagnostic programmes, were merely rehabilitation units.

4.2.6.1   Structure of the building and diagnostic facilities
Camus described an appropriate unit, its building, the site and components: theatre, linen room, 25 bed wards + a single bed isolation room (for the disturbed patient), sterilisation room, electro-therapy and massage room. The decoration of the room and a pleasant environment were recognised, because these long-term patients easily become despondent and demoralised. It was important for the patients to go in the open air so the unit should be on the ground floor or in a building with lifts.

4.2.6.2   Nursing equipment
The equipment was quite advanced with air cushions, cushions made of horse hair and fine straw and leather, air and water mattresses, special bed tables and protective linen, recycling buckets to sort the cotton from the dressing and bed cradles to relieve pressure from the weight of blankets. Special equipment was recommended for paralysed patients with contractures of the muscles.

Camus used wheelchairs or trolleys, monkey poles, and crutches or long sticks to help the patient walk, because it was important for the patient to be able to move about independently.

4.2.6.3   Physiotherapy
The speciality of physiotherapy did not exist at that time but treatment with massage and electricity, was available in the units. Some equipment was used with patients in a sitting position, such as the Pied de Gautier (sitting aid). Small trolleys were used to hold all the equipment required to treat spinal injury patients, and could be taken from patient to patient.

It was believed that patients with cauda equina lesions would benefit from traction equipment using springs, which lifted the foot and kept it in the correct position. Mme Dejerine stressed the importance for rehabilitation of the position of the patient, and his legs and feet for incomplete lesions. She described in detail rehabilitation and mobilisation:

> "paraplegics should be encouraged to stand and try and walk with the help of two nurses and then with sticks."

> "They should stand at the back of their bed, holding on to the bar and flex knees and ankles on demand and stand on the tip of their toes. As soon as possible, gymnastics will be carried out and after that the patient will be sent to the countryside where he will be able to do gardening." (Camus, 1917)

4.2.6.4 Hydrotherapy

They recommended manipulation whilst the patient was immersed in a bath. They described the use of hot air baths and vapour baths. Turkish baths were primarily stimulants of the cutaneous functions both glandular and circulatory. Massage douche was a soothing and gentle procedure. They warned against the use of water under pressure. Hyperthermal whirlpool baths were useful to prepare the patient for massage and movement and at lower temperature, promote cleansing and healing of wounds and the separation of dead tissue. They could be used in substitution for massage and to assist the mechanical treatment of injured limbs. They warned against the dangers of using too high temperatures in cases of nerve injuries because of the anaesthesia or partial anaesthesia of the skin, which could result in scalding without the patient being aware of this. It was recognised that in paralysis from injuries to nerves no direct benefit could be obtained from electrical stimulation and that the treatment should be supportive in the forms of baths, massage and electricity to improve the circulation.

They described gunshot wounds affecting the vertebral column with intrathecal haemorrhage or concussion of the spinal cord often causing extensive paralysis, which sometimes gradually cleared up. In some cases the irritative condition of groups of muscles persisted which easily threw them into painful contraction. In such cases sedative pool baths or the warm low-pressure douche with soothing massage was preferable to stimulant surface treatment.

4.2.6.5 Electricity

Camus suggested that doctors should have facilities for electrical diagnosis and treatment. Indeed, electricity in the form of faradisation was used not only for diagnosis, but also for stimulation of the perineal region to help sphincter re-education.

4.2.7   Vocational training and reintegration

Camus stated that if patients have normal power in their upper limbs, they should be given equipment to carry out some work, which would help their functional, and later on their professional, rehabilitation. He urged that the injured should be returned to their original occupation whenever possible, especially if it was agriculture. In his book, *Physical & Occupational Re-education of the Maimed,* translated into English in 1918, Camus describes how he devised a large number of artificial aids to help with the various tasks required to cultivate the land, such as an agricultural arm, a pruner's hand, a rein holder etc... He tried to adapt the patient to the implement and the implement to the patient (Camus, 1918). He clearly pioneered the concept of rehabilitation.

In his book *Physical Remedies for Disabled Soldiers* 1917, Fortescue Fox describes how the training, carried out in special centres, was for the most part voluntary and varied in character. Unfortunately, the section on spinal injury does not give any detail of rehabilitation, and we can only assume that they probably died and therefore never made use of the special centres.

4.2.8   Operative management of the spine

The only doctors to discuss operation on the spine were Guillain and Barré. Having first discussed the pathology, they noted that spinal lesions could affect the soft tissues and the bones and they recommended that the wound be examined as early as possible. There should be a débridement of the entry wound with removal of all fragments of clothing and foreign parts. The wound should be dealt with like any other compound injury. They recognised that strong antiseptics could damage the cord. They harked back to fears that Brown-Séquard had recognised, and dismissed, of the temperature of the operating theatre affecting the spinal cord. General anaesthesia could be dangerous so they recommended local anaesthesia or delaying operation for several days. They were aware of the dangers of opening the dura mater and were opposed to exploring the spinal cord itself when trying to remove fragments.

Roussy and Lhermitte also recommended that operations on recently wounded patients should be avoided because they were still in a state of "shock" and might not recover from the anaesthetic. A patient should be left alone for a while after admission to the specialised unit so that he could recover from this state of shock, and then procedures such as débridement could be contemplated. They did not recommend laminectomy unless it would be risk free and straightforward. They detailed how the laminectomy should be performed if it was absolutely necessary due to compression. They also described how the dura could be repaired and the severed cord could be sutured together.

4.2.9   Psychological aspects

Camus gives the first account of psychological reactions to injury. He recommended a firm handling of patients, isolating patients away from the ward if they became demoralised and aggressive, and destroyed the atmosphere of the unit. Guillain and Barré observed that some cachectic patients stayed euphoric to the end: they were often surprised by patients' resigned and uncomplaining attitudes, presumably due to the lack of physical pain. Patients were to be taken outside to the open air and had diversionary therapy.

4.2.10   Statistics

Guillain and Barré gave one statistic of the outcome of spinal injury based on 100 spinal injury patients, 82% of them died immediately and the others died within 22 days (Table 7). They recognised that if the soldiers had wounds of the chest, the cervical spine or the abdomen, they would die of their injuries and would never arrive at the spinal units so were not included in the statistics. Guillain and Barré, never saw patients with cervical lesions, and implied that these died immediately. There are no figures of the total number of spinal injury patients treated in relation to the other wounded soldiers, and as with the American and the British literature, they have to be estimated. Nevertheless, many articles suggest that there were large numbers of such patients.

Table 7. Statistical data by Guillain & Barré (1916)

Total number of spinal injury soldiers treated	100
Immediate death	82
Later death within a maximum of 22 days	18
Patients improving spontaneously (outcome fatal?)	2
Patients improving after surgery (outcome fatal?)	2

4.2.10.1   Patients being discharged

Though there is no information on patients being discharged, Mme Dejerine referred to patients' prolonged stay at the Invalides or at the Salpêtrière so that they left hospital after treatment. This is supported by the description of the patients in her paper: three cases of heterotopic calcification were seen after nearly two years for patient 1 (injury 9 March 1916-last report 20 January 1918), nearly one year for patient 2 (injured 16 April 1917 – last description 25th March 1918), and over three years for patient 3 (injured 18th December 1914 - last description 30 January 1918). Clearly her patients survived considerably longer than those described by Guillain and Barré. Guillain and Barré described a high acute mortality partly from intercurrent injuries.

Mme Dejerine talked about long-term rehabilitation of paraplegics, especially those with cauda equina lesions and compares that situation favourably with an amputee who has lost both his legs (Camus, 1917). Camus mentioned that patients resisted the idea of professional rehabilitation because they had been hospitalised for so long that they did not believe in working anymore. He mentioned benefactors who lent their country houses so that partially handicapped patients, whether with spinal injuries, shellshock or epilepsy, could practice gardening, growing plants, rearing animals and working with leather, as part of convalescence. Some were in wheelchairs, and Bellot (1917) described a patient who survived 18 months after a spinal injury and recovered completely only to die from an infection in the site where the bullet was lodged.

Marie does not mention any patient being discharged, but claimed that the prognosis was serious but not life threatening, with soldiers having a better prognosis than civilians, perhaps propaganda to maintain morale. With complete cord lesions, life expectancy was brief, but as Roussy and Lhermitte also found, patients with incomplete or cauda equina lesions, could improve and even be cured if they did not develop pressure sores. Thus Roussy and Lhermitte (1918) described two cachectic patients who were treated and recovered, their general state being maintained for 18 and 19 months.

4.2.10.2   Clinical descriptions of diseases

The French neurologists naturally made careful clinical descriptions of various syndromes, such as acute meningitis due to the compound nature of a gunshot wound or when the pressure sores penetrated through to the spinal cord. Fatal ascending purulent meningitis was described. Bellot reported on the development of syringomyelia in a soldier with an incomplete lesion, who was discharged home and eighteen months later developed syringomyelia from a compound wound (Silver, 2001). Mme Dejerine wrote a classic description of heterotopic calcification due to a cord lesion, secondary changes or primary trauma to the muscles and joints (Dejerine & Cellier, 1918). Patients developed pneumonia from an inability to cough because of paralysed intercostal muscles. Marie attributed the infrequent injuries to the cervical and dorsal parts of the spine to a protective effect of the rucksack, but it is probably due to death of soldiers wounded in the higher part of the back (Marie, 1915).

The wealth of French First World War neurological literature, the documentation and detail is remarkable, as is the emphasis on the principles of treatment. They recognised that one doctor should be in charge who should take a comprehensive approach to the management of the patient. They were aware of the importance of early transfer to specialised centres and prevention of complications and were conservative in the management of the spine. These principles were probably not incorporated into routine management and were then largely forgotten and had to be re-learned subsequently after the Second World War.

5.   BETWEEN THE WARS

After the First World War, there are no French reviews or reports on spinal injury management. By contrast, in the United Kingdom, the United States of America and Germany, there were accounts, which have been described in other chapters. There was a continuing population of spinal injury patients from the First World War at the Royal Star & Garter in Richmond

There is no such material from France, either in textbooks, libraries or journals. The leading French spinal injury consultants, Marc Maury at Garches, Paul Dolfus at Mulhouse, and Alain Rossier in Switzerland have all assured me that there was nothing relevant in the French literature, that spinal injury management started again after the second World War at the polio unit at Garches with Grossiord, and that modern treatment started only after they visited Stoke Mandeville Hospital and learned Guttmann's methods (1950-1960). The sections on the spine in the standard French textbooks merely refer to scoliosis secondary to tuberculosis of the spine. Merle d'Aubigné should have the last word of this section:

> "It is amazing to note how my country was isolated during the 1920's. Perhaps on account of France's brilliant contribution to the progress of surgery before 1914 and during World War I, our masters were not very interested in the work from foreign countries. We were trained to believe that French surgery was the best but as I did not find any satisfactory answer to my problem, I was not so convinced." (d'Aubigné, 1982)

Chapter 8

Discussion

1. PRINCIPLES OF TREATMENT

Injury of the spinal cord has been known since antiquity. There is no means of repairing the spinal cord. The basis of treatment of these injuries consists of preventing complications (pressure sores and urinary tract infection) until the vertebral fracture has stabilised. It is essential to avoid manipulation of the vertebrae that could further damage the cord, so that it has the optimum chance of recovery. When the fracture has stabilised, the patient can be rehabilitated to a wheelchair life, using the parts of the body that are not paralysed to compensate for the parts that are.

Faced with such a catastrophic injury, surgeons have concentrated upon carrying out an immediate operation, hoping that it would cure the patient. While the surgeons were concentrating upon vertebral and spinal cord injuries, the patient was succumbing rapidly to intercurrent complications such as pressure sores and urinary tract infections. There could be no rehabilitation of the patients, as they died shortly after injury from complications so long-term studies could not take place.

In the past, some visionary doctors such as Wagner pioneered effective treatment but his teachings were not adopted, have been forgotten and had to be relearned.

Treatment has to be evaluated in terms of what was available at the time. Surgery on the spinal column could only take place when there was effective anaesthesia. Catheter drainage required modern non-irritant catheter materials and rehabilitation needed modern wheelchairs.

Until now this monograph has evaluated the contribution that an individual has made under his country of origin. An attempt is now made to correlate these ideas and apportion credit and priority of discovery.

2.   PRIORITY OF DISCOVERY AND APPORTIONING CREDIT

Table 8 is a list of authors who have reviewed the history of spinal injuries.

Table 8. Historical Review of the Literature

Author	Date	Publication Type	Analysis of personalities or treatment	Time period covered
Brown-Séquard	1852	Part of textbook	√	To 1852
Markham	1951	Part of textbook	√	To 1951
Benes	1968	Part of textbook	√	To 1965
Bennett	1964	Part of textbook	√	To end of 19th century
Guttmann	1973	Part of textbook	√	To 1973
Comarr	1983	Munro memorial lecture	√	1930 onwards
Krueger	1984	Munro memorial lecture	√	1930 onwards
Hughes	1987	Article: Historical account		To 1918
Ohry	1989	Monograph: Historical account	√	To end of 19th century

2.1   What recognition did they receive at the time and was it accepted as mainstream treatment? Did subsequent investigators acknowledge the priority of discovery?

Investigators concentrate on their own work, and occasionally refer to work from their own country. Thus in the United States, priority is given exclusively to the American contributions that Munro and Bors made, and in Britain, priority is given to Guttmann. Scant acknowledgement is made of contributions from other countries, and French work is forgotten.

Before and during the 19th century, doctors were more broadly educated and had an international outlook. Paris was recognised as the centre of scientific and medical work and English doctors had to travel there. Bell acknowledged the work of Magendie and doctors in the 19th century acknowledged the work of Dupuytren, Charcot and Brown-Séquard.

In the 20th century doctors acknowledged the work of Wagner and Stolper. From the beginning of the First World War, medicine became polarised and parochial. The development of the Internet whereby all knowledge should be accessible to research workers has made the situation worse not better. If the information is not available on the Internet, which applies only to modern literature, it is completely ignored. Older literature is lost sight of and mistakes are copied from one paper to another.

3.   HISTORICAL REVIEW OF THE LITERATURE

Few people have written books or articles on the history of the treatment of spinal injury. The majority are straightforward historical accounts and the few who have attempted to establish priority of discovery are largely hagiographies (Table 8).

No comprehensive monograph has been written on the history of the treatment of spinal injury but articles have described fragments. The article by Frankel (1971) on intermittent catheterisation gives a historical review of bladder management, as does Guttmann in his textbook on spinal cord injuries (Guttmann, 1973).

The history of the management of the fracture is well covered in numerous books, Markham (1951), Bennett (1964), Guttmann (1973) and Ohry (1989). Ohry's book only covers the 19th century. Brown-Séquard (1852) gave elegant and detailed descriptions of the surgical approach to the spine but these contemporaneous accounts were lost track of.

Benes (1968), Comarr (1983), and Krueger (1984) are the only authors to try and analyse the different contributions made by Munro, Guttmann and Bors but as Bors was still alive and Munro and Guttmann had died only recently, not enough time had passed for the contributions to be evaluated. The accounts were very short and part of the Donald Munro Memorial address. Comarr and Krueger, who worked in the Veterans' Hospitals, both attributed the development of the treatment of spinal injuries to Munro. They were antagonistic towards Guttmann describing him as a self-advertiser.

In this work, statements have been verified by referring back to original documents whenever possible, and for the 20th century, by interviewing surviving patients and doctors from the early era.

3.1   Management of the fracture

Definitions
1.   Postural Reduction: Reducing the fracture by manipulation.

2.   Operative reduction: Reducing the fracture by surgery on the vertebrae (without exposing the cord).

3.   Laminectomy: Removing the bone to view the spinal cord and possibly operate upon it.

Fracture of the spine has been recognised from the time of Hippocrates. The first account of injury of the spinal cord and paraplegia was five thousand years ago.   Hippocrates in Ancient Greece was the first to recognise and discuss reduction of the dislocated spine. He recommended reduction of the dislocation by manual means. It is suggested that Paul of Aegina, in the 7th Century was the first to suggest decompression of the spine.

In the 16th century, Paré, performed surgical decompression of the spine but also described methods of reduction by direct pressure. Petit in the 18th century and Dupuytren in the 19th century reiterated the desirability of postural reduction. Dupuytren recognised the dangers of manipulation since it would cause an increase in deformity of the spine and damage the cord.

At the beginning of the 19th century, there was controversy amongst British surgeons. Cooper was in favour of operating on the fracture to decompress the spinal cord no matter how risky the procedure. Bell was opposed to this. His views were accepted by Charcot in France, but Charcot's contemporary, Brown-Séquard, was in favour of surgery upon the spine and wrote chapters in a textbook on the subject, recognising the contrasting views of Cooper and Bell but still coming down in favour of operating on the spine and decompression, a policy based largely on animal experiments.

Early operation was favoured until the end of the 19th century and the advent of Wagner. Wagner was opposed to operation, favoured conservative treatment and recommended immobilisation in bed until the fracture was united.   His views were accepted as authoritative throughout not just Germany but also the English-speaking world.

In the First World War, the role of surgery upon the spine was again a major source of controversy. Many of the wounds were compound wounds of the spinal column where debridement was necessary but even then, there was no unanimity. Cushing and Symonds were in favour of surgery, but all the French surgeons opposed surgery apart from Calot who advocated postural reduction.

With regard to the United Kingdom, the views of the MRC monograph was extremely conservative. Extra medullary haemorrhage of sufficient degree to cause compression of the cord was almost unknown although pressure on the cord is frequently exerted by a missile or in-driven fragment of bone. This compression is not an active or progressive process and therefore does not call for immediate surgical intervention. On the other hand, the presence of a foreign body, or a vertebral deformity may retard the recovery of a contused cord, and in such cases early, though not immediate operation may be indicated. It was easier to put arguments against rather than for an operation although the presence of septic wounds required attention. In the United States, Frazier was opposed to surgery and followed the cautious approach of Bell.

There was little change between the wars and the English surgeons, Jefferson and Watson-Jones, and Böhler in Austria, favoured the conservative approach in the form of manual reduction. All were opposed to laminectomy, believing it could do little good and much harm.

Munro followed these conservative views and believed that treatment of the spine was only of secondary importance and no effort should be made to reduce a fracture by operation; gentle traction should be used to replace the vertebrae, under X-ray control. He was not in favour of decompressive laminectomy and showed a reduction of 30% mortality of cervical cases after laminectomies were abandoned. Munro was very early in the field and more importantly his views were accepted by the neurosurgeons who worked in military hospitals around the world during the Second World War (Munro, 1952). Unfortunately, at a later stage, neurosurgical residents in the United States were put under great pressure to perform laminectomies during their training (they had to carry out a certain number of operations to achieve Board recognition) and patients were under pressure to have operations until their insurance money was used up. As a result, Munro's views were ignored in the United States.

In the United Kingdom, Guttmann was fiercely opposed to laminectomy showing that it could only do harm. His views were accepted because he produced statistical evidence that no benefit had been shown to accrue and also because there was a shortage of neurosurgeons. Neurosurgeons were therefore happy to accept that damage occurred at the time of injury and there was no benefit in carrying out a laminectomy at any stage.

Surgery upon the spinal column to reduce the fracture came into prominence with the work of Nicoll (1948, 1949) and Holdsworth (1953, 1963) who described the problems with spinal column stability and advocated the treatment of the fracture. These views were not adopted because of Guttmann's strenuous opposition to any form of operation upon the vertebrae. The views of Nicoll and Holdsworth have recently become orthodox treatment in the United Kingdom and there is a more open-minded approach. Even at the spinal unit, Stoke Mandeville Hospital, the 'Mecca' of the conservative management of spinal injuries, with Guttmann's retirement and the appointment of a neurosurgeon and a spinal surgeon, spinal surgery is now an accepted part of the treatment (Silver & Henderson, 1992).

3.2 The prevention of pressure sores

Pressure sores have been known since antiquity but they were regarded as an inevitable occurrence that killed the patient. The first person to discuss their prevention was Petit (1726), who recognised their dangers and exhorted the surgeon in charge to keep the patient in as proper a position as possible, lifting and visiting them often in order to prevent pressure sores. Tissot, Charcot and Brown-Séquard recognised the importance of lifting and turning patients and preventing maceration of the skin. Wagner saw that the patients should be turned and described a bucket underneath the bed and special sheets and cushions to prevent sores. Marie described in detail how the patients should be turned; the doctor had to inspect the sores himself, and not rely on the nursing staff. This policy was accepted during the First World War but not implemented. The first person to rigorously implement it was Munro who stressed that the turning had to be done on the hour rigorously and the doctor had to monitor that it was done.

Pressure sores were exacerbated by the unfortunate use of plaster beds, which had been used successfully for patients with tuberculosis of the spine. With tuberculosis of the spine, there was often no loss of sensation and plaster beds could be used successfully. With spinal injury patients, plaster beds gave rise to severe contractures, pain and pressure sores.

Munro was the first to describe prevention of pressure sores. His work achieved widespread recognition and was implemented by Guttmann who abolished plaster beds and instituted regular turning with signatures to be obtained from the nursing staff for each turn. As a result of the staff from the Middlesex Hospital relocating to Stoke Mandeville, their massage school (the precursor of the physiotherapy department) was also based at this hospital. These physiotherapists aimed to make patients fit, active and able to look after themselves. Guttmann acknowledged their contribution at the time. This was the beginning of rehabilitation of patients with spinal injuries in the United Kingdom.

3.3 Management of the bladder

Following spinal injury, the bladder is paralysed and has to be drained. This was done initially by intermittent catheterisation. Although Bell gave a detailed description of this methodology (Bell, 1807), little else was written, other than describing how the catheter was inserted and then removed. Later discussion was concerned with overwhelming infection which supervened in the bladder when there was retention of urine. The pus would inevitably be absorbed into the blood stream causing septicaemia and backpressure upon the kidneys. The bladder would then have to be drained by an indwelling catheter (catheter à demeure). Brodie, Bell and Charcot performed intermittent catheterisation. There was no distinction made between these forms of catheterisation until Wagner (who favoured intermittent catheterisation) and Kocher (who favoured continuous drainage with antiseptic precautions).

In the First World War initial management of the bladder became a subject of controversy. The bladder was initially managed by intermittent catheterisation but during transport, this could not be carried out regularly and soldiers developed severe ascending infections due to failure to drain the bladder. It was recognised that during transport an indwelling catheter should be inserted. To obviate this problem altogether a suprapubic catheter was inserted or, in a small number of cases, the bladder was expressed manually. This issue remained controversial until the end of the war, and the question also arose as to when the bladder should be washed out. Sadly, it was universally accepted that infection was inevitable and was caused by the catheter. The infection manifested itself with attacks of shivering and sweating and local abscesses leading to fistulae in the scrotum. During the First World War, soldiers died of acute ascending pyelonephritis, and after the war survivors suffered from chronic pyelonephritis with renal and bladder calculi. The few who survived the First World War had incomplete lesions and minimal interference with their bladder (Frankel, 1971).

The breakthrough came with Munro who argued that patients should neither have pressure sores nor sepsis of the renal tract. Munro's solution was a tidal drainage apparatus. This apparatus became accepted as the way of preventing urinary sepsis and was widely adopted throughout the United States and by Guttmann when he opened the spinal unit at Stoke Mandeville. It was recognised that if the bladder was carefully monitored and meticulously managed, infection was not inevitable. Although Riches, urological surgeon to the unit, favoured suprapubic catheterisation (Riches, 1943) (as did the United States Forces for transport), Guttmann rapidly switched newly arrived acute patients to intermittent catheterisation. Doctors and orderlies were specially trained to do all the catheterisations.

3.4   Total health of the patient

While nothing can be done to heal the spinal cord, the complications of paralysis can be avoided, such as gross sepsis arising from pressure sores, and urinary tract infection leading to septicaemia and anaemia. Anaemia secondary to pressure sores and renal failure is due to toxic depression of the bone marrow and is resistant to protein feeding and vitamin supplements and will respond only to repeated and massive blood transfusions. This picture of the emaciated 'Buchenwald patient' was common at the end of the Second World War.

3.5   Maintenance of nutrition

During the first six weeks after injury, patients would be in a catabolic state with rapidly breaking down tissues. They would naturally have a poor appetite and if in addition they developed pressure sores and suffered overwhelming sepsis, they would loose considerable amounts of protein from the pressure sores. The need for high protein feeding to counteract this was recognised in the United States, Canada and In the United Kingdom.

3.6   Blood transfusion

Blood transfusion has two main roles in the treatment of spinal injuries: Spinal injury does not occur in isolation. 90% of patients have severe intercurrent injuries. Blood is essential in restoring and resuscitating the severely surgically shocked patient and is particularly useful for managing acute injuries where there is associated trauma of the chest and abdomen and limb fractures.

Blood transfusion also plays an essential role in improving the patients' nutrition in cases of chronic anaemia due to sepsis as this does not respond to antibiotics. Blood transfusions were not available until the Second World War. It was not of paramount importance since both Wagner and Munro were able to restore patients to health without the use of blood transfusion.

During the Second World War, blood transfusions became freely available with the setting up of blood banks in the United Kingdom and the United States and the establishment of large banks of blood to deal with acute trauma caused by air raids. Because the shelf life of blood was finite, there was no resistance for it to be used to maintain the nutrition of paraplegics in dealing with chronic sepsis. Thus blood transfusions were freely given to these patients rather than the blood being discarded.

In Germany there were no blood banks and no paraplegics.

3.7   Antibiotics

The role of antibiotics is controversial. It is believed that their development and administration enabled patients with spinal injuries to be kept alive. Facts presented in this book would suggest otherwise since Wagner, at the end of the 19th century, and Munro until 1945, rehabilitated spinal patients successfully without the use of antibiotics. They stressed and showed that the best treatment for urinary tract infection was to ensure free drainage of the bladder and no blockage of the catheters. Riches and Bors agreed with this. Antibiotics could be of value in dealing with overwhelming infection and septicaemia from the urinary tract but the source of the infection has to be eliminated first.

Antibiotics were given to patients with pressure sores to establish a sterile field and deal with any septicaemia when bacteria became disseminated around the body. Prevention was the most important aspect when dealing with pressure sores, regular turning was paramount. However when a severe sore developed this had to be dealt with by the removal of necrotic tissue and when there was septicaemia, antibiotics would be life saving.

The other important aspect was dealing with chest infection, particularly in patients with high cord transactions and tetraplegia. Here again the prevention of infection by physiotherapy and postural drainage was more important than the use of antibiotics though when overwhelming infection developed, antibiotics could be life saving. The evidence suggests that successful management of the spinal patient resulted from understanding the fundamental principles: prevention of infection of the renal tract by free drainage; prevention of pressure sores by regular turning; prevention of chest infections by postural drainage; and regular physiotherapy. Antibiotics are no substitute for these. There is no doubt that when overwhelming sepsis develops from pyonephrosis in the kidney, a pressure sore with cellulitis, or pneumonia, that antibiotics can be life saving but by then the battle has largely been lost. Antibiotics were not critical in the development of effective treatment.

3.8 Early admission to specialised centres

Spinal patients had to be admitted early to a specialised centre. Munro, Holdsworth and Watson-Jones recognised that the real solution to the treatment of these patients was the early admission to a spinal unit, before complications could occur.

> "If he is competent and familiar with his own necessary deficiencies... he [the general surgeon] will promptly recognize that ....such patients that they should be promptly transferred to a neurosurgical centre." (Munro, 1952)

In the United Kingdom, Watson-Jones stated that in 1955 Sheffield was receiving acute admissions and this was the solution for the optimum care of a spinal patient since they would not develop preventable complications. Holdsworth, an orthopaedic surgeon, was in charge of the acute orthopaedic unit at Sheffield Infirmary and transferred patients at a later stage to Wharncliffe. In 1953, in a paper on the management of spinal fractures, he described 68 patients of whom 47 were treated from the beginning and emphasised that much better results were achieved by admitting the patients straight away.

"Bad initial treatment results in a host of other complications such as gross angulation of the spine, stiffness of joints, contractures and deformities, which seriously delay or even prevent late rehabilitation." (Holdsworth, 1953)

The unit in Sheffield pioneered acute admissions. Hardy, who was in charge of the unit at Wharncliffe from 1948, has confirmed this to me (Hardy, personal communication, 1990).

Guttmann (1954) emphasised that cases should be admitted early and I tried to determine how quickly after injury patients were admitted to Stoke Mandeville. I went through the notes of the living survivors, representing only 1 in 10 of the original patients, and I could not find any acute admissions before the end of 1955. Guttmann recognised the vital need for the patients to come in early before complications had developed:

"The sooner the paraplegic can be admitted to a spinal unit or hospital equipped with all necessary facilities, the greater is his chance for speedy and complete rehabilitation." (Guttmann, 1954)

But admitted that:

"The majority of paraplegics were admitted at later dates, following onset of paraplegia." (Guttmann, 1954)

Whilst it is possible that there were occasional acute admissions between 1944 and 1951, in two early papers (Guttmann & Frankel, 1966, Frankel, 1969), there were no acute spinal injuries reported before 1951. In the paper on intermittent catheterisation by Guttmann and Frankel (1966), 1954 was taken as the starting point of acute admissions. Acute cases were not admitted consistently until 1954-55, mainly because Stoke Mandeville was not regarded as an acute unit. At Stoke Mandeville by 1956 there were a large number of acute admissions and a regular catheter round was carried out by the resident doctors throughout the day to drain the bladders.

3.9   Specialised staff and facilities

Dupuytren (1846) and Wagner (1898) emphasized the need for specialised treatment. During the First World War specialised units were set up in France and are described in detail by Camus *et al* (1917).

Holmes looked after patients in base hospitals in France who were later transferred to the London hospital, then on to the Empire Hospital, and eventually to the Royal Star and Garter Home. The need for specialised facilities was recognised and in the 1916 Annual Medical Report of the Royal Star and Garter Home, they discussed the needs of paraplegics:

"They need many special and costly appliances, the services often of a male nurse as well as of a female nurse, massage, electrical treatment and unremitting medical and surgical attention. This cannot be obtained in a cottage or even in a cottage hospital."

Apart from the Royal Star and Garter Medical Report and the 1924 MRC monograph from the committee upon injuries of the nervous system (whose members included Head, Riddoch, Sargent, Buzzard, Trotter and Bristow) which advocated transfer to a specialised unit, patients with spinal injuries were not sent to specialised units. These patients were scattered around hospitals such as Queen Square London, where there was a high mortality from pressure sores.

The necessity for setting up specialised units was not recognised until Munro approached the insurance companies and saw that all traumatic spinal cases came to his neurosurgical unit at Boston.

"It was soon apparent that whenever such paralysed patients could be brought together and handled in a ward or in a group of hospital rooms constituting, as it were a special service with specially trained hospital nurses and attendants for them, the need for the special nurses was reduced or eliminated entirely in a matter of weeks...Furthermore, a comparison with our earlier experience demonstrated the value of moving such cases into specialized surgical clinics for paraplegics, where all the diagnostic and surgical services described in this volume were applied and where a co-ordinated and all-out program for the rehabilitation of the patient was instituted. The length of hospitalisation was shortened, the incidence of complications reduced to a minimum, permanent morbidity was done away with and life expectancy increased with elimination of the need for future hospitalisation, attendant care at home and the like. Thus the costs were reduced at a fairly early date and were maintained at a low level as time went on, not only without detriment to the patients but usually to his considerable benefit." (Munro, 1952)

Insurance companies accepted his recommendations, which benefited both the patients and themselves.

When the United States entered the war in 1941, the American Forces accepted the need for specialised spinal units. Initially, some 1400 patients were gathered in neurosurgical units but they saw the necessity for specialised teams of dedicated neurosurgeons, neurologists, psychiatrists and physical medicine consultants. The key person was the doctor in overall charge of the patients. The need for adequate numbers of specialised staff at all levels, doctors, physiotherapists, nurses, orderlies and remedial gymnasts or masseurs, was recognised.

Wagner gave a very detailed description of how the fracture should be managed and how incontinence should be prevented but one cannot tell whether there were specialised nursing staff and equipment. It may be that Wagner's unit had such facilities but he did not document it.

The need for specialised staff was first documented by the French, (Camus, 1917), during the First World War. They gave detailed recommendations on the setting up of a specialised unit, the equipment required, the staffing requirements, the medical care to be given to such patients (bladder and bowel management, pressure sores management), and functional and professional rehabilitation.

While very detailed care was described in the 1924 MRC monograph, there are again no specific descriptions of transfer to a specialised unit or its facilities. There are descriptions of facilities at the Royal Star and Garter Home where specialised techniques were carried out.

Special sheets and bladder management equipment were described by Wagner and the French used monkey poles, wheelchairs, trolleys, special linen, Dupont beds, air mattresses, foot rests, cushions, etc... The MRC monograph did not describe specialised equipment in any detail but Munro documented callipers and rehabilitation equipment.

When the units opened in the United Kingdom in 1940, they were short of equipment and only had old-fashioned heavy wooden wheelchairs and metal bedpans. The squabbling and shifting of responsibility between the central supplies body, the Ministry of Pensions and the local health authorities exacerbated this situation.

Whilst the Everest and Jennings lightweight metal chair for paraplegics was invented in 1936, Franklin Roosevelt never wished to be seen in a wheelchair for reasons of personal vanity and this delayed its acceptance (Tremblay, personal communication, 2000). In the United Kingdom the heavy Travaux chairs were still being used until the United States wheelchair basketball team visited Stoke Mandeville for the Paraplegic Games for the Disabled in 1948. Athletes from the United Kingdom were unable to compete against their American counterparts and as a result lightweight chairs were introduced, initially for sport, and subsequently for general use.

3.10   Physiotherapy and functional rehabilitation

Physiotherapy and rehabilitation are two comparatively recent terms. One looks in vain for such descriptions at the time of Bell but treatment was carried out on patients, although under different names. The techniques of physiotherapy have been used since antiquity. They were derived from various popular but dubious practices: massage, hydrotherapy, electro-therapy, physical re-education and exercise. 'Physiotherapy' as a term was not used until the end of the First World War, and 'rehabilitation' did not appear until the Second World War. Thus the concept of reintegration or returning a person to society developed during the 20th century.

There have been no textbooks dedicated exclusively to the history of the treatment of spinal injury and information has been derived from primary sources, papers and journals. In contrast, there is a rich literature in the form of books and chapters in books on the history of exercise, hydrotherapy, electrotherapy, and massage as methods of treatment. In the past these different therapeutic regimes have been appropriated by charlatans at different times in history and fallen into disrepute. It is difficult to appreciate the changes in treatment when one sees the scientific dedicated professional physiotherapists of today in contrast with the dubious practices of the past. Their contribution has proved to be beneficial to the total care of the paraplegic patient, and is an integral part of the modern therapeutic regime.

A few individual patients who survived for a year or two were described prior to the First World War. During the First World War a few patients with incomplete lesions or cauda equina lesions survived long enough to go home.

In France there are no accounts of patients being rehabilitated and sent home and although Mme Dejerine (1918) alluded to a rehabilitation centre at the Conference Interalliée, there is no evidence that paraplegic patients were treated there.

In the United States, a few patients survived. Frazier (1918) described 75 patients being discharged out of a total of 208 cases and one in four of these were healthy.

I have seen one or two survivors from the First World War and Frankel described 66 survivors (Frankel, 1971). Many of the British survivors went to the Royal Star and Garter Home where they led an institutionalised life. Patients received various forms of treatment such as electricity, and massage. They were ambulated with callipers, mobilised in their wheelchairs and given diversional therapy. One patient travelled round Europe. Some married and a certain number returned home. This has to be contrasted with the rather bleak view presented by Gowlland (1934) and Allen (1964/5) of the residents just being bathed and cared for.

It was through Munro's vision and his fundamental work that rehabilitation progressed. He believed that if patients had a good pair of arms and could manage their bladders, they could be discharged home.

During and immediately after the Second World War the Americans pursued a collaborative programme and set up a highly organised system of spinal care, but only in the Veterans Hospitals (Straus 1998). The Veterans Hospitals were transformed from old soldiers' and sailors' homes into advanced research centres. Resources and money were made available for research and treatment and a superb hospital system providing comprehensive care was instituted. Soldiers were mobilised, taught to walk and discharged home. Deaver presented a graduated programme of exercises, taught patients to walk and to transfer from bed to chair and chair to bed. By 1946 a third of patients were being mobilised and a third were being discharged home. Kessler and Abrahamson (1950) recognised that this programme of mobilisation was valuable not just for psychological reasons but also because it prevented demineralisation of the bones thus reducing stones in the renal tract.

The Canadians took this a stage further. Both civilians and children were treated on the spinal unit. Jousse visited both Deaver and Munro and set up an integrated programme based on Munro's principles. Munro acknowledged that the Canadians were responsible for setting in motion the rehabilitation of spinal cord casualties from the Second World War (Munro, 1952).

Jackson Burrows told me that Guttmann and Holdsworth visited the United States where they learnt Munro's methods, which they brought back and practised in the United Kingdom. I cannot find a record of Guttmann travelling to the United States during the war. He went soon after the war but this was after he had established the spinal unit at Stoke Mandeville, was already treating spinal patients and established a reputation for excellence. His secretary, Miss Scruton, confirmed to me that he had the highest regard for Munro but he did not visit the United States until after the war. Again, I cannot find any record of Holdsworth going to the United States though there is a record of Nicoll going in both 1947 and 1948. Jackson Burrows' statement is therefore incorrect. Nevertheless, Guttmann was profoundly influenced by Munro's work. He knew of the work of Deaver and Munro which preceded his own. He certainly used Munro's tidal drainage equipment and was aware of its use in American service hospitals. In Guttmann's copy of Munro's textbook, he underlined his work 25 times and in his monograph (Guttmann, 1953), quoted Munro 10 times. He set up programmes of rehabilitation and physiotherapy following the same principles as the Americans, but he was less aggressive in his approach to physiotherapy. He did not want patients to be taught how to fall, as he was concerned that they might injure themselves and he had different techniques. It is to his credit, and because there was a comprehensive health service in the United Kingdom, that by 1948 a programme of rehabilitation was established. Patients were returning to their own homes or to places such as the Kytes Estate (a hospital estate specifically for paraplegics).

During the First World War Robert Jones set up disabled workshops. These continued until the Second World War and paraplegic patients were taken to Egham and Leatherhead to pursue vocational training and watch making. A considerable amount of this rehabilitation was patient driven, patients demanded it and even if they did not insist on walking, they demanded to be independent, to go home and to look after themselves.

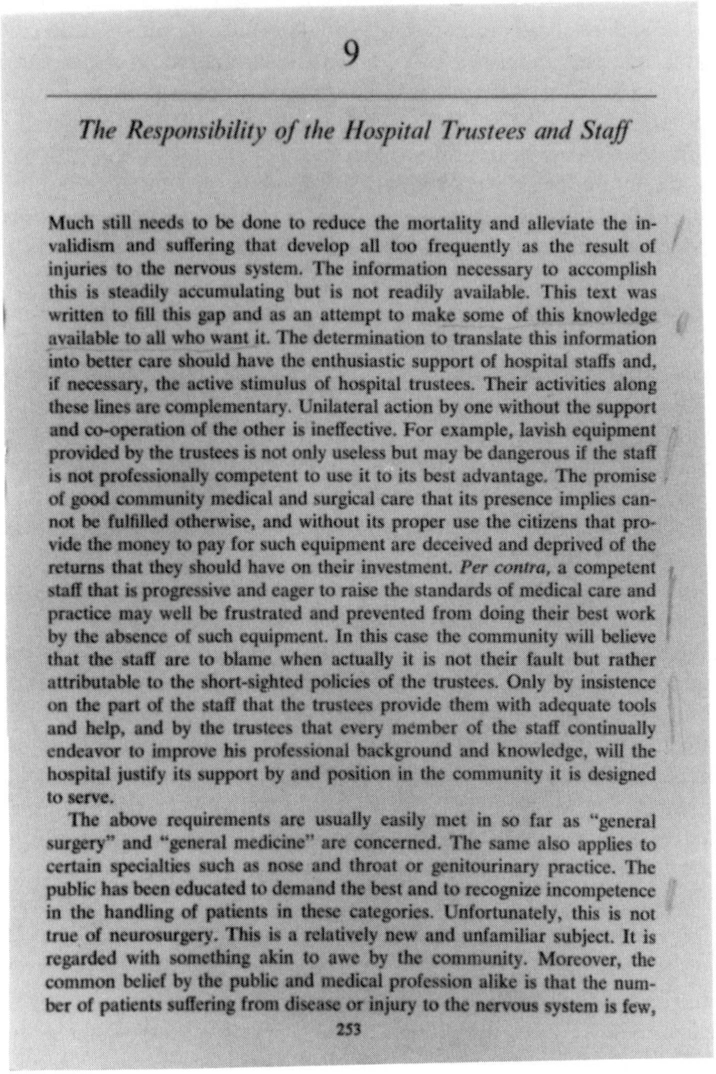

9

The Responsibility of the Hospital Trustees and Staff

Much still needs to be done to reduce the mortality and alleviate the invalidism and suffering that develop all too frequently as the result of injuries to the nervous system. The information necessary to accomplish this is steadily accumulating but is not readily available. This text was written to fill this gap and as an attempt to make some of this knowledge available to all who want it. The determination to translate this information into better care should have the enthusiastic support of hospital staffs and, if necessary, the active stimulus of hospital trustees. Their activities along these lines are complementary. Unilateral action by one without the support and co-operation of the other is ineffective. For example, lavish equipment provided by the trustees is not only useless but may be dangerous if the staff is not professionally competent to use it to its best advantage. The promise of good community medical and surgical care that its presence implies cannot be fulfilled otherwise, and without its proper use the citizens that provide the money to pay for such equipment are deceived and deprived of the returns that they should have on their investment. *Per contra*, a competent staff that is progressive and eager to raise the standards of medical care and practice may well be frustrated and prevented from doing their best work by the absence of such equipment. In this case the community will believe that the staff are to blame when actually it is not their fault but rather attributable to the short-sighted policies of the trustees. Only by insistence on the part of the staff that the trustees provide them with adequate tools and help, and by the trustees that every member of the staff continually endeavor to improve his professional background and knowledge, will the hospital justify its support by and position in the community it is designed to serve.

The above requirements are usually easily met in so far as "general surgery" and "general medicine" are concerned. The same also applies to certain specialties such as nose and throat or genitourinary practice. The public has been educated to demand the best and to recognize incompetence in the handling of patients in these categories. Unfortunately, this is not true of neurosurgery. This is a relatively new and unfamiliar subject. It is regarded with something akin to awe by the community. Moreover, the common belief by the public and medical profession alike is that the number of patients suffering from disease or injury to the nervous system is few,

253

Figure 19. This is one of 25 passages marked by Guttmann in his copy of Munro's book *The Treatment of Injuries to the Nervous System* (1952). Reprinted with permission from Elsevier.

Camus pioneered the idea of rehabilitation in France. Among the ex-servicemen there were many millions who were wounded and crippled. He realised that the crippled and disabled should be discharged home and return to work. He published a book about rehabilitating all the disabled including the blind and amputees, showing how splints could be used to aid them to plough and garden. He described in detail equipment and implements and showed how they could be trained to work gainfully. There is little evidence that spinal patients survived long enough to participate in the programme. No record exists of paraplegics who survived in France after the First World War, comparable to the records of the Royal Star and Garter Home in the United Kingdom.

Unfortunately, Duchenne's revolutionary work on electrical stimulation, which delineated the action of the muscles, and his use of active splints with springs, seemed to have been forgotten completely by the outbreak of the First World War, only to be rediscovered within the last twenty years.

The German approach was different. Frenkel realised, that the normal part of the nervous system had to compensate for the parts that were damaged. Tabetic patients had lost posterior column function. He devised a series of exercises whereby patients compensated with their eyes for the loss of the posterior column function. His work was adopted throughout Europe and is quoted in British textbooks. Foerster worked with Frenkel and continued Frenkel's work at a time when descriptive neurology was in the ascendant but therapeutic neurology was sterile. Foerster was committed to rehabilitation but this all appeared to die out with the advent of the Nazis and whilst spinal rehabilitation was being carried out in Austria, this was not the case in Germany. Nevertheless, Guttmann had seen how patients were being rehabilitated in a comprehensive way in the German peripheral nerve injury units and he brought these ideas to the United Kingdom and developed them at the spinal unit, Stoke Mandeville Hospital in order to deliver total care to the patients. In particular he used Frenkel's exercises to enable the patients to compensate with their eyes for the loss of proprioception from the paralysis of the lower limbs. Guttmann's ideas on rehabilitation were adopted by other spinal units and pioneered the rehabilitation role of the physiotherapist in the United Kingdom.

3.11   Vocational training

In the past, it was thought that the crippled should be locked away unseen in an institution. With the advent of the First World War, there were so many of them and they were so hideously deformed such as 'the Grands Mutilés' who went out in masks, that Camus said that they should be reintegrated into society and go home. This clamour for the rights of the disabled for proper facilities started after the war. Very well equipped workshops were set up for the disabled in France and Great Britain although in France, no account could be found of patients with spinal injuries surviving.

Records of spinal patients going to Egham and other centres during the Second World War have been found. There were workshops in Roehampton for amputees. At the spinal unit, Stoke Mandeville Hospital vocational training was pursued both at the hospital and at a radio factory in Aylesbury. In the United States, there were vocational workshops where patients could earn a living.

3.12   Reintegration

In the United States, due both to a more aggressive approach to treatment and because money was not available to keep patients in hospital indefinitely, patients were sent home. Munro recognised that the Canadians were ahead of him as they pioneered a programme of discharging patients home to lead independent and integrated lives in the community. The Canadians encouraged their spinal patients to participate in sports such as bowling and moose shooting with the able-bodied rather than leaving them segregated in institutions.

In the United Kingdom, immediately after the Second World War, servicemen received pensions. Buildings were expensive but labour was cheap and patients stayed in hospital for a long time. There was no pressure to discharge them.

It was thought that patients with spinal injuries should live in permanent institutions (such as Lyme Green and the "doghouse." (Duchess of Gloucester House)) and indeed some of the first patients stayed for years at Stoke Mandeville (Sheppard-Jones, 1958) and then they were to be discharged to large 'long-term homes' where there was nursing provision for them. Subsequently, they began to live at home. This may have started when patients married nurses or physiotherapists and set up home together. The Kyte's Estate was established for the disabled. Since that time, the clamour from the disabled has led to even tetraplegic patients on ventilators demanding to live in the community as a right, the fundamental principle of rehabilitation. They want to organise their own care rather than wait for nurses and carers to come in and they want to pay for it themselves.

3.13   Research, both applied and fundamental

3.13.1   Applied research

Whilst spinal injury has been known since antiquity it is only since Wagner's work at the end of the 19th century that patients survived and there was an opportunity for research.

3.13.1.1   First World War

In the First World War in the United Kingdom, different forms of bladder management were assessed: expression, intermittent catheterisation and suprapubic catheterisation. Head and Riddoch and Holmes wrote a classic series of papers on the neuro-physiology of the paralysed bladder and how the patient should be treated.

Further applied research, as detailed in First World War papers, investigated whether a laminectomy was of any advantage in the treatment of spinal injury.

The French contribution was descriptive neurology and the only major research work was that of Mme Dejerine on heterotopic calcification where she established its relationship with paralysed parts of the body.

3.13.1.2   Between the wars

Between the wars, some seminal research work was carried out by Denny-Brown and Robertson, using the spinal patient as a physiological preparation to study bladder and bowel function.

3.13.1.3   Second World War

During the Second World War, the Americans carried out systematic statistical research on treatment and mortality. They instituted combined meetings and conferences with the hospitals where patients were treated to present their experience on different aspects of treatment (Kennedy, 1946). Abramson carried out elegant work on calcium metabolism (1948). In the United Kingdom all the research on spinal treatment was carried out by Guttmann who produced a large series of papers on the practical management of the patient, the pathogenesis of pressure sores, the management of the bladder, physiotherapy and operative intervention to alleviate spasms.

3.13.2   Fundamental research

It is very difficult to keep an animal with paraplegia alive and like humans they require a great deal of care and attention to prevent sepsis. When patients were kept alive in good health, then fundamental research on the autonomic function could be carried out using the patient as a spinal preparation free of sores and urinary tract infection enabling studies for spinal cord function to be carried out   This was initiated by Riddoch and Head in the First World War, followed by Denny-Brown and Robertson and then by Guttmann who published a series of papers in collaboration with Whitteridge (Guttmann and Whitteridge, 1947) at the department of physiology in Oxford and later on the spinal unit at Stoke Mandeville Hospital.

3.14 Statistics

The mortality figures and the causes of death are an ultimate arbiter of the success or failure of treatment. In Germany, Wagner described some patients surviving after injury, but unfortunately, he gave no figures.

3.14.1 First World War mortality

In the United States, of the servicemen who sustained spinal cord injuries, 80% died immediately, and the few who returned home virtually all died within a few weeks. Frazier described survival. Out of a total of 228 cases (not necessarily all servicemen or under his care), 75 patients were discharged and when he followed them up he found that 1 in 4 were well, 1 in 2.5 were partially incapacitated and 1 in 9 died later.

In the United Kingdom, the death rate from spinal injury is difficult to ascertain but it was very high, at over 60%. The only survivors were those who went to the Royal Star and Garter Home and amongst those, the mortality was around 18% at the beginning of the war and declined significantly thereafter. It must be noted though that not all the patients at the Royal Star and Garter Home were traumatic paraplegics and a large proportion were suffering from disseminated sclerosis. Thomson-Walker described an 82% death rate in the First World War.

In France, Guillain and Barré stated that 82% of soldiers with spinal cord injury died immediately and the remaining died within 22 days. They never saw patients with cervical lesions, which implies that these patients died immediately.

Detailed mortality figures are not available for France and Germany for either of the World Wars.

3.14.2 Second World War mortality

In the Second World War, patients were being kept alive and 1400 spinal injury patients returned to the United States. Munro analysed the causes of death of 100 patients of whom 16 had bedsores. He found that 10% died within 24hrs of admission to hospital, and the total death rate in hospital was of 38%. Another 4 patients died after discharge, bringing the overall morality rate to 42%, still a much lower death rate than that experienced in Europe at the time. Munro updated his figures in 1954 when, for a total of 445 patients, the mortality had fallen to 34% (which is not really significant).

In the United Kingdom, mortality in spinal units other than Stoke Mandeville was quite appalling (Dick, 1949, Nicoll, Nov-48) but Guttmann had already demonstrated good results (Winner, 1949). These were late admission. Presumably all the patients with an acute spinal injury had died.

By 1946, Guttmann published figures showing that out of a total of 176 patients, 164 survived (this included patients still alive after 1 to over 7 years) (Guttmann, 1946).

3.15   Sport

Literature on the use of sport for rehabilitation of disabled people goes back to Greenwich Hospital where in 1796 a cricket match took place between the One Armed and the One Legged (Lloyd & Coulter, 1961). During the First World War, the French used sport to rehabilitate amputees; they played quoits, and bowls in a glasshouse. In the United Kingdom, swimming was used as a mode of exercise and after the First World War there are accounts of wheelchair bound patients at the Royal Star and Garter Home playing competitive sports during a sports day. In Germany, the amputees and the blind were participating in sport. In America, there were competitive wheelchair sports at the Veterans Hospitals. In contrast, the Canadians believed that disabled should compete alongside the able bodied in such sports as bowling and moose shooting.

It is to Guttmann's credit that he could think laterally. He was a keen observer who could assimilate ideas from different disciplines possibly because he had worked in neurology, neurosurgery, neuropathology and psychiatry, and in different countries.

He obtained ideas on sport from Germany and possibly from the Royal Star and Garter Home while he was a visiting consultant and started the wheelchair games, which became such a feature of the rehabilitation of patients at Stoke Mandeville. Sport taught patients to be independent. When the United Kingdom wheelchair athletes saw the lighter wheelchairs that the United States used, these became incorporated into daily use. They were no longer expected to sit on the side of the sports field, people came to watch them perform. It is a moving and humbling experience to see the Olympic stadiums at Barcelona and more recently in Sydney in the year 2000 full of able-bodied people cheering on the wheelchair athletes and having daily reports on television and in the newspapers with headlines as to the number of medals being achieved by the wheelchair sportsmen and women. The wheelchair athlete is not permitted to compete against the able-bodied in the marathon since they can cover the distance at a faster speed. Today, sport is not only carried out by patients with spinal injury, but also by people with other forms of disability. The able-bodied have found the equipment and the sports so attractive to them that competitions are being devised for the able-bodied using wheelchairs like any other piece of sporting equipment.

Chapter 9

Conclusion

Logically, in view of the primacy of German medicine, the modern treatment of spinal injuries should have developed in Germany but this did not happen. Intellectually there was a fine neurological tradition and medically there was a high standard of medical care in university hospitals. Bismarck had set up the first social security system. Wagner had shown by meticulous studies how spinal injuries could be treated at the end of the 19th century. During the First World War, the treatment of spinal injuries was similar in Germany, France, America and Britain. In 1933 the Nazis came to power and their ideas permeated all aspects of life and decimated German medicine. Jewish doctors were expelled from their appointments, the Neurological Association was dissolved, and ideas on rehabilitation were rejected because mentally retarded and severely physically and mentally disabled people were institutionalised and killed.

In France, despite the advanced work by Camus and the Dejerines during the First World War, the treatment of spinal injury patients after the war was discontinued for political and economic reasons. There was no healthcare or social security and medicine between the wars, particularly orthopaedics, was stagnant.

The real father of the ideas on the treatment of spinal injuries was Munro in America. He was a brilliant writer, forceful, thoughtful and didactic and is quoted extensively because most of his ideas were so well explained. Both the American Forces and the American Veterans' Association adopted his doctrine. No man is a prophet in his own country and credit is now given to Bors as the founder of comprehensive spinal injury units in the United States. Bors said when he set up the spinal unit at Long Beach in 1950 that he only had two of Munro's papers to look at. Guttmann put Munro's ideas into practice in the United Kingdom.

Despite the firm foundation set out by Munro in 1936, when he demonstrated that patients with spinal injury could and should be kept alive, and the magnificent work in the American Army and Veterans Hospitals, ideas on the treatment of spinal injuries did not permeate outside these hospitals and treatment was restricted to veterans. There are many reasons for the opposition to there being a comprehensive social security system in the United States which involve political and economic factors.

In Canada, a large country with a small population, looking both to the United Kingdom and America, with a high standard of living and medical care, comprehensive service evolved rapidly and civilians of all ages as well as ex-servicemen were treated.

Spinal injury treatment reached its full development in the United Kingdom. Just as in the United States and France, patients with spinal injuries had been treated in the First World War at the Royal Star and Garter Home but this was very much on a custodial basis, with little therapeutic treatment. The spinal units, which were set up for a short while in the United Kingdom between 1940 and 1944, were failures, with a high mortality and morbidity and patients were no better after three years than they were on arrival.

The successful treatment of spinal injuries in Europe can largely be attributed to the influence of one man: Ludwig Guttmann. He would not have succeeded in his medical approach had it not been for the advent of the National Health Service. He was working for a Ministry of Pensions Hospital sited at an EMS Hospital. The systems of care and financing with full time staff were forerunners of the National Health Service. The Health Service allowed patients to be admitted for treatment at the hospital that was appropriate for their care without there being a financial penalty. While the principle is excellent, the implications are still being addressed in the United Kingdom because eventually everything has to be paid for. With the establishment of the Health Service all patients could be admitted for specialised treatment although it took longer for this to be implemented for women and children. There was no financial penalty on the patient and doctors were willing to refer such disastrous cases to specialised centres. The role of the Health Service cannot be under estimated. Despite the fact that the United Kingdom was impoverished, having paid for a long expensive war, the founding of the Health Service in 1948 was a visionary step and provided both comprehensive medical care in re-equipped hospitals and social security for the whole population including the disabled.

Charitable foundations played an important role from the outset. Then, as now, they served as pump primers. The Rockefeller Foundation funded Foerster, Queen Square, Munro, Guttmann and, even to this day, Bracken at Yale. It is sad to relate that they also sponsored the Kaiser-Wilhelm Institute which was responsible for the eugenic work in Germany. The Royal Star and Garter Home was built in 1916 thanks to worldwide fund raising by the Women of the Empire, a charitable organisation.

Why did Guttmann have such a profound effect on spinal injury treatment? He was a German Jewish outsider. The term 'Outsider' was coined by Colin Wilson. In fact, the term 'ethical outsider' originated in 1870 in Germany where it referred to Jews. Jews were excluded from professional careers so they were well accustomed to working against prejudice, which, no doubt, had a stimulating effect.

When Guttmann came to Stoke Mandeville in 1944, which was the only job he could get, he seized on this chance. He had not been able to do the work that he wanted for 12 years and during this period he had time to formulate his ideas. It is not known what he had learned from Wagner but certainly from Foerster he had gained some remarkable ideas about physiotherapy and operations on the spinal cord and nerve roots to relieve spasticity.

All these factors Guttmann seized upon and incorporated into his practice. For problems he was not familiar with such as the management of the fractured spine and the paralysed bladder, he adopted a very simple form of treatment. For the spine he used postural reduction, which amounted to no treatment at all and for the bladder he used the method of intermittent catheterisation. He effectively did not carry out laminectomies because this treatment had been shown by Wagner, Frazier and by Munro to be useless and positively harmful. His opposition to surgical stabilisation of the spine was less profitable.

He insisted that he was consultant in charge and concentrated all knowledge and power in his hands. Such authoritarianism is not necessarily a bad thing in the early days of management because he set up an excellent method of treatment, but it could be repressive. When he got things right they went really well; when he got things wrong they went dramatically wrong.

A reflection of the concept of the outsider was that Guttmann was unwilling to have the unit moved to Oxford or any university centre. If the unit had gone to Oxford, it would have been incorporated into the University.

Interestingly, Foerster, although the outstanding neurologist in Europe between the wars, was unwilling to take up a post in Berlin. He stayed where he was, (just as Wagner stayed in a small town in Silesia), and eventually the Rockefeller Foundation built a research institute for him because until then he had been financing all the research himself. Although recognised as being an outstanding neurologist in Germany, he was not part of the university establishment. Because he was such a disagreeable man and no one would work with him, he left no school of neurology. Foerster venerated another outsider: Duchenne de Boulogne. Duchenne was a sad lonely figure with no appointment in the Paris hospitals, no patients and no beds. All his research was done on other consultants' patients.

Outsiders work beyond the mainstream of medicine and their behaviour is not necessarily accepted. What is behaviour of the outsider? It was said of Disraeli by Lord Stanley: "Mr Disraeli has had to make his position, and men who make their positions will say and do things which are not necessarily to be said or done by those for whom positions are made." Guttmann and Foerster were clearly such outsiders.

The fact that Ludwig Guttmann had to withdraw from clinical work to do research work for five years may have been of great benefit. He was able to study and he had a great thirst to succeed when he was appointed. In a traditional clinical career in the United Kingdom, newly appointed doctors often work so hard clinically that by the time they reach the age of 45 or 50, they are burnt out or they devote themselves to private practice and have no time for research. From 1933 to 1939 Guttmann was unable to do academic work and could only treat Jewish patients and from 1939 to 1945 he was unable to treat any patients at all. This isolation meant he could devote all his energies to the unpromising field of spinal injuries. Maybe he felt sympathy for the paraplegics who had been abandoned by the Nazis and, like the Jews, despised and regarded as less than human.

Bors, a Jew, was also an outsider away from his native country of Czechoslovakia. He was very well trained in three separate disciplines: as an anatomist, general surgeon and as an urologist. He was a very energetic man and worked in a Veterans Hospital.

Other Jews, such as Remak, Oppenheim and Ehrlich, could not achieve recognition by the establishment because of their religion.

In 1944 when Guttmann set up his unit, managing spinal patients represented a new challenge. Orthopaedics and neurosurgery were new disciplines.

Guttmann emphasised that the clinical notes must be written up meticulously because they were to be used for research. He believed that the work that was being done was first rate. You identified with him and the work and when he said you would do a research project on a particular aspect, you felt that you were in the forefront of medicine. All the staff on the unit were proud to participate. He was unsparing in his demands and would never accept second best. This was the way he inspired people. He was a dynamic, charismatic figure as was Foerster.

Thus far, we have looked at the role of Guttmann as an outsider and Guttmann as a Jew but what was his role as a German scientist?

English medicine at the time was based on the honorary system whereby consultants were given honorary appointments and visited hospitals on a weekly basis. However this was 'more honoured in the breach than in the observation' and sometimes consultants did not go near their patients for weeks at a time (Schurr, 1997). Junior doctors, who were few and far between, had the responsibility of treating the patients on the wards and consultants were only consulted when the junior doctors needed their expertise. They would perhaps visit the hospital once a week. All the information had to be assembled for them at the weekly ward round and decisions about treatment were necessarily delayed from one week to another because the only people who could take the major decisions were the consultants. As such, they took little responsibility or interest in what the nurses did so that the prevention of pressure sores was looked on as the prerogative of the nursing staff. Their appointments, even at teaching hospitals, in many cases, were not taken seriously and the whole emphasis was on private practice (Horder, 1966).

In 1954 ten years after Guttmann set up his unit, specialisation was in an interim position. Arthur Porritt (1900-1993), a general surgeon at St Mary's, was still dealing with fracture cases and neurosurgery was being carried out by general surgeons. This was the same hospital where penicillin was discovered.

The contrast with the dedication in the old County Council Hospitals such as the Central Middlesex was striking. Medical students made regular pilgrimages and fought to do their clinical training at the Central Middlesex where the consultants were full time, working frequently throughout the night alongside the junior staff, showing what dedication and professionalism could do. There was an MRC unit in gastroenterology, the first in the country. The fundamental work on epidemiology of smoking and carcinoma of the bronchus was done there by Richard Doll. It was a powerhouse of ideas and treatment.

Attempts had been made before the war to institute a full time system at the London and Middlesex Hospitals as in the continental University Hospitals. There were one or two consulting rooms at the Middlesex where consultants could consult their private patients on the premises and be available for their voluntary practice geographically full time and this was the practice at the London Hospital. The consultants there had to be geographically full time but this was necessarily fragmented and never succeeded, as they preferred to spend their time in Harley Street.

In contrast Guttmann set up a service whereby he saw every patient on admission, saw every patient every week, did ward rounds in the physiotherapy/occupational therapy department, was constantly available to direct treatment and concentrated research, treatment, and teaching all into his own hands. He insisted that the nurses, physiotherapists, cleaners or anyone who breathed or moved on the spinal unit should be entirely subservient to him and took orders from him as he said it was part of the medical treatment. He was meticulous and hard working, studying patients and supervising their treatment. He set up a German academic unit.

Although there are disadvantages to this hierarchical system which stifled initiative, the assembly of large numbers of spinal patients enabled the benefit of various forms of treatment to be appreciated, as opposed to the London teaching hospitals which were virtually cottage hospitals where each consultant would pursue a different policy with regard to anticoagulant therapy on his patients with such a common condition as coronary thrombosis. Standardisation was impossible so that results could not be evaluated.

Guttmann's attitude to work is part of the German scientific tradition as epitomised by Ehrlich:

> "After working at home in the early morning, Ehrlich used to arrive at his laboratory shortly after 10am. He would then immediately visit all the different sections of both his Institutes, with the exception of those which could work independently, such as the 'Section for Control of the Serum Preparations for Human and Animal Treatment', which was run according to State regulations." (Marquardt, 1949)

Ehrlich controlled all current experiments of the Chemical and Biological Sections of the George Speyer-Haus, and the Cancer Section of the Serum Institute, and gave instructions for new experiments and methods.

Guttmann could treat patients very well based on his knowledge, his ability, his psychological insight and his sympathy but he was very autocratic (Sheppard-Jones, 1958). He stated that a patient did not become a saint as soon as they became a paraplegic and if they were not an ideal patient and did not get on with him, they could be banished from the unit.

Guttmann had the ability not only to learn a great deal, but also to think laterally. However, he was jealous of his knowledge. He would push a question aside and say: "send the patient to me for treatment." Nevertheless questioning him was very interesting because first he would give you a superficial answer, then you went away and read up papers and came back and questioned him again with contrary views and he would give you a much more studied answer which showed that he was aware of the literature, had thought about it and could answer your question. Learning from him was a difficult and extremely painful process.

There was the contrast that Guttmann could inspire great loyalty and people were willing to identify and work with him but at the same time people who knew him well evinced a great dislike of the personal traits he showed in his professional world. It is recognised that some very successful people are extremely difficult, with socially unattractive traits, being egotistical, stubborn, disagreeable, underhand, manipulative and bullies.

Unquestionably Guttmann put ideas together. Few of them were original. They were all in existence before and being practiced by Wagner and Munro. It was his drive, his energy, his enthusiasm, his intolerance of carelessness, refusal to accept inefficiency and low standards of treatment, which wedded them together in a comprehensive treatment programme. He did not merely give instructions and depart. Within half an hour he would come back and see how much progress had been made and would return again two hours later and by then if the job had not been started there would be a row.

Guttmann glamorised the work. He ran the unit like an academic unit with its propaganda and theoretical and practical research and teaching. People came to see the unit and respected both the unit's work and the spinal patients.

The setting up of specialised units and the early transfer of patients under one consultant who could take all the decisions was backed up by full therapeutic treatment where all specialities were available. This was the cornerstone of spinal injury management.

It is apparent that Wagner and Kocher had initiated these ideas and shown how it could be carried out but their ideas, possibly due to the advent of the First World War, were not continued. Foerster, apart from his great physiological work, incorporated physical methods of treatment, which was revolutionary. Munro at the City Hospital, Boston, Guttmann at Stoke Mandeville and Bors at the Long Beach Veterans Hospital demonstrated how the treatment could be successfully carried out. The credit for the development of the treatment lies with Munro who was the first to practice it. Munro set out a clear programme of treatment and arranged with the insurance companies to receive the spinal cases at his hospital. Unfortunately, he only had 10 beds but his publications were extremely influential, particularly with doctors treating American spinal injury casualties from the Second World War and with Ludwig Guttmann. Whilst Munro showed the way, it is Guttmann in the United Kingdom who instituted an integrated programme of treatment, facilitated by the favourable structure of the Health Service.

Bibliography

Abramson AS. Bone Disturbancies in Injuries to the Spinal Cord and Cauda Equina (paraplegia). *The Journal of Bone and Joint Surgery* 1948; 30:982-987.

Adams Captain E. Gunshot Wounds of the Spine. *The Lancet* 1916; 1:677-678.

Allen D. Spinal Unit at the Star and Garter Home. *The Cord* 1964/5; 17:14-16.

Aly G, Chroust P, Pross C. *Cleansing the Fatherland*. The John Hopkins University Press: Baltimore & London, 1994.

Aminoff MJ. *Brown-Séquard A Visionary of Science*. Raven Press: New York, 1993.

Armour Lieutenant-Colonel D. Gunshot Wounds of the Spine. *The Lancet* 1916; 1:677-678.

Bamji AN. The Macalister Archive: Records from the Queen's Hospital Sidcup 1917-1921. *Journal of Audiovisual Media in Medicine* 1993; 16:76-84.

Barclay Dr J. *In Good Hands -The History of the Chartered Society of Physiotherapy 1894-1994*. Butterworth Heinemann: Oxford, 1994.

Barnes JK. *The Medical and Surgical History of the War of the Rebellion (1861-1865)*. 2nd edn. Government Printing Office: Washington, 1875.

Barton LG. The reduction of fracture dislocations of the cervical vertebrae by skeletal traction. *Surg. Gynec. & Obst.* 1938; 67:94-69.

Bearsted H. *The Edwin Smith Surgica Papyrus*. Vol 1. Chicago, 1930.

Beecher HK, Altschule MD. *The First Three Hundred Years, Medicine at Harvard*. University Press of New England: New Hampshire, 1977.

Bell Sir C. *Essays on the Anatomy of Expression in Painting*. Longman, Rees, Hurst, Orme: London, 1806.

Bell Sir C. *A System of Operative Surgery founded on the Basis of Anatomy*. Longman, Hurst, Rees and Orme: London, 1807.

Bell Sir C. *Observations on injuries of the spine and of the thigh bone*. Thomas Tegg: London, 1824.

Bell Sir C. *Institutes of Surgery in two volumes*. Vol 1. Adam & Charles Black: Edinburgh; Longman, Orme, Brown, Green & Longmans: London, 1838.

Bellot V. Balle de Fusil dans La Queue de Cheval. *Bulletin Acad. De Med.* 1917; 77:749-753.

Benes V. *Spinal Cord Injury*. Balliere, Tindall & Cassell: London, 1968.

Bennett G. Historical Chapter. In: Howorth MB, Petrie JG (eds). *Injuries of the Spine*. Williams & Wilkins Co: Baltimore, 1964.

Böhler L. *The Treatment of Fractures translated by EW Hey Groves.* 4th edn. Wright: Bristol, 1935.

Borchard A et al. Gunshot Injuries of the Spinal Cord. *Medical Supplement* 1919; 142-149.

Bors E. The Spinal Cord Injury Center of the Veterans Administration Hospital, Long Beach California, U.S.A. *Paraplegia* 1967-8; 5:126-130.

Bors E, Comarr AE. *Neurological Urology.* S. Karger: Basel,München,Paris, New York, 1971.

Botterell EH, Jousse AT. Paraplegia Following War. *Canad. M.A.J.* 1946; 55:249-259.

Braune W, Fischer O. *The Human Gait translated by P Maquet & R Furlong.* Springer-Verlag: Berlin 1987.

Brockliss L, Jones C. *The Medical World of Early Modern France.* Clarendon Press: Oxford, 1997.

Brodie Sir BC. *Pathological and Surgical Observations on the Diseases of the Joints.* Longman, Brown, Green & Longmans: London, 1850.

Brodie Sir BC. *Diseases of the Urinary Organs, The Works of Benjamin Collins Brodie collected and arranged by Charles Hawkins.* Vol 2. Longman, Green, Longman, Roberts, & Green: London, 1865.

Brown-Séquard E. Experimental Researches applied to Physiology and Pathology. *The Medical Examiner and Record of Medical Science* 1852; 92:481-503.

Brown-Séquard E. *Course of Lectures on the Physiology and Pathology of the Central Nervous System.* Collins: Philadelphia, 1860.

Brown-Séquard E. *Lectures on the Diagnosis and Treatment of the Principal Forms of Paralysis of the Lower Extremities.* Williams & Norgate: Edinburgh, 1861.

Burleigh M. *Death and Deliverance - 'Euthanasia' in Germany 1900-1945.* Cambridge University Press: Cambridge, 1994.

Burleigh M. *The Third Reich.* Macmillan: London, 2000.

Burrell HL. A Summary of all the Cases of Fracture of the Spine (224) which were treated at the Boston City Hospital from 1864 to 1905. *Trans. Am. Med. Assoc.* 1905; 223:66-92.

Buzzard EF. Memoranda: Swimming in the Treatment of Paralysis. *The British Medical Journal* 1919; 1:610.

Buzzard EF. Gunshot Wounds and Injuries of the Spinal Cord. *The Lancet* 1916; 1:711-716.

Calot F. *Traitment de la Paralysie, L'Orthopédie indispensable aux praticiens.* A.Maloine et fils: Paris, 1923.

Cameron JE. War wounds of the spinal cord. *J.A.M.A.* 1945; 128 No.2: 152-165.

Campbell Munro A. Report on Paraplegia with reference to Newcastle Hospital. *Public Record Office* 23-Apr-1945; PIN15/2392.

Campbell Munro A. Letter to the Medical Superintendent Childwall Hospital regarding Mr J. Sykes' visit to Stoke Mandeville. *Public Record Office* 18-Jul-1945; PIN15/2392.

Campbell Munro A. Letter to Dr J. Prideaux. *Public Record Office* 23-Aug-1945; PIN15/2392.

Camus Jean. *Physical and Occupational Re-education of the Maimed translated by WF.Castle.* Bailliere Tindall & Cox: London, 1918.

Camus Jean. *Conférence Interalliée pour l'Etude de la Rééducation Professionnelle et des questions qui intéressent les Invalides de la Guerre.* Vol 3. Imprimerie Chaix: Paris, 1919.

Caplan, AL. How did Medicine go so wrong? In: Caplan AL (ed). *When medicine went mad.* Humana Press: Totowa, New Jersey, 1992.

Carr W. *A History of Germany 1815-1945.* 2nd edn. Edward Arnold Ltd: Bath, 1979.

Charcot Jean Martin. *Lectures on The Diseases of the Nervous System translated by George Sigerson.* The New Sydenham Society: London, 1877.

Charcot Jean Martin. *Lectures on the Diseases of the Nervous System translated by Sigerson.* 2nd Series. New Sydenham Society: London, 1881.

Charcot Jean Martin. *Charcot on Diseases of the Nervous System translated by Thomas Savill .* Vol 3. The New Sydenham Society: London, 1889.

Christopher F. Compression Fractures of the Spine. *American Journal of Surgery* 1930; 9:423-429.

Claude H, Lhermitte J. Sur un cas de séction anatomique complète de la moelle dorsale. Suture de la moelle. Survie de huit mois. *Bulletin et Mem Soc. Med. des Hopitaux de Paris* 1918; 11:1051-1057.

Cloward RB. Treatment of acute fractures of the cervical spine. *J Neurosurg* 1961; 18:201-209.

Collier J. Gunshot Wounds and Injuries of the Spinal Cord. *The Lancet* 1916; 1:711-716.

Comarr AE. First Donald Munro Memorial Lecture presented at the 29th Annual Meeting of the American Paraplegia Society 1983. Unpublished typescript sent to me by Dr I. Eltori.

Commissioner of Medical Services Scotland Region. Letter to the Ministry of Pensions regarding Dr Ferguson's visit to Stoke Mandeville. *Public Record Office* 29-Nov-1944; PIN15/2392.

Connors JF, Nash IE. The management of urologic complications in injuries to the spine. *American Journal of Surgery* 1934; 159-167.

Cooper Sir Astley. *A Treatise on Dislocations and on Fractures of the Joints.* Longman, Hurst, Rees, Orme & Brown: London, 1823.

Cooper AP, Cline H. Of Wounds of the Scalp. *The Lancet* 1824; 1:393-398.

Cooter R. *Surgery and Society in Peace and War.* The Macmillan Press Ltd: London, 1993.

Couvreur Médecin-Major. *Conférence Interalliée pour l'Etude de la Rééducation Professionnelle et des questions qui intéressent les Invalides de la Guerre.* Vol 3. Imprimerie Chaix: Paris, 1919.

Cranford RE. How did Medicine go so wrong? In: Caplan AL (ed). When medicine went mad. Humana Press: Totowa, New Jersey, 1992.

Critchley MacDonald. *The Divine Banquet of the Brain.* Raven Press: New York, 1979.

Crutchfield WG. Skeletal traction for dislocation of the cervical spine - Report of a case. *Southern Surgeon* 1933; 2:156-159.

Crutchfield WG. Fracture-dislocations of the cervical spine. *Am. J. Surg.* 1937; 38:592-598.

Crutchfield WG. Treatment of injuries of the cervical spine. *Journal of Bone & Joint Surgery* 1938; 20:696-704.

Cumming IE. Structural and Functional changes in Urinary Tract following Focal Cord Lesions. *Journal American Medical Association* 1932; 1198-2004.

Curling T.B. Essay on affection of the bladder in paraplegia. *London Medical Gazette* 1833; 13:76-80.

Curling T.B. Further observations on affection of the bladder in paraplegia. *London Medical Gazette* 1836; 18:325-331.

Cushing Harvey. *From a Surgeons' Journal 1915-1918.* Constable and Co Ltd: London, 1936.

Cushing H. Neurosurgery. In: Ireland MW. *The Medical Department of the United States Army in the World War.* Vol 11. Government Printing Office: Washington, 1927.

D'Aubigné Merle Surfing the Waves : Fifty years in the Growth of French Orthopedic Surgery. *Clinical orthopedics and research* 1982; 171:1-23.

Deaver GG, Brown ME. The Challenge of Crutches - Methods of Crutch Management. *Archives of Physical Medicine* 1945; 397-403.

Deaver GG, Brown ME.   The Challenge of Crutches - Crutch Walking: Muscular Demands and Preparation.   *Archives of Physical Medicine* 1945; 515-525.

Deaver GG, Brown ME.   The Challenge of Crutches - Standard Crutch Gaits and How to Teach Them.   *Archives of Physical Medicine* 1945; 573-582.

Deaver GG, Brown ME.   The Challenge of Crutches - Prescribing Crutch Gaits for Orthopaedic Disabilities.   *Archives of Physical Medicine* 1945; 747-753.

Deaver GG, Brown ME.   The Challenge of Crutches - Daily Activities on Crutches.   *Archives of Physical Medicine* 1946; 141-157.

Deaver GG, Brown ME.   The Challenge of Crutches - Living with Crutches and Canes.   *Archives of Physical Medicine* 1946; 683-703.

Dejerine Mme JMJ, Cellier A.   Para-ostéo-arthropathies des paraplégiques par lésion médullaire   *Annales de Médecine* 1918; 5:497-535.

Dejerine Mme JMJ, Cellier A.   Trois cas d'ostéomes-ossifications périostes juxta-musculaires et interfasciculaires chez des paraplégiques par lésion traumatique de la moelle épinière.   *Société de Neurology* 1918; 159-172.

Dick TBS.   Rehabilitation in Chronic Traumatic Paraplegia - A clinical study.   A thesis presented to the Victoria University of Manchester for the Degree of Doctor or Medicine, 1949.

Dick TBS.   Traumatic Paraplegia Pre-Guttmann.   *Paraplegia* 1969-70; 7:173-178.

Doherty WB, Runes D.   *Rehabilitation after Injuries to the Central Nervous System, Rehabilitation of the War Injured.*   Chapman & Hall Ltd: London.

Duchenne de Boulogne Guillaume.   *De l'éléctrisation localisée et de son application à la pathologie et à la thérapeutique.*   3rd edn. Librairie J.B. Bailliere et Fils: Paris, 1872.

Duchenne de Boulogne Guillaume.   Duchenne de Boulogne – Obituary.   *Gazette Hebdomadaire de Medecine et de Chirurgie* 1875; 12:622-623.

Duchenne de Boulogne Guillaume.   *The Physiology of Movement translated by EB Kaplan.*   WB Saunders & Co: USA, 1959.

Dunn Lieut.Colonel CL.   *The Emergency Medical Services.*   Vol 1. Her Majesty's Stationery Office: London, 1952.

Dupuytren Guillaume.   *On the Injuries and diseases of bones translated and edited by F. Le Gros Clark.*   The Sydenham Society: London, 1846.

Eiselberg A. Freih v.   Gehirn- und Nervenschüsse insbesondere Spätchirurgie.   Vehr. d. 2. Kriegschirurgentag. 26 und 27 April 1916.   *Bietr.z.kin.Chir.* 1916; 101:59-122.

Elsberg CA.   *Diagnosis and Treatment of Surgical Diseases of the Spinal Cord and its Membranes.*   W.B.Saunders & Co:Philadelphia & London, 1916.

Fagge CH, Pye Smith PH.   *Textbook of the Principles and Practices of Medicine.* 3rd edn. Vol 2. J. & A. Churchill: London, 1891.

Feasby WR.   *Official History of the Canadian Medical Services 1939-1945.*   Vol 2. Edmond Cloutier: Ottawa, 1953.

Foerster O, Frenkel HS.   Les troubles de la sensibilité dans le tabes.   *Rev. neurol.* 1899; 7:822-826.

Foerster O, Frenkel HS.   Untersuchungen über der Störungen der Sensibilität bei der Tabes dorsalis.   *Arch. Psychiat. Nervenkr.* 1900; 33:108-158,450-520.

Foerster O.   *Handbuch der Neurologie.*   Vol 11, Part 3. Otto Julius Springer: Berlin, 1927-1936.

Fortescue Fox R.   *Physical Remedies for Disabled Soldiers.*   Bailliere Tindall & Cox: London 1917, 200-236.

Fraenkel G.J.   *Hugh Cairns.*   Oxford University Press: New York, 1991.

Frankel HL. et al.   The value of postural reduction in the initial management of closed injuries of the spine with paraplegia and tetraplegia.   *Paraplegia* 1969; 7:179-192.

Frankel HL. Development of the method of intermittent catheterization in the treatment of the bladder in acute paraplegia. *Proceedings of the eighteenth veterans administration - Spinal Cord Injury Conference* 1971; 132-138.

Fraser F. Letter on Ureters and Their Orifices in Gunshot Wounds of the Spine. *British Medical Journal* 1919; 1:293.

Fraser FR. Letter regarding staffing at Park Prewett and referring to Guttmann's ability. *Public Record Office* 26-Jun-43; MH76/142.

Frazier CH, Allen AR. *Surgery of the spine and the spinal cord.* Appleton: New York & London, 1918.

Frenkel Dr H.S. *The Treatment of Tabetic Ataxia by means of Systematic Exercise translated and edited by L. Freyberger.* Rebman Ltd: London, 1902.

Friedländer S. *Nazi Germany and the Jews.* Orion Books, London, 1997.

Fulton JF. *Harvey Cushing - A biography.* Charles C.Thomas: Springfield Illinois, 1946.

Gask GE. Letter to Fraser praising Guttmann's ability. *Public Record Office* 15-Jul-44; MH76/142.

Gilbert M. *The First World War.* Harper Collins: London, 1995.

Go BK, DeVivo MJ, Richards JS. In: Stover SL, DeLisa JA, Whiteneck GG (eds). *Spinal Cord Injury.* Aspen Publishers: Gathersburg Maryland,1995.

Goodman S. *The Spirit of Stoke Mandeville.* Collins: London, 1986.

Gowlland EL The After Treatment of Paraplegia Following Spinal Injuries and of Disseminated Sclerosis. *The Medical Press and Circular* 1934; 81-84.

Guillain George, Barré J-A. Les Plaies de la Moelle Epinière par Blessures de Guerre. *La Presse Médicale* 1916; 62:497-501.

Guillain G. *J-M. Charcot 1825-1893 His Life - His Work, translated by P. Bailey.* Pitman Medical Publishing Co: London, 1959.

Gull W. Cases of paraplegia. *Guy's Hospital Reports* 1856; 2:143-187.

Gull W. Cases of paraplegia. *Guy's Hospital Reports* 1858; 4:169-208.

Günther HFK. *The racial elements of European History translated by G C Wheeler.* 2nd edn. Methuen & Co Ltd: London, 1927.

Guttmann L. Discussion on Rehabilitation after Injuries to the Central Nervous System. *Proceedings of the Royal Society of Medicine* 1941; 35:305-308.

Guttmann L. New Hope for Spinal Cord Sufferers. *Medical Times* 1945; 318-326.

Guttmann L. Rehabilitation after Injuries to the Spinal Cord and Cauda Equina. *The British Journal of Physical Medicine and Industrial Hygiene* 1946; 130-137.

Guttmann L. Rehabilitation after Injuries to the Spinal Cord and Cauda Equina. *The British Journal of Physical Medicine and Industrial Hygiene* 1946; 162-171.

Guttmann L, Whitteridge D. Effects of Bladder Distension on Autonomic Mechanisms after Spinal Cord Injuries. *Brain* 1947; 70:361-404.

Guttmann L. The Treatment and Rehabilitation of Patients with Injuries of the Spinal Cord. In: Cope Z Sir (ed). *Surgery.* Her Majesty's Stationery Office: London, 1953.

Guttmann L. Statistical Survey on One Thousand Paraplegics and Initial Treatment of Traumatic Paraplegia. *Proceedings of the Royal Society of Medicine* 1954; 47 No 12:1099-1109.

Guttmann L. The National Spinal Injuries Centre Stoke Mandeville Hospital, Aylesbury, Bucks. *Monthly Bulletin of the Ministry of Health and Public Health Laboratory Service* 1962; 21:60-70.

Guttmann L, Frankel HL. The value of intermittent catheterisation in the early management of traumatic paraplegia and tetraplegia. *Paraplegia* 1966; 4:63-84.

Guttmann L. *Spinal Cord Injuries - Comprehensive Management and Research.* Blackwell Scientific Publications: Oxford, 1973.

Haymaker W, Schiller F. *The Founders of Neurology.* 2nd edn. Charles C Thomas: Springfield Ilinois, 1970.

Hays Major General SB. Neurosurgery. In: Coates JB (ed). *Surgery in World War II.* Vol 2. Office of the Surgeon General Department of the Army: Washington DC, 1959.

Head H, Thompson T. The grouping of afferent impulses within the spinal cord. *Brain* 1906; 29:537.

Head H, Riddoch G. The automatic bladder, excessive sweating and some other reflex conditions in gross injuries of the spinal cord. In: *Studies in Neurology.* Vol 2. Oxford Medical Publications: London, 1920.

Heinemann-Grüder A. In: Renneberg M, Walker M (eds). *Science, Technology and National Socialism.* Cambridge University Press: Cambridge, 1994.

Hobson EPG. *Physiotherapy in Paraplegia.* J. & A. Churchill Ltd: London, 1956.

Holden W. *Shell Shock.* MacMillan Publishers Ltd: London,1998.

Holdsworth FW, Hardy S. Early Treatment of Paraplegia from Fractures of the Thoraco-Lumbar Spine. *Journal of Bone and Joint Surgery* 1953; 35B No 4:540-550.

Holdsworth FW. Fractures Dislocations and Fracture Dislocations of the Spine. *Journal of Bone and Joint Surgery* 1963; 45B No 1:6-20.

Holmes G, Edinger L, Wallenberg A. Untersuchungen über das Vorderhirn der Vogel. In: Edinger L. *Untersuchungen über die vergleichende Anatomie des Gehirnes.* 1903, 415-427.

Holmes G. Observations on The Paralysed Bladder. *Brain* 1933; 56:383-396.

Holmes G. On Spinal Injuries of warfare - Goulstonian Lectures. *British Medical Journal* 1915; 2:769-774,815-821,855-861.

Horder M. *The Little Genius.* Duckworth: London, 1966.

Hughes JT. Historical Review of Paraplegia before 1918. *Paraplegia* 1987; 25:168-171.

Hugonet Médecin Aide-Major. *Conférence Interalliée pour l'Etude de la Rééducation Professionnelle et des questions qui intéressent les Invalides de la Guerre.* Vol 3. Imprimerie Chaix: Paris, 1919.

Hulke JW. *The Bradshaw Lecture to the Royal College of Surgeons of England, On Fractures and Dislocations of the Vertebral Column.* Harrison & Sons: London, 1892.

Hutchinson J. On Dislocations and Fractures of the Spine - A Clinical Lecture. *London Hospital Reports* 1866; 3:357-372.

Jefferson G. Discussion on Spinal Injuries - Section of Orthopaedics. *Proceedings of the Royal Society of Medicine* 1927; 625-648.

Jefferson G. The treatment of Spinal Injuries. *The Practitioner* 1933; 130:332-341.

Jefferson G. Concerning Injuries of the Spinal Cord. *British Medical Journal* 1936; 2:1125-1130.

Jefferson G. *Selected Papers.* Pitman Medical Publishing Co. Ltd: London, 1960.

Kater MH. Doctors under Hitler. The University of North Carolina Press: Chapel Hill & London, 1989.

Katz J. How did Medicine go so wrong? In: Caplan AL (ed). *When medicine went mad.* Humana Press: Totowa, New Jersey, 1992.

Kaviraj Kunja Lal Bhishagratna. *Sushruta Samhita.* Vol. II. Calcutta, 1911.

Keegan J. *The First World War.* Random House (UK) Ltd: London, 1998.

Kennedy RH. The New Viewpoint Toward Spinal Cord Injuries. *Annals of Surgery* 1946; 124 No 6:1057-1065.

Kessler H, Abramson AS. Rehabilitation: The rehabilitation of the paraplegic. *New York State Journal of Medicine* 1950; 43-47.

Knight G. War Injuries of the Spine and Spinal Cord. *Proceedings of the Royal Society of Medicine* 1938; 32:247-255.

Kocher TJ. Die Verletzungen Der Wirbelsäule Zugleich als Beitrag zur Physiologie des menschlichen Rückenmarks. *Mittheilungens.d.Grenzgeb.d.Medicin.u. Chir.* 1896; 416-659.

Krueger EG. Second Donald Munro Lecture presented at the 30th Anniversary Conference of the American Paraplegia Society 1984. Unpublished typescript sent to me by Dr I. Eltori.

Lawrie RS, Nathan PW. Automatic Tidal Drainage of the Bladder. *The Lancet* 1939; 2:1072.

Le Vay D. *The History of Orthopaedics*. Parthenon Publishing Group Inc: New Jersey, 1990.

Licht SL. *Therapeutic Exercise*. Elizabeth Licht: New Haven Connecticut, 1965.

Liddell Hart BH. *History of the Second World War*. William Clowes Ltd: London, 1971.

Lifton RJ. *The Nazi Doctors*. Basic Books Inc: New York, 1986.

Ljunggren B, Buchenfelder M. Wilhelm Wagner (1848-1900) A Centennial Commemoration of a Forgotten Pioneer Neurosurgeon. *Sydvenska medicinhistoriska sällskapets årsskrift* 1989; 139-155.

Lloyd C, Coulter J. *Medicine and the Navy 1200-1900*. Vol 3. E & S Livingstone Ltd: Edinburgh & London, 1961.

Macklin R. How did Medicine go so wrong? In: Caplan AL (ed). *When medicine went mad*. Humana Press: Totowa, New Jersey, 1992.

MacPherson WG. *Medical Services General History. History of the Great War Based on Official Documents*. Vol 1. His Majesty's Stationery Office: London, 1921.

Makins GH. *Surgical Experiences in South Africa 1899-1900*. Henry Frowde & Hodder & Stoughton, Oxford University Press: London, 1913.

Manuel DE. *Marshall Hall (1790-1857), Science and Medicine in Early Victorian Society*. Editions Rodopi BV: Amsterdam-Atlanta, 1996.

Marburg O, Ranzi E. Die Kriegsbeschädigung des Rückenmarks und ihre operative Behandlung. *Arch. f. clin. Chir. Berl.* 1918; 72-282.

Marburg O, Ranzi E. Gunshot Injuries of the Spinal Cord. *Medical Supplement* 1919; 142-149.

Marburg O. Traumatic Injuries of the Spinal Cord. In: *Handbuch der Neurologie* by Foerster O. Vol 11, Part 3. Otto Julius Springer: Berlin, 1927-1936.

Marie P. *Lectures on Diseases of the Spinal Cord translated by M Lubbock*. Vol 152. New Sydenham Society: London, 1895.

Marie P. *Bulletin de L'Académie de Médecine*. 2nd edn. Masson et Cie: Paris, 1915.

Markham JW. Surgery of the Spinal Cord and Vertebral Column. In: Walker AE (ed) *A history of Neurological Surgery*. Balliere, Tindall & Cox: London, 1951.

Marquardt M. *Paul Ehrlich*. William Heinemann: London, 1949.

Mayer L. *The Orthopaedic Treatment of Gunshot Injuries*. WB Saunders: Philadelphia & London, 1918.

McAlpine DWC. et al. Special Surgery in Wartime - Diagnosis and Treatment of Spinal Cord Injuries. *The Practitioner "Booklets"* 1940; 11:17-28.

McAlpine D et al. Discussion of the Treatment and Prognosis of Traumatic Paraplegia. *Proceedings of the Royal Society of Medicine* 1947; 40:219-232.

McHenry LC. *Garrison's History of Neurology*. Charles C Thomas: Springfield, Illinois, USA, 1969.

McKenzie Kenneth G. Fracture, Dislocation, and Fracture-Dislocation of the Spine. *Canad. M.A.J.* 1935; 32:263-269.

Medawar J, Pyke D. *Hitler's Gift.* Richard Cohen Books, London, 2000.

Medical Research Council Privy Council. *Injuries of the Spinal Cord and Cauda Equina.* His Majesty's Stationery Office: London, 1924.

Medical Superintendent. Letter to Dr Murchie or Group Captain Cooper at the Ministry of Health regarding staffing problems at Stoke Mandeville. *Public Record Office.*08-Oct-45; MH76/143 .

Mennell JB. *Massage : Its Principles and Practice.* J A Churchill: London, 1917.

Mitchell SW. Fat & Blood – and How to Make Them. Lippincott: Philadelphia 1877.

Mitchell JK. Remote Consequences of Injuries of the Nerves and their Treatment. Lea Brothers & Co: Philadelphia, 1895.

Mitchell TJ. *Official History of the War - Medical Services - Casualties and Medical Statistics. History of the Great War based on Official Documents.* The Imperial War Museum Department of Printed Books: London, 1931.

Morton D, Wright G. *Winning the Second Battle: Canadian Veterans and the Return to Civilian Life. 1915-1930.* University of Toronto Press: Toronto, 1987.

Müller-Hill Benno *Murderous Science.* Oxford University Press: Oxford, 1988.

Munro D. The Cord Bladder Its Definition Treatment and Prognosis When Associated With Spinal Cord Injuries. *Journal of Urology* 1936;36:710-729.

Munro D. Care of the Back Following Spinal Cord Injuries - A consideration of Bed Sores. *The New England Journal of Medicine* 1940; 223 No 11:391-398.

Munro D. Thoracic and Lumbosacral Cord Injuries - A Study of Forty Cases. *The Journal of the American Medical Association* 1943; 122 No 16:1055-1063.

Munro D. The Rehabilitation of Patients Totally Paralyzed below the Waist, with Special Reference to Making them Ambulatory and Capable of Earning their Living. *The New England Journal of Medicine* 1945; 233 No 16:453-461.

Munro D. *The Treatment of Injuries to the Nervous System.* WB Saunders: Philadelphia & London, 1952.

Munro D. The Rehabilitation of Patients Totally Paralyzed Below the Waist, with Special Reference to Making them Ambulatory and Capable of Earning their Own Living. *The New England Journal of Medicine* 1954; 250:4-14.

Murchie F. Letter from the Ministry of Health regarding staffing at Stoke Mandeville. *Public Record Office* 22-Jan-1943; MH76/142.

Murchie F. Letter to Dr F. Herrald confirming Guttmann's employment at Stoke Mandeville. *Public Record Office* 08-Dec-1943; FD1/6555.

Nicoll EA. Closed Fractures of the Spine. *The Journal of Bone and Joint Surgery* 1948; 30B:725-728.

Nicoll EA. Copy of typescript of records from the Miners' Welfare Commission: Meeting held in November 1948 - Report on Wharncliffe paraplegic unit.

Nicoll EA. Fracture of the Dorso-Lumbar Spine. *The Journal of Bone and Joint Surgery* 1949;31B No 3:376-394.

Ohry A, Ohry-Kossoy K. *Spinal Cord Injuries in the 19th Century.* Churchill Livingstone: Edinburgh, 1989.

O'Malley CD, Saunders JB de C. *Leonardo da Vinci on the human body.* Henry Schuman Inc: New York, 1952.

Oppenheim H. *Textbook of nervous diseases for physicians and students translated by Alexander Bruce.* 5th edn. Vol 1. Otto Schulze & Co: Edinburgh,1911.

Owen ARG. *Hysteria, Hypnosis and Healing the work of J.M. Charcot.* Dobson Books Ltd: Bristol, 1971.

Paré Ambroise. *The Works of that Famous Chirurgion Ambroise Paré* (1649) *translated by T Johnson.* R Cotes & W Dugard: London, 1702.

Petit J-L. *A Treatise of the Diseases of the Bones translated from the French version of 1705*. T. Woodward: London, 1726.

Poore GV. *Selection from the Clinical Works of Dr Duchenne (De Boulogne)*. The New Sydenham Society: London, 1858.

Porter R. *The Greatest Benefit to Mankind*. Harper Collins: London, 1997.

Powell E. Lloyd Roberts Lecture. *Proceedings of the Royal Society of Medicine* 1962; 55:1-6.

Prather GC. Spinal Cord Injuries; Care of the Bladder. *Journal of Urology* 1947; 57:15-28.

Preuss J. *Biblical & Talmudic Medicine translated by F. Rosner*. Jason Aronson Inc: New Jersey, 1993.

Proctor RN. How did Medicine go so wrong? In: Caplan AL (ed). *When medicine went mad*. Humana Press: Totowa, New Jersey, 1992.

Pross C. Nazi Doctors, German Medicine and Historical Truth. In: Annas GJ, Grodin MA (eds). *The Nazi doctors and the Nuremberg Code*. Oxford University Press: London, 1992.

Public Record Office documents 1940-1944. Correspondence relating to the setting up of spinal units, MH76/142.

Public Record Office documents 1942-1944. Correspondence relating to the setting up of the South of England spinal unit with special reference to Stoke Mandeville and the role of Seddon, MH76/142.

Public Record Office documents 1945-1959. Correspondence relating to the supply of equipment to paraplegics, PIN15/2392 & MH58/653 .

Richardson H. *English Hospitals 1660-1948*. BPC Wheatons Ltd: Exeter, 1998.

Riches EW. Suprapubic Catheterisation for Paralysis of the Bladder in Spinal Injury. *The Lancet* 1943; 2:128-130.

Riches EW. The Methods and Results of Treatment in Cases of Paralysis of the Bladder following Spinal Injury. *The British Journal of Surgery* 1943; 31:135-146.

Riddoch G. The Reflex Functions of the Completely Divided Spinal Cord in Man, Compared with those Associated with Less severe Lesions. *Brain* 1917; 60:264-402.

Riddoch G. Letter to Fraser regarding the follow up of patients with spinal injuries. *Public Record Office* 12-Aug-1943; MH76/142.

Riddoch G. Letter from Riddoch to Herrald commenting on Guttmann's work. *Public Record Office* 15-Mar-1945; FD1/6555.

Romberg MH. *A Manual of the Nervous Diseases of Man translated by EH Sieveking*. Vol 1 & 2. The Sydenham Society: London, 1853.

Rows RG. Neurasthenia and War Neuroses. In: Macpherson WG et al (eds). *Medical Services Surgery of the War. History of the Great War Based on Official documents*. Vol 2. His Majesty's Stationery Office: London, 1923

Roussy G, Lhermitte J. *Blessures de la Moelle & de la Queue de Cheval*. Masson & Cie: Editeurs, 1918.

Royal Star and Garter Annual Medical Reports 1916-1940.

Sandifer P, Guttmann L. The Early Treatment of Traumatic Paraplegia. *Middlesex Hospital Journal* 1944; 44:67-70.

Sargent Lieutenant-Colonel P. Gunshot Wounds of the Spine. *The Lancet* 1916; 1:677-678.

Saunders JB.deC, O'Malley CD. *The illustrations from the works of Andreas Vesalius of Brussels*. The World Publishing Co: Cleveland & New York, 1950.

Schurr PH. *So that was life. A biography of Sir Geoffrey Jefferson*. Royal Society of Medicine Press Ltd: London, 1997.

Schwartz O. Ueber Störungen der Blasenfunktion nach Schussverletzungen des Rückenmarks. *Mitt. a. d. Grenzgeb. d. Med. u. Chir.* 1916; 29:174-227.

Sector Hospital Officer. Letter from Leatherhead Hospital to Sir Claude Frankau at the Ministry of Health regarding transportation of patients to Queen Elizabeth Training College. *Public Record Office* 17-Jul-1945; MH76/142.

Sheppard-Jones E. *I walk on wheels.* Geoffrey Bles:London, 1958.

Sherren James *Injuries of Nerves and their Treatment.* James Nisbet & Co. Ltd: London, 1908.

Sherrington Charles S. *The integrative action of the nervous system.* Yale Univ. Press: New Haven, 1906.

Sigerist Henry E. *Civilization and Disease.* Cornell University Press: Ithaca, New York, 1943.

Silver J. Duchenne: Neurologist dogged by misfortune. *General Practitioner* 1971; Nov-12:11.

Silver JR. A History of Paraplegia. *History of Medicine* 1974; 6:18-22.

Silver JR. Sir Charles Bell – Artist and Surgeon *Update* 1975; July:151-152.

Silver JR, Henderson NJ. Conservative Management of Spinal Injury. In: Findlay G & Owen R (eds). *Surgery of the Spine.* Vol 2. Blackwell Scientific Publications: London, 1992.

Silver JR. The British Contribution to the Treatment of spinal injuries. *J. Hist. Neurosci.* 1993; 2:151-157.

Silver JR. Early Autonomic Dysreflexia. *Spinal Cord* 2000; 38:229-233.

Silver JR. The History of Guttmann's and Whitteridge's discovery of autonomic dysreflexia. *Spinal Cord* 2000; 38:581-596.

Silver JR. History of post-traumatic syringomyelia: post traumatic syringomyelia prior to 1920. *Spinal Cord* 2001; 39:176-183.

Silver J.R. The earliest case of cauda equina syndrome caused by manipulation of the lumbar spine under a general anaesthetic. *Spinal Cord 2001;* 39: 51-53.

Silver J.R. The decline of German medicine, 1933-45. *J R Coll Physicians Edinb.* 2003; 33: 54-66.

Silver J.R. History of Infarction of the Spinal Cord. *Journal of the History of the Neurosciences. Due to be published 2003.*

Stookey B. Air-Cushion Reduction of Incomplete Vertebral Fracture Dislocations. *American Journal of Surgery* 1934; 26 No 3:513-515.

Straus E. *Rosalyn Yalow.* Helix Books:Cambridge Massachusetts, 1998.

Strümpell Dr A. *A Textbook of Medicine translated by H. Vickery.* H K Lewis: London, 1888.

Symonds CJ. Laminectomy in Gunshot Injuries of the Spinal Cord. *The Lancet* 1917; 1:93-98.

Symonds C. Studies in Neurology. Oxford Medical Publications: London, 1970.

Taylor AS. Fracture Dislocation of the Cervical Spine. *Ann Surg.* 1929; 90:321-340.

Thomson EH. *Harvey Cushing.* Henry Schuman: New York, 1950.

Thomson Walker JW. The Bladder in Gunshot and Other Injuries of the Spinal Cord. *The Lancet* 1917; 1:173-179.

Thomson Walker JW. The Treatment of the Bladder in Spinal Injuries in War. *Proceedings of the Royal Society of Medicine* 1937; 30, Part II:1233-1240.

Thorburn W. *A Contribution to the Surgery of the Spinal Cord.* Griffin: London, 1889.

Thorburn W, Richardson G. The Pathology of Gunshot Wounds of the Spinal Cord. *The British Journal of Surgery* 1918; 6:481-493.

Thorburn W. The Pathology of Gunshot Wounds of the Spinal Cord. *The British Journal of Surgery* 1920-1; 8:202-218.

Thorburn W. Injuries to the spine. In: MacPherson WG. et al (eds). *Medical Services Surgery of the War. History of the Great War Based on Official documents.* Vol 2. His Majesty's Stationery Office: London, 1922.

Tissot J-C. *Gymnastique médicinale et chirurgicale, ou essai sur l'utilité du mouvement, ou des différents exercices du corps, et du repos dans la cure des maladies.* Bastien: Paris, 1780.

Tremblay M. The Canadian Revolution in the Management of Spinal Cord Injury. *Canadian Bulletin for the History of Medicine* 1995; 12:125-155.

Tribe CR, Silver JR. *Renal Failure in Paraplegia.* Pitman Medical Publishing Co Ltd: London, 1969.

Vellacott PN, Webb-Johnson AE. Spinal Injury with Retention of Urine-The Avoidance of Catheterisation. *The Lancet* 1919; 1:733-737.

Vital D. *A People Apart.* Oxford University Press: New York, 1999.

Wagner W, Stolper P. Die Verletzungen der Wirbelsäule und des Ruckenmarks. Verlag von Ferdinand Enke: Stuttgart, 1898.

Watson-Jones R. The Treatment of Fractures and Fracture Dislocations of the Spine. *Journal of Bone and Joint Surgery* 1934; 16:34-45.

Watson-Jones R. Mr Freston's note of the 'General Discussion' with Dr Winner - Meeting of the Executive Committee of the Miners. *Public Record Office* 18-Mar-1949; MH58/653.

Watson-Jones Sir R. *Fractures and Joint Injuries.* 4th edn. E & S Livingstone Ltd: Edinburgh & London, 1955.

Weale A. *Science and the Swastika.* Macmillan Publishers: London, 2001.

Weindling P. *Health, Race and German Politics between National Unification and Nazism 1870-1945.* Cambridge University Press, 1993.

White Captain JC, Hamm Captain WG. Primary Closure of Bedsores by Plastic Surgery. *Annals of Surgery* 1946;124:1136-1145.

Wilson SAJ. *Neurology.* Edited by AN Bruce. E Arnold: London, 1940.

Winner A. Report on Spinal Units for the Ministry of Health. *Public Record Office* 1949; MH 58/653 Appendix A and B.

Winter JM. *The Great War and the British People.* MacMillan: London, 1985.

Wong K Chimin, Wu Lien-Teh. *History of Chinese Medicine.* The Tientsin Press: Tientsin, 1932.

Woodhall B. Historical Note, The Zone of Interior, The Management of Paraplegic Patients. In: Coates JB (ed). *Surgery in World War II.* Vol 2. Medical Department, United States Army. US Government Printing Office: Washington, 1959.

Young HH, Davis DM. *Young's Practice of Urology.* WB Saunders: Philadelphia, 1926.

Glossary

Alternating stepping reflex – a reflex of the lower limbs where the whole lower limb moves in a step

Anuria – a condition in which no urine is voided

Ataxia – loss of coordination

Atlas – the first cervical vertebra

Autonomic dysreflexia – a reflex of the cardiovascular system resulting in high blood pressure when the bladder or other organ is stimulated

Bradycardia – slow heart beat

Calvaria – the skull cap or vault of the head

Cauda equina – a collection of nerve roots from the lumbar sacral and coccygeal spinal nerves that run down inside the spinal column until they leave through their respective openings

Cervical – neck.

Clonus - a succession of intermittent muscular relaxations and contractions

Closed reduction – manipulation of the vertebral column usually under an anaesthetic without opening

Compression fracture – the front-part of a vertebral body is compressed to half or less of its normal height

Conservative treatment of a spinal injury – just leaving the vertebral column to unite in any position

Computed tomography (CT) can distinguish soft tissues from cysts or fat

Continuous catheterisation – leaving the catheter in situ continuously to drain the bladder

Contracture – the abnormal fixation or limitation of range of any joint, caused by muscle imbalance, muscle shortening as a result of bad positioning or insufficient physiotherapy.

Cordotomy – the surgical operation of cutting the antero-lateral tracts of the spinal cord to relieve otherwise intractable pain

Crura cerebri – part of the brain

Cystitis – inflammation of the bladder

Cystogram - x ray picture of the urinary bladder with contrast media

Cystotomy – cutting into the urinary bladder

Decubitus ulcers – bed sores

Dermatome – skin segment corresponding to a nerve supply

281

Detrusor contraction – reflex contraction of the bladder

Dislocation – of vertebrae may occur without fracture (especially in the cervical spine) but is usually combined with fractures at all levels of the spine. Vertebrae may be displaced backwards, forwards or sideways.

Dorsal – upper back. Also called thoracic.

Dysphagia – difficulty in swallowing

Dyspnoea – difficulty in breathing

Epiphysis – the spongy extremity of a bone, attached to it for the purpose of forming a joint with the similar process of another bone

Erysipelas – a disease characterised by diffuse inflammation of the skin and fever.

Eschar – a piece of the body killed by heat or caustics

Excision of sore – The black and greenish necrotic tissue covering the depth of the sore is excised. Intact skin and bleeding granulations are preserved.

Expression – method of emptying the bladder by compressing the abdominal wall

Fistula – an unnatural narrow channel leading from some natural cavity to the surface or a communication between two cavities where none should exist

Flaccid – The form of paralysis of muscle in which it loses all tone. Reflexes are absent.

Fracture-dislocation – in addition to compression of the body of a vertebra, there is also dislocation of one vertebra relative to another with tearing of ligatures and sometimes fracture of the bony walls of spinal canal

Gibbus – deformity of the spine

Haematomyelia – blood in the spinal cord

Haematuria – blood in the urine

Haemoptysis – the spitting up of blood from the lower air passages

Hemiplegia – paralysis limited to one side of the body

Heterotopic calcification – abnormal calcification around joints and bones in paralysed parts of the body

Hyperaesthesia - oversensitiveness of a part

Hypertrophy – the increase in size of an organ as the result of an increased amount of work demanded of it by the body

Hypoglossal – 12th cranial nerve

Ileus – stoppage of peristalsis due to paralysis of the bowels

Inanition – exhaustion through lack of food

Incomplete lesion – paraplegia due to partial damage of the spinal cord in which, below its upper level, there are remnants of active movement or sensation.

Intermittent catheterisation – placing a catheter in the bladder at regular intervals, draining the urine and then removing the catheter

Intravenous pyelogram (IVP) – a procedure for getting x rays of the urinary tract by injection of contrast medium intravenously

Laminectomy – Neurosurgical operation in which selected spinous processes and part of the laminae of vertebrae are removed and the spinal canal opened from an incision on the back.

Lesion – general term for damage to the spinal cord.

Level of a lesion – The upper limit of the paralysed area, described according to the uppermost segment of the cord involved.

Lumbar – lower back

Luxation – another name for dislocation

MRI – Magnetic Resonance Imaging

Mass reflex – reflex of the whole of the paralysed part of the body, described by Head

Meteorism – the distension of the abdomen by gas produced in the intestines (flatulence)

Microcephaly – abnormal smallness of the head

Myelography – injection of a radio-opaque substance into the cerebrospinal fluid of the spinal cord to assist in diagnosis

Nephrosis – The chronic form of kidney damage due to either vascular disease or persistent infection

Open reduction – open reduction of the vertebral column usually under anaesthetic

Osteomyelitis – Infection and creeping destruction of bone underlying neglected pressure sores.

Papillitis – inflammation of any papilla

Paraparetic – partial paralysis

Paraplegia – paralysis of the lower limbs [Greek]

Paresis – a state of partial paralysis

Periosteum – the membrane surrounding a bone

Polyuria – excessive urine

Postural reduction – reducing the fracture by manipulation

Pott's disease – the angular curvature of the spine which results from tuberculous disease

Priapism – erection

Pyaemia – a form of blood poisoning in which abscesses appear in various parts of the body

Pyelonephritis – inflammation of the kidney

Pyuria – Pus in the urine

Quadriparetic – paralysis of all four limbs [Latin]

Reflux – Normally the ureter is a one way passage, pumping urine from the kidneys into the bladder. In certain conditions bladder pressure causes urine to run back up the ureter.

Rhizotomy – the surgical operation of cutting a nerve root, for example, to relieve pain

Sagittal – the term applied to a structure or section running from front to back in the body

Somatic – relating to the body as opposed to the mind

Sphincter ani – anal sphincter

Spinal shock – the initial stage after injury to the spinal cord in which all function ceases in the cord below the level of the lesion.

Stenosis – unnatural narrowing in any passage or orifice of the body

Suprapubic catheterisation – catheters are passed into the bladder via an incision in the lower abdominal wall to allow urine to drain or wash out an infected bladder

Surgical treatment of a spinal injury – placing the vertebrae in alignment under an anaesthetic and possibly fixing them

Synergist – a muscle that works in concert with an agonist muscle to perform a certain movement

Syringomyelia – a rare disease affecting the spinal cord in which are found irregular cavities surrounded by an excessive amount of connective tissue of the central nervous system.

Tabes dorsalis – locomotor ataxia

Tetraplegia (also known as quadriplegia) – paralysis of all four limbs [Greek]

Theca – a sheathlike structure enclosing the brain and spinal cord

Tidal drainage – method for giving continuous bladder washouts with antiseptic solution

Traction – used with skull callipers to reduce and maintain in alignment fracture-dislocations of the cervical spine

Uraemia – the clinical state that arises from renal failure

Urethritis – inflammation of the urethra

About the Author

John Russell Silver was born in London in 1931. His father was a general practitioner who later specialised in psychiatry.

John Silver received his schooling at University College School, Hampstead, and trained in medicine at the Middlesex Hospital. He graduated in 1954 and after two house jobs worked as a registrar for Sir Ludwig Guttmann for a year at the National Spinal Injuries Centre. During this time he worked for a spell in the Hungarian refugee camps after the 1956 revolution. After his National Service in orthopaedics in the Royal Air Force, he continued his training in spinal injuries spending 3½ years in the neurology, neurosurgery and physiology departments of the Middlesex Hospital. He returned to the National Spinal 'Injuries Centre for 3 years in a research post until appointed consultant in charge of the Liverpool Centre and Lecturer in Surgery in 1965. In 1970 he returned to Stoke Mandeville as a consultant in spinal injuries during which time he served as Chairman of the Division until he retired from clinical practice in 1993. Since that time he has continued his research work and medico-legal work.

He has written 4 books and over 200 medical papers, his particular interest being medical history, the treatment of spinal injuries, vascular disease of the spinal cord and sporting accidents causing spinal injuries. As a result of these researches he was responsible for a change in the laws of rugby union following which there was a reduction in serious spinal injuries.

He described a new disease, familial spastic paraplegia with amyotrophy of the hands, which is eponymously named after him.

He is a Fellow of the College of Physicians of Edinburgh and London, and wrote his M.D. on the history of the treatment of spinal injuries upon which this book is based. He has been Chairman and President of the Tissue Viability Society and President of the Sports Medicine section of the Royal

Society of Medicine, and also council member of the History of Medicine section of the Royal Society of Medicine. He has been a council member of the International Medical Society of Paraplegia and on the editorial board of Paraplegia.

He is married to Marilyn who is a psychiatric social worker. He has two sons, one of whom is a dentist, the other is a solicitor.

His hobbies are reading, historical research, tennis and swimming.

Index

287